T0263193

Genitourinary Imaging

Guest Editors

PAUL NIKOLAIDIS, MD
NANCY A. HAMMOND, MD

RADIOLOGIC CLINICS OF NORTH AMERICA

www.radiologic.theclinics.com

Consulting Editor
FRANK H. MILLER, MD

March 2012 • Volume 50 • Number 2

SAUNDERS an imprint of ELSEVIER, Inc.

W.B. SAUNDERS COMPANY
A Division of Elsevier Inc.

1600 John F. Kennedy Boulevard • Suite 1800 • Philadelphia, Pennsylvania 19103-2899

http://www.theclinics.com

RADIOLOGIC CLINICS OF NORTH AMERICA Volume 50, Number 2
March 2012 ISSN 0033-8389, ISBN 13: 978-1-4557-4464-0

Editor: Sarah Barth
Developmental Editor: Donald Mumford

© 2012 Elsevier Inc. All rights reserved.

This journal and the individual contributions contained in it are protected under copyright by Elsevier, and the following terms and conditions apply to their use:

Photocopying
Single photocopies of single articles may be made for personal use as allowed by national copyright laws. Permission of the Publisher and payment of a fee is required for all other photocopying, including multiple or systematic copying, copying for advertising or promotional purposes, resale, and all forms of document delivery. Special rates are available for educational institutions that wish to make photocopies for non-profit educational classroom use. For information on how to seek permission visit www.elsevier.com/permissions or call: (+44) 1865 843830 (UK)/(+1) 215 239 3804 (USA).

Derivative Works
Subscribers may reproduce tables of contents or prepare lists of articles including abstracts for internal circulation within their institutions. Permission of the Publisher is required for resale or distribution outside the institution. Permission of the Publisher is required for all other derivative works, including compilations and translations (please consult www.elsevier.com/permissions).

Electronic Storage or Usage
Permission of the Publisher is required to store or use electronically any material contained in this journal, including any article or part of an article (please consult www.elsevier.com/permissions). Except as outlined above, no part of this publication may be reproduced, stored in a retrieval system or transmitted in any form or by any means, electronic, mechanical, photocopying, recording or otherwise, without prior written permission of the Publisher.

Notice
No responsibility is assumed by the Publisher for any injury and/or damage to persons or property as a matter of products liability, negligence or otherwise, or from any use or operation of any methods, products, instructions or ideas contained in the material herein. Because of rapid advances in the medical sciences, in particular, independent verification of diagnoses and drug dosages should be made.

Although all advertising material is expected to conform to ethical (medical) standards, inclusion in this publication does not constitute a guarantee or endorsement of the quality or value of such product or of the claims made of it by its manufacturer.

Radiologic Clinics of North America (ISSN 0033-8389) is published bimonthly by Elsevier Inc., 360 Park Avenue South, New York, NY 10010-1710. Months of issue are January, March, May, July, September, and November. Periodicals postage paid at New York, NY and additional mailing offices. Subscription prices are USD 421 per year for US individuals, USD 659 per year for US institutions, USD 202 per year for US students and residents, USD 491 per year for Canadian individuals, USD 827 per year for Canadian institutions, USD 606 per year for international individuals, USD 827 per year for international institutions, and USD 290 per year for Canadian and foreign students/residents. To receive student and resident rate, orders must be accompanied by name of affiliated institution, date of term and the signature of program/residency coordinatior on institution letterhead. Orders will be billed at individual rate until proof of status is received. Foreign air speed delivery is included in all *Clinics* subscription prices. All prices are subject to change without notice. **POSTMASTER:** Send address changes to *Radiologic Clinics of North America*, Elsevier Health Sciences Division, Subscription Customer Service, 3251 Riverport Lane, Maryland Heights, MO63043. **Customer Service: Telephone: 1-800-654-2452** (U.S. and Canada); **1-314-447-8871** (outside U.S. and Canada). **Fax: 1-314-447-8029. E-mail: journalscustomerservice-usa@elsevier.com** (for print support); **journalsonlinesupport-usa@elsevier.com** (for online support).

Reprints. For copies of 100 or more of articles in this publication, please contact the Commercial Reprints Department, Elsevier Inc., 360 Park Avenue South, New York, New York 10010-1710. Tel.: (+1) 212-633-3812; Fax: (+1) 212-462-1935; E-mail: reprints@elsevier.com.

Radiologic Clinics of North America also published in Greek Paschalidis Medical Publications, Athens, Greece.

Radiologic Clinics of North America is covered in *MEDLINE/PubMed (Index Medicus), EMBASE/Excerpta Medica, Current Contents/Life Sciences, Current Contents/Clinical Medicine, RSNA Index to Imaging Literature, BIOSIS, Science Citation Index,* and *ISI/BIOMED.*

Printed and bound by CPI Group (UK) Ltd, Croydon, CR0 4YY

Transferred to Digital Print 2012

Contributors

CONSULTING EDITOR

FRANK H. MILLER, MD
Professor of Radiology; Chief, Body Imaging
Section and Fellowship Program and GI
Radiology; Medical Director MRI,
Department of Radiology, Northwestern
University Feinberg School of Medicine,
Chicago, Illinois

GUEST EDITORS

PAUL NIKOLAIDIS, MD
Associate Professor in Radiology,
Department of Radiology, Northwestern
University, Feinberg School of Medicine,
Chicago, Illinois

NANCY A. HAMMOND, MD
Assistant Professor in Radiology,
Department of Radiology, Northwestern
University, Feinberg School of Medicine,
Chicago, Illinois

AUTHORS

RICHARD BELLAH, MD
Radiology Attending, Director of Ultrasound
and Student Programs, Department of
Radiology, The Children's Hospital of
Philadelphia, University of Pennsylvania,
Philadelphia, Pennsylvania

PUNEET BHARGAVA, MD
Assistant Professor, Department of Radiology,
VA Puget Sound Health Care System,
University of Washington, Seattle, Washington

DAVID D. CASALINO, MD
Professor of Radiology, Department of
Radiology, Northwestern University,
Chicago, Illinois

CARLOS CUEVAS, MD
Assistant Professor, Department of Radiology,
University of Washington Medical Center,
Seattle, Washington

KASSA DARGE, MD, PhD
Radiology Attending, Chief, Division of Body
Imaging, Department of Radiology, The
Children's Hospital of Philadelphia, University
of Pennsylvania, Philadelphia, Pennsylvania

MANJIRI K. DIGHE, MD
Associate Professor, Department of Radiology,
University of Washington Medical Center,
Seattle, Washington

JOEL FLETCHER, MD
Professor of Radiology, Department
of Radiology, Mayo Clinic, Rochester,
Minnesota

AJIT H. GOENKA, MD
Clinical Fellow, Section of Abdominal
Imaging, Imaging Institute, Cleveland Clinic,
Cleveland, Ohio

SHAWN HAJI-MOMENIAN, MD
Association of Alexandria Radiologists,
Alexandria, Virginia

NANCY A. HAMMOND, MD
Assistant Professor in Radiology,
Department of Radiology, Northwestern
University, Feinberg School of Medicine,
Chicago, Illinois

ROBERT HARTMAN, MD
Assistant Professor of Radiology, Department of Radiology, Mayo Clinic, Rochester, Minnesota

JEFFREY C. HELLINGER, MD
Radiology Attending, Associate Professor of Radiology and Pediatrics, Department of Radiology, Stony Brook University Medical Center, Stony Brook, New York

JEAN HWA LEE, MD
Assistant Professor, Department of Radiology, University of Washington Medical Center, Seattle, Washington

NALINI KANTH, MD
Residency Program Director; Director, Genitourinary Radiology, Department of Radiology, Nassau University Medical Center, East Meadow, New York

AKIRA KAWASHIMA, MD, PhD
Professor of Radiology, Department of Radiology, Mayo Clinic, Rochester, Minnesota

SHUAI LENG, PhD
Assistant Professor of Medical Physics, Department of Radiology, Mayo Clinic, Rochester, Minnesota

CYNTHIA MCCOLLOUGH, PhD
Professor of Biomedical Engineering and Medical Physics, Department of Radiology, Mayo Clinic, Rochester, Minnesota

FRANK H. MILLER, MD
Professor of Radiology; Chief, Body Imaging Section and Fellowship Program and GI Radiology; Medical Director MRI, Department of Radiology, Northwestern University Feinberg School of Medicine, Chicago, Illinois

BRANDON MIROCHNIK, MD
Radiology Resident R2, Department of Radiology, Nassau University Medical Center, East Meadow, New York

SAMDEEP MOULI, MD, MS
Department of Radiology, Northwestern University, Chicago, Illinois

PAUL NIKOLAIDIS, MD
Associate Professor in Radiology, Department of Radiology, Northwestern University, Feinberg School of Medicine, Chicago, Illinois

ERICK M. REMER, MD
Professor of Radiology, Section of Abdominal Imaging, Imaging Institute, Cleveland Clinic, Cleveland, Ohio

POOJA RENJEN, MD
Pediatric Radiology Attending, Department of Radiology, Hackensack Radiology Group, Hackensack University Medical Center, Hackensack, New Jersey

SHETAL N. SHAH, MD
Assistant Professor of Radiology; Co-director, Center for PET and Molecular Imaging, Section of Abdominal Imaging, Imaging Institute, Cleveland Clinic, Cleveland, Ohio

ALVIN SILVA, MD
Associate Professor of Radiology, Department of Radiology, Mayo Clinic, Scottsdale, Arizona

MYLES TAFFEL, MD
Assistant Professor of Radiology, Department of Radiology, George Washington University Medical Center, Washington, DC

NAOKI TAKAHASHI, MD
Associate Professor of Radiology, Department of Radiology, Mayo Clinic, Rochester, Minnesota

RANU TANEJA, MD
Staff Radiologist, Department of Radiology, Changi General Hospital, Singapore

TERRI VRTISKA, MD
Assistant Professor of Radiology, Department of Radiology, Mayo Clinic, Rochester, Minnesota

CAROLYN WANG, MD
Assistant Professor, Department of Radiology, University of Washington Medical Center, Seattle, Washington

Contents

This article discusses modern dual-energy computed tomography (DECT) and the unique material-specific information these scanners can provide. A description of the technical aspects of the various DECT techniques is provided. Specific clinical applications in urologic imaging, including chemical composition of urolithiasis, evaluation of renal masses, detection of urothelial neoplasms, and adrenal adenoma imaging, are discussed. The unique postprocessed image sets, including virtual noncontrast, iodine overlay, and stone composition, are described.

Diagnostic imaging of pediatric urologic disorders is continuously changing as technologic advances are made. Although the backbone of pediatric urologic imaging has been ultrasound, voiding cystourethrography, and radionuclide scintigraphy, newer and advanced modalities are becoming increasingly important. This article discusses the techniques and clinical applications of three such imaging modalities as they pertain to pediatric urologic disorders: (1) MR urography; (2) advanced ultrasound (harmonic imaging, three-dimensional, and voiding urosonography); and (3) CT angiography.

The discovery of an incidental adrenal mass (adrenal incidentaloma) continues to rise with the increasing use of cross-sectional imaging. Although most adrenal lesions are benign and asymptomatic, radiologists should guide evaluation of these lesions, whether benign or malignant. This article reviews the various imaging techniques used to evaluate adrenal masses and their relative strengths and weaknesses. It focuses on the most prevalent adrenal pathologies and their typical imaging characteristics, and concludes with a brief discussion of developing techniques, including diffusion-weighted imaging and dual-energy CT.

As an increasing number of imaging examinations are performed, a greater number of incidental renal lesions are detected. Apart from the usual cysts and solid renal cell carcinomas, a variety of unusual benign and malignant renal lesions exist. Imaging is invaluable in characterizing these lesions and is confirmatory in some benign lesions. Renal cell carcinoma remains the diagnosis of exclusion; however, assessment of the imaging pattern in the appropriate clinical context can improve

Imaging of the Retroperitoneum

Ajit H. Goenka, Shetal N. Shah, and Erick M. Remer

The retroperitoneum is the compartmentalized space bounded anteriorly by the posterior parietal peritoneum and posteriorly by the transversalis fascia. It extends from the diaphragm superiorly to the pelvic brim inferiorly. This article discusses clinically relevant anatomy of the abdominal retroperitoneal spaces, their cross-sectional imaging evaluation with computed tomography and magnetic resonance imaging, and the imaging features of common retroperitoneal pathologic processes.

GOAL STATEMENT

The goal of the *Radiologic Clinics of North America* is to keep practicing radiologists and radiology residents up to date with current clinical practice in radiology by providing timely articles reviewing the state of the art in patient care.

ACCREDITATION

The *Radiologic Clinics of North America* is planned and implemented in accordance with the Essential Areas and Policies of the Accreditation Council for Continuing Medical Education (ACCME) through the joint sponsorship of the University of Virginia School of Medicine and Elsevier. The University of Virginia School of Medicine is accredited by the ACCME to provide continuing medical education for physicians.

The University of Virginia School of Medicine designates this enduring material activity for a maximum of 15 *AMA PRA Category 1 Credit*(s)™ for each issue, 90 credits per year. Physicians should only claim credit commensurate with the extent of their participation in the activity.

The American Medical Association has determined that physicians not licensed in the US who participate in this CME enduring material activity are eligible for a maximum of 15 *AMA PRA Category 1 Credit*(s)™ for each issue, 90 credits per year.

Credit can be earned by reading the text material, taking the CME examination online at http://www.theclinics.com/home/cme, and completing the evaluation. After taking the test, you will be required to review any and all incorrect answers. Following completion of the test and evaluation, your credit will be awarded and you may print your certificate.

FACULTY DISCLOSURE/CONFLICT OF INTEREST

The University of Virginia School of Medicine, as an ACCME accredited provider, endorses and strives to comply with the Accreditation Council for Continuing Medical Education (ACCME) Standards of Commercial Support, Commonwealth of Virginia statutes, University of Virginia policies and procedures, and associated federal and private regulations and guidelines on the need for disclosure and monitoring of proprietary and financial interests that may affect the scientific integrity and balance of content delivered in continuing medical education activities under our auspices.

The University of Virginia School of Medicine requires that all CME activities accredited through this institution be developed independently and be scientifically rigorous, balanced and objective in the presentation/discussion of its content, theories and practices.

All authors/editors participating in an accredited CME activity are expected to disclose to the readers relevant financial relationships with commercial entities occurring within the past 12 months (such as grants or research support, employee, consultant, stock holder, member of speakers bureau, etc.). The University of Virginia School of Medicine will employ appropriate mechanisms to resolve potential conflicts of interest to maintain the standards of fair and balanced education to the reader. Questions about specific strategies can be directed to the Office of Continuing Medical Education, University of Virginia School of Medicine, Charlottesville, Virginia.

The faculty and staff of the University of Virginia Office of Continuing Medical Education have no financial affiliations to disclose.

The authors/editors listed below have identified no financial or professional relationships for themselves or their spouse/partner:

Sarah Barth, (Acquisitions Editor); Richard Bellah, MD; Puneet Bhargava, MD; Kassa Darge, MD, PhD; Manjiri K. Dighe, MD; Ajit H. Goenka, MD; Shawn Haji-Momenian, MD; Nancy A. Hammond, MD (Guest Editor); Robert Hartman, MD; Jeffrey C. Hellinger, MD; Jean Hwa Lee, MD; Nalini Kanth, MD; Akira Kawashima, MD, PhD; Shuai Leng, PhD; Frank H. Miller, MD (Consulting Editor); Brandon Mirochnik, MD; Samdeep Mouli, MD, MS; Paul Nikolaidis, MD (Guest Editor); Erick M. Remer, MD; Pooja Renjen, MD; Alvin Silva, MD; Myles Taffel, MD; Naoki Takahashi, MD; Ranu Taneja, MD; Terri Vrtiska, MD; and Carolyn Wang, MD.

The authors/editors listed below have identified the following financial or professional relationships for themselves or their spouse/partner:

David D. Casalino, MD is an industry funded research/investigator for Eli Lilly.
Carlos Cuevas, MD is an industry funded research/investigator for Merck.
Joel Fletcher, MD receives grant support from Siemens Healthcare.
Klaus D. Hagspiel, MD (Test Author) is an industry funded research/investigator for Siemens Medical Solutions.
Cynthia McCollough, PhD is an industry funded research/investigator for Siemens Healthcare.
Shetal N. Shah, MD is a consultant for Dendreon Corp.

Disclosure of Discussion of Non-FDA Approved Uses for Pharmaceutical Products and/or Medical Devices

The University of Virginia School of Medicine, as an ACCME provider, requires that all faculty presenters identify and disclose any off-label uses for pharmaceutical and medical device products. The University of Virginia School of Medicine recommends that each physician fully review all the available data on new products or procedures prior to clinical use.

TO ENROLL

To enroll in the Radiologic Clinics of North America Continuing Medical Education program, call customer service at 1-800-654-2452 or sign up online at http://www.theclinics.com/home/cme. The CME program is available to subscribers for an additional annual fee USD 245.

Radiologic Clinics of North America

THE CLINICS ARE NOW AVAILABLE ONLINE!

Access your subscription at:
www.theclinics.com

Radiologic Clinics of North America

FORTHCOMING ISSUES

Pancreatic Imaging
Desiree Morgan, MD, and
Koenraad Mortele, MD, Guest Editors

Imaging of the Spine
Timothy Maus, MD, Guest Editor

Imaging of Lung Cancer
Ella Kazerooni, MD, MS, and
Baskaran Sundaram, MBBS, MRCP, FRCR,
Guest Editors

RECENT ISSUES

November 2011
Imaging of Bone and Soft Tissue Tumors
G. Scott Stacy, MD, Guest Editor

January 2012
Emergency Radiology
Jorge A. Soto, MD, Guest Editor

THE CLINICS ARE NOW AVAILABLE ONLINE!

Access your subscription at
www.theclinics.com

Preface

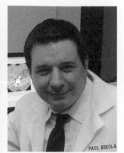
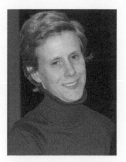

Paul Nikolaidis, MD   Nancy A. Hammond, MD
Guest Editors

It was our great pleasure to compile this issue of *Radiologic Clinics of North America* devoted to genitourinary (GU) imaging. We are deeply indebted to all of the authors for their expertise, hard work, and dedication to this project. Their proficiency in GU radiology is evident in each and every article in this issue.

In recent years, numerous technological advances have occurred in our field, employing state-of-the-art imaging modalities and newer imaging processing techniques. One such notable development involves dual-energy CT platforms along with innovative scanning techniques with great promise in the diagnosis and characterization of renal masses, urinary tract stone disease, and adrenal lesions. The technical aspects of dual-energy scanning along with specific advantages conferred in imaging the GU tract are presented in this issue.

Diagnostic imaging of pediatric urologic disorders is continuously changing as technological advances are made. In the field of pediatric urologic imaging, in addition to ultrasound, voiding cystourethrography, and radionuclide scintigraphy, newer and advanced modalities are becoming increasingly important. Cutting edge techniques including magnetic resonance urography, advanced ultrasound (harmonic imaging, 3D, voiding urosonography), and computed tomographic angiography as they pertain to pediatric urologic disorders are presented in this issue.

The detection of incidental adrenal masses continues to rise with the increasing use of cross-sectional imaging. A comprehensive article on adrenal imaging reviews all currently available imaging techniques employed in evaluating adrenal masses. The strengths and weaknesses of more conventional modalities and a review of developing

techniques, including diffusion weighted imaging and dual-energy CT, are discussed.

In addition to these newer developments, we have included comprehensive, state-of-the art review articles on almost all components of the GU tract: the kidneys, ureters, bladder, retroperitoneum, and scrotum. The wonderful images that accompany these articles nicely complement the text, creating a useful overview in each topic.

We would like to thank Frank Miller, MD, the series editor for *Radiologic Clinics of North America*, for the opportunity to develop this issue. We would also like to thank Eric Russell, MD, our department chair, for his enduring support, and our colleagues at Northwestern Memorial Hospital for their encouragement. We would like to acknowledge the hard work by David Botos, who was provided with the arduous task of processing numerous images in a very short timeframe.

We are also greatly indebted to Sarah Barth at Elsevier for her invaluable assistance, constant availability, and consistent communication during the preparation of this issue. Last, we would be remiss not to thank our families for their love, encouragement, and support.

Paul Nikolaidis, MD

Nancy A. Hammond, MD
Department of Radiology
Northwestern University
Feinberg School of Medicine
676 North Saint Clair, Suite 800
Chicago, IL 60611, USA

E-mail addresses:
p-nikolaidis@northwestern.edu (P. Nikolaidis)
NHammond@nmff.org (N.A. Hammond)

Radiol Clin N Am 50 (2012) xi
doi:10.1016/j.rcl.2012.02.010
0033-8389/12/$ – see front matter © 2012 Elsevier Inc. All rights reserved.

Applications of Dual-Energy CT in Urologic Imaging: An Update

Robert Hartman, MD[a,*], Akira Kawashima, MD, PhD[a],
Naoki Takahashi, MD[a], Alvin Silva, MD[b], Terri Vrtiska, MD[a],
Shuai Leng, PhD[a], Joel Fletcher, MD[a],
Cynthia McCollough, PhD[a]

KEYWORDS

- Computed tomography (CT) • Dual-energy CT (DECT)
- Urinary tract stones • Renal neoplasms • Adrenal adenoma

Computed tomography (CT) imaging is a vital tool in the evaluation of suspected abnormalities of the kidneys and urinary tract. In recent years, the development of dual-energy CT (DECT) platforms and innovative scanning techniques has provided additional tools for the diagnosis and characterization of renal masses, urolithiasis, and disorders of the uroepithelium. This article discusses the technical aspects of dual-energy scanning and its specific utility in imaging of the kidneys and urinary tract.

In CT, measured CT number is related to the linear attenuation coefficient of scanned material, which is a function of x-ray beam energy, material density, and material atomic number. Therefore, CT number is not material specific and 2 different materials can have the same CT numbers if the difference of atomic number is compensated by the difference of material density. In conventional CT, data are measured at one given tube potential (kV) and material-specific information is not available. DECT is an imaging technique that acquires 2 CT data sets at 2 different beam spectra, from which material-specific information can be obtained by exploring the energy dependence of attenuation coefficient for each material.

DECT TECHNIQUES

Different techniques and hardware platforms have been explored to achieve DECT capabilities. There are mainly 3 implementations currently available from 3 different manufacturers using dual-source, fast-kV switching, and dual-layer detector techniques. Other emerging DECT techniques include using photon-counting detectors and performing 2 consecutive scans on a standard CT scanner. Each DECT technique has its advantages and disadvantages compared with other implementations.[1,2]

For a dual-source CT scanner (dsDECT), 2 independent x-ray tube and detector systems are mounted together on the CT gantry, spaced approximately 90° apart.[3,4] Dual-energy scans are achieved by operating the 2 x-ray tubes at different tube potentials (eg, 140 kV and 80 kV) to simultaneously acquire 2 data sets corresponding to 2 different beam spectra.[5] Because the 2 tube-detector systems can be operated independently, there is flexibility to adjust tube current (mA) of each tube to optimize image quality. Another advantage of the dual-source system is that independent beam filtration can be applied to the 2 x-ray tubes. It has been demonstrated that an extra-thin layer of tin filter added to the 140-kV beam improves image quality and material decomposition capability because of the further separation between the low-energy and high-energy spectra.[6–10] This allows DECT to differentiate more materials (eg, different types of non-uric acid renal stones) or potentially allow for differentiation of materials that could not be differentiated

[a] Department of Radiology, Mayo Clinic, 200 First Street SW, Rochester, MN 55905, USA
[b] Department of Radiology, Mayo Clinic, 13400 East Shea Boulevard, Scottsdale, AZ 85259, USA
* Corresponding author.
E-mail address: Hartman.robert@mayo.edu

Radiol Clin N Am 50 (2012) 191–205
doi:10.1016/j.rcl.2012.02.007
0033-8389/12/$ – see front matter © 2012 Elsevier Inc. All rights reserved.

before (eg, iron and calcium).[7,11,12] Because of the spectral shift generated by the tin filter, 100 kV can be used as the low-energy beam while still maintaining sufficient spectral separation for material decomposition. This allows better penetration than the 80-kV beam and is especially beneficial for large-size patients. One limitation of a dsDECT system is the limited field of view (FOV). Because of the space limit inside the CT gantry, the second detector is smaller in the axial plane compared with the primary detector, which consequently limits the in-plane FOV to 26 cm for the first-generation dual-source scanners. The FOV has been enlarged to 33 cm for second-generation dual-source scanners, which is sufficient to cover the internal organs for most patients. Because of the 90° difference in the data acquisition for low-kV and high-kV data, dual-energy processing is conducted in image space for dual-source CT systems. Because 2 tubes are operated together, cross scatter from one tube is measured by the other tube, but correction algorithms have been developed for this effect.

Another implementation is fast-kV switching on a single-source scanner (ssDECT), which involves rapid alternation of tube potentials between 80 and 140 kV during the gantry rotation.[13–15] A single tube and detector system is used, similar to conventional CT, although modification of the generator, detector, and data acquisition system (DAS) is required to accomplish the rapid switching of tube potentials. A FOV of 50 cm can be achieved on this system, the same as single-energy CT (SECT). As low-kV and high-kV projection data are acquired at essentially the same location and time, the fast-kV switching technique enables projection-based dual-energy data processing. This has the potential to eliminate beam-hardening artifacts. One limitation of ssDECT is the inability to change tube current (mA) while simultaneously switching the tube potential. For this reason, tube current modulation is currently not available.[14]

Because low-energy photons are attenuated more than high-energy photons, a higher tube current is required for the low-kV beam than for the high-kV beam, or other approaches need to be used to compensate for this difference, such as increasing the number of views for the low-kV beam.[14] The goal is to balance the image quality between the 2 image sets and avoid inferior image quality of the low-kV images. Another limitation of this approach is that beam filtration has to be the same for low and high kV, as they share the same tube. Therefore, the spectral separation is maybe limited.

A third DECT technique is the use of a dual-layer detector.[16–20] A single x-ray tube (usually operated at high tube potential, eg, 140 kV) is used during the data acquisition. Two data sets are generated with lower-energy photons mainly detected by the upper-layer detector and high-energy photons detected by the lower-layer detector. The principle used in this approach is that low-energy photons are more attenuated and deposit the most energy in the upper-layer detector, whereas the high-energy photons are less attenuated and capable of penetrating the upper-layer detector. The data-acquisition procedure is similar to the standard single-energy CT scan and a full FOV is achievable. The low-energy and high-energy data sets are acquired at exactly the same time and location, without any mismatch in temporal or spatial domain. A major limitation of this approach is the potential significant spectral overlap between the low-energy and high-energy data sets that might compromise material decomposition capability of this system. It might also be challenging to match the image quality of the low-energy and high-energy data sets on this system.

Recently, the development of photon-counting detector techniques provides another option to achieve DECT and multi-energy (spectral) CT.[21–23] Conventional CT detectors integrate the charges generated by x-ray photon interactions and record a signal proportional to the total energy deposited by all x-ray photons without any information of individual photons. In contrast, photon-counting detectors process each photon individually. X-ray photons are sorted into multiple bins based on their energy, which provides energy-dependent data sets for multi-energy CT. The advantage of this system is that data from each energy set are acquired at exactly the same time and location, theoretically with no spectral overlap. Prototype micro-CT and clinical-CT systems have been built using photon-counting detectors, although more investigation is needed to overcome technical challenges, such as maximal photon flux and detector stability before deployment to clinical practice.

Use of 2 consecutive axial or spiral scans, each acquired at different tube potentials, has also been investigated to achieve DECT.[24,25] The advantage of this approach is that it can be performed on a standard single-source, single-detector CT system, which is more widely available than the other DECT approaches that are available only on high-end scanners. A major challenge of this approach is the time delay between the 2 scans, which makes the study susceptible to patient motion. In one study on renal stone differentiation, regions of interest (ROIs) were manually drawn on the low-energy and high-energy images separately to ensure proper registration of the target stones and avoid mismatch caused by patient motion.[24] A more-elegant solution is to use image registration techniques to align the 2 image sets before the dual-energy processing.[25] In general, this approach should be applied only to applications with limited patient motion.

DECT IMAGES

In DECT, because the 2 data sets are acquired at different beam energies and different processing techniques can be applied, multiple-image data sets can be obtained from a single examination.

Non–Material-Specific Images

Images corresponding to the low-energy and high-energy data sets can be directly obtained, similar to standard single-energy images. In general, the low-energy images usually have a higher contrast and improved lesion visualization in contrast scans owing to higher attenuation coefficients of iodine at lower energy; however, the low-energy images are also associated with higher image noise (Fig. 1). On the other hand, high-energy images usually have lower-image noise but also lower image contrast. Although higher-

contrast noise ratio can be obtained using low-energy images in small patients, image noise and artifacts increased dramatically for large-size patients.[26] Although either low-energy or high-energy images alone can be used in routine clinic diagnosis, image noise tends to be higher than a standard single-energy scan because of the dose split between the 2 data sets. To fully use all delivered x-ray photons, mixed images are usually generated to mimic an image data set that is similar to a routine single-energy scan. Several blending techniques, linear or nonlinear, have been investigated to generate the mixed images. Using a linear blending technique, it has been shown that image quality of the mixed images depends on both the assigned weighting factors and the dose partition between the high-energy and low-energy beams. At the same radiation dose, similar image quality as a standard 120-kV single-energy scan can be obtained using optimal weighting factors.[27] For nonlinear blending techniques, weighting factors are assigned to each individual pixel, instead of the whole image, to optimize the image quality of the mixed images. This approach takes advantage of the high enhancement in the low-energy beam for image regions with iodine contrast and the

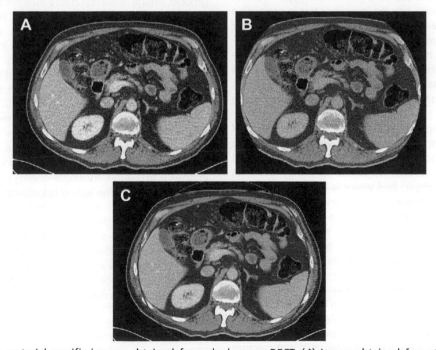

Fig. 1. Non–material-specific images obtained from dual-source DECT. (*A*) Image obtained from 100-kV tube demonstrates increased noise in the image but higher contrast from the iodine in the vessels. (*B*) Image obtained from the 140-kV tube demonstrates less noise and contrast in the image. (*C*) Mixed image obtained by blending the 100-kV and 140-kV data. The image approximates an image obtained on SECT at 120 kV.

low noise in the high-energy beam for regions without iodine.[28]

Material-Specific Images and Material Decomposition Methods

The main benefit of DECT is its capability to generate material-specific images. By exploring the energy dependence of x-ray attenuation, materials can be differentiated or quantified based on the measured dual-energy data. To differentiate 2 materials, eg, uric acid (UA) from non-UA renal stones, a threshold of CT number can be applied. To eliminate a certain material, eg, bone, a weighted subtraction between the 2 energy data sets can be performed. To quantify the mass fraction of given materials, eg, amount of iodine absorbed in a lesion, sophisticated material decomposition algorithms are needed.[29]

In the energy range of diagnostic x-rays, 2 reaction mechanisms account for most x-ray attenuation: photoelectric and Compton effects. The linear attenuation of any given material can be expressed as a combination of 2 base materials. With 2 measurements in DECT, the fraction of each base material can be numerically solved and material-specific images obtained.[30] Alternatively, the linear attenuation coefficient can also be modeled as a function of material density (ρ), atomic number (Z), and photon energy.[31] Both of these methods can be implemented in projection space (before reconstruction) or image space (after reconstruction).[5] In principle, DECT can differentiate only 2 materials with the 2 distinct measurements. With an additional constraint, such as volume conservation or mass conservation, it has been shown that 3 materials can be identified using DECT.[32]

Depending on the imaging targets and clinical applications, different base materials can be selected. Iodine and water are commonly used as base materials, as iodine is widely used as imaging contrast, and water is the major component of the human body. One example is the DECT urogram, in which iodine and water images are generated from contrast scan.[33] The water images generated in these scans are usually referred to as virtual noncontrast (VNC) or virtual nonenhanced images, which can be used for stone detection by removing the iodine signal. With this, the noncontrast scan can be eliminated. Another common base material in DECT is calcium, which is the major component of bones and plaques. Effective bone removal and calcium removal using DECT have been demonstrated in neurological, cardiac, and vascular imaging. The appropriate selection of base materials can be appreciated in the following sections with specific clinical examples given.

Energy-Specific Images

In CT, polychromatic x-rays are used and CT number represents the linear attenuation coefficient of x-ray photons at the effective beam energy. In DECT, the mass fraction of each base material is quantified after the material decomposition. With mass attenuation coefficients for different elements found at the National Institute of Standards and Technology,[34,35] virtual monochromatic images can be synthesized. These images represent the attenuation map at a given photon energy (keV), instead of a wide energy spectrum. Similar to the material-specific images, virtual monochromatic images can be synthesized using either projection-based or image-based methods.[36] Using projection-space computed monochromatic images, curves of the CT numbers, in Hounsfield units (HU), of different materials can be displayed over a range of 101 discrete energies (40–140 keV).[14] Projection-based methods may reduce beam-hardening artifacts. Virtual monochromatic images provide users with the flexibility to select appropriate keVs to highlight features of interest.[15,37,38] For imaging tasks involving iodine contrast, lower keV images have brighter iodine signals and higher contrast relative to the background. Image noise first decreases with increasing keV up to the effective keV of the high-energy beam, and then increases with keV. An optimal keV exists for virtual monochromatic images that maximize the contrast-to-noise ratio (CNR).[36,37] The image quality (eg, CNR) of virtual monochromatic images at optimal keV can be superior to standard 120-kV single-energy images.[37] Because of the brighter iodine signal and higher CNR, the amount of iodine contrast can be potentially reduced for certain clinical applications. An alternative approach to dual-energy monochromatic images is to use low-kV single-energy scans, which can also improve the iodine brightness and iodine CNR. It has been demonstrated that in smaller patients 80-kV single-energy images have a better CNR than the dual-energy monochromatic images given the same radiation dose.[36] A low-kV single-energy CT scan is a better alternative to a DECT scan with virtual monochromatic images if material specific imaging is not required.[39]

RADIATION DOSE IN DECT AND DOSE-REDUCTION METHODS

Although 2 measurements are made in DECT, the radiation dose used to acquire each measurement alone is lower and therefore the total radiation dose is not necessarily higher than single-energy CT. The mixed images are generated by blending the low-energy and high-energy images, therefore fully using all x-ray photons and radiation dose. It has been demonstrated that similar image quality and radiation dose can be obtained using a linear blending technique on a dsDECT system.[27]

In DECT, the low-energy and high-energy images are usually noisier than the standard single-energy images given the same radiation dose, owing to the dose split between the 2 measurements. These 2 image sets are usually treated independently; however, substantial correlation exists, as they measure exactly the same anatomic region. By exploring the redundancy information in energy domain, a noise-reduction algorithm dedicated to DECT and multi-energy CT has been developed.[40] Image noise of low-energy and high-energy images can be reduced to the level of mixed image, which uses all x-ray photons. This algorithm can also be applied to material-specific images before or after material decomposition.

CLINICAL APPLICATIONS
Renal Stone Characterization Using DECT

Additional information about renal stone characterization beyond their size and location has been a goal of CT acquisitions since the early 1980s,[41] but has only been fully realized beginning in 2006 with the innovative development of simultaneous DECT acquisitions.[3] In the past, SECT provided an initial significant step in the care of the growing number of patients with renal stone disease, estimated at 13% of men and 5% of women,[42] by allowing radiologists and clinicians to precisely detect stones and determine treatment based on location, size, and associated complications[43–47]; however, SECT technology could not consistently characterize stones into specific subtypes based on attenuation values at a single-energy x-ray.[48–56] DECT takes advantage of the unique absorption characteristics of urinary stone subtypes at high-energy and low-energy x-rays, allowing composition characterization, as well as benefiting patient care by directing treatment at the time of initial stone detection, potentially reducing billions of dollars in renal stone treatments each year.[42,57]

Characterization of stone subtypes is an invaluable tool in patient management, as more than 50% of patients will experience recurrent stone disease after treatment.[58] Advances in the treatment of stone disease range from medical management to a variety of noninvasive and invasive urologic techniques. The correct classification of the stone composition before intervention leads to the most favorable treatment choice.[59,60] Previously, stone type characterization has often required a lengthy series of imaging, laboratory, and pathology examinations.

The dsDECT system offers a rapid characterization tool at the time of initial imaging evaluation. This was first achieved by differentiation between UA and non-UA (commonly calcium-containing) renal stones. Because UA calculi comprise approximately 10% of stone disease and are typically treated medically, using urinary alkalization with stone dissolution, separating this specific subtype of stone disease provides a potential first management step in a renal stone treatment algorithm. Differentiation of UA from non-UA stones using dsDECT was first performed using in vitro models with high sensitivity and accuracy (88%–100%).[61–67] This differentiation was further improved after the addition of tin filtration for the high-energy x-ray tube,[7,11,65] given the better spectral separation, which improves stone characterization using dual-energy ratios. Subsequent in vivo studies for stone characterization also demonstrated high accuracy for separating UA and non-UA stones. Separation of UA and non-UA stones has been performed using a low-dose protocol,[67] with sensitivity of 100% and specificity of 97%. Accurate separation of cystine as a unique stone subtype has also been performed in vivo.[17,67,68] Most recently, 5 subtypes of renal stones (uric acid, cystine, struvite, calcium oxalate monohydrate/calcium oxalate dihydrate/brushite, and hydroxyapatite/carbonate apatite) have been accurately differentiated in vitro using dsDECT with tin filtration.[11] A non-commercially available data processing technique with voxel-by-voxel analysis has also identified 5 unique renal stone subtypes both in vitro[61] and in vivo[69] (UA, cystine, struvite, calcium oxalate/calcium phosphate, and brushite). The characterization of additional stone types other than UA is important to patient management, because stones known to be resistant to extracorporeal shock wave lithotripsy, including brushite, cystine, and calcium oxalate monohydrate, can be directed to management by percutaneous or endoscopic stone removal. Moreover, characterization of struvite stones directs the surgeon to total stone removal rather than allowing for small residual fragments that may result in persistent symptoms and recurrent stone growth.

The most frequently used tool for depiction of renal stone subtype characterization on dsDECT uses a 3-material decomposition algorithm that assumes every voxel includes a component of water, calcium, and/or UA. The voxels are then color coded based on the quantity of each of these components (Syngo Kidney Stone, Siemens Healthcare,

Forchheim, Germany). The processing time using this tool is rapid, requiring only several minutes, resulting in display of UA stones with a red overlay and non-UA (typically calcium stones) with a blue overlay (**Fig. 2**).

Although dsDECT acquisitions often do not increase the radiation dose when compared with routine SECT, renal stone CTs, especially in the recurrent stone former, who may require multiple exams over their lifetime, are often acquired with low radiation dose acquisitions. Alternatively, a tailored approach to characterize urinary calculi could use a low-dose unenhanced CT of the urinary system, followed by limited unenhanced dual-energy acquisitions of the urinary tract containing a visible calculus. Recent studies[70] characterized 24/24 of ureteral calculi larger than 3 mm as UA, calcium salt, or combined UA–calcium salt using stone-targeted DECT with 100% specificity. It is important to note that only one-third of calculi are considered pure stones composed of a single component, whereas 44% contain 2

components and nearly 25% contain 3 or more components.[71] Initial studies demonstrate that accurate classification of mixed stone types is more challenging than pure stone types.[68] Further research is needed to depict the distinctive portions of stone disease containing more than 1 component.

The method for renal stone characterization on ssDECT makes use of projection data, which allows for estimation of the atomic number of specific materials. This has the potential to differentiate stones that are composed primarily of UA, calcium oxalate, cystine, or struvite.[17] These data can be viewed as a separate display (Effective-Z), or overlaid onto the monochromatic images.[72] For ssDECT, renal stone characterization is as yet a work-in-progress; however, our preliminary investigations suggest that a multiparametric approach using material base pairs, computed monochromatic attenuation with spectral HU graph, and effective-z analysis has potential for the discrimination of various renal calculi (**Fig. 3**).

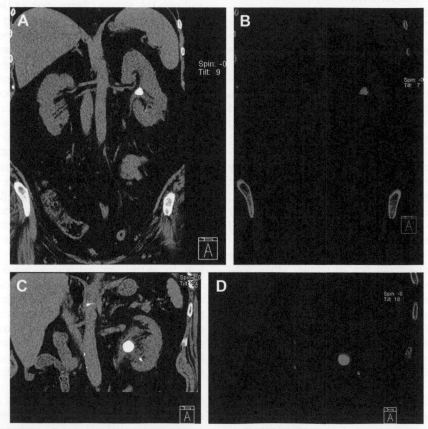

Fig. 2. (*A*) A 63-year-old woman with a left renal calculus and history of ileostomy secondary to Crohn disease. (*B*) The red coding is consistent with a UA stone, due to high concentrations of UA in acidic urine combined with low urine volume. (*C*) A 45-year-old man with a left renal calculus and urinary tract dilatation. (*D*) The blue coding is consistent with a non-UA, calcium oxalate stone.

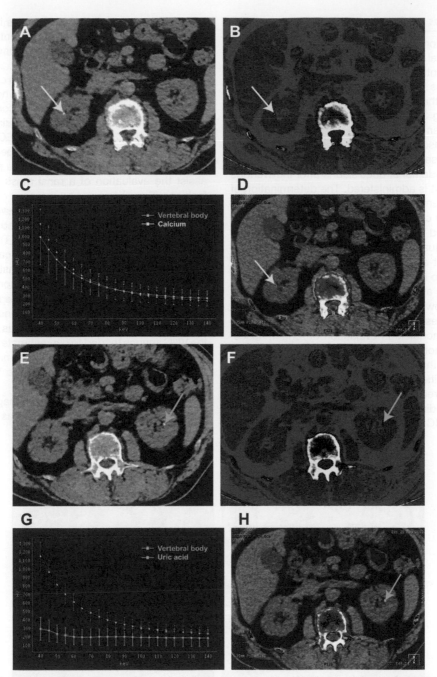

Fig. 3. Calcium-containing versus UA stone. (*A, E*) DECT water-density (VNC) images show a hyperdense stone in the right kidney (*A; gold arrow*), and a similar-size hyperdense stone in the left kidney (*E; green arrow*). On these virtual noncontrast images, these are otherwise indeterminate for calcium versus UA stones. (*B, F*) DECT material-specific iodine images show that the calcium-containing stone remains visible (*B, gold arrow*), mimicking the color overlay hue of other calcium-containing structures (ie, vertebral body and ribs); however, the UA stone is not perceptible on the same display (*F, green arrow*), as it does not contain calcium. (*C, G*) DECT spectral HU plot shows an upward-sloping curve at lower keV (*C, gold curve*) for the calcium stone, similar to the upward-sloping curve for bone (*C, peach curve*); however, UA stones generally have a relatively flatter curve (*G, green curve*). (*D, H*) Effective-Z and material-specific iodine data can be overlaid on the monochromatic display for easy discrimination of calcium-containing (*D; gold arrow;* note: similar hue as vertebral body and ribs) and UA stones (*H; green arrow*).

Renal Mass Evaluation

The detection and characterization of renal masses is an integral part of genitourinary CT. Specifically, the differentiation between a benign cyst and a solid mass is a necessity of any renal CT protocol. Typically, the determination of a cystic or solid mass using SECT relies heavily on the detection of enhancement within the center of the lesion. For this reason, most renal mass CT protocols require a baseline unenhanced CT acquisition followed by additional acquisitions after intravenous (IV) contrast is administered. The determination of enhancement relies on the measurement of the CT number centrally within the mass on the unenhanced and enhanced acquisitions. An increase in the attenuation of the mass of more than 20 HU on contrast-enhanced acquisitions is used as the threshold to identify a solid enhancing mass.[73,74]

DECT's ability to produce material-specific images allows for the identification of iodine within body tissues. This has the potential to allow for single CT acquisition evaluation of renal masses. If the technology and scanning techniques can be optimized, the necessity for a baseline unenhanced CT acquisition could be eliminated, leading to significant reductions in radiation dose to patients.

DECT iodine identification allows for postprocessed VNC, and material-specific iodine image sets to be produced. The VNC series is achieved by removing the attenuation from identified iodine within the body structures to reproduce the baseline unenhanced attenuation.

The material-specific iodine images can be used to produce iodine overlay images where a color map, showing the location and/or concentration of iodine within body tissues, is superimposed on the gray-scale CT image. With dsDECT, another image set depicting only iodine can be produced. These additional image sets have the potential to assist the evaluation of a renal mass in different fashions (Fig. 4).

Similar to current single-energy evaluation of a mass, the VNC images can be used to replace the true unenhanced CT acquisition. The attenuation of the lesion on the VNC series can serve as a baseline to compare with the contrast-enhanced series. Neville and colleagues[75] demonstrated no statistically significant difference in the attenuation of renal lesions between true unenhanced images and the VNC images; however, it was noted that the VNC images tended to overestimate the attenuation relative to the true unenhanced images. Graser and colleagues[76] have shown the VNC to be useful for mass evaluation.

Alternatively, the iodine-specific image sets obtained on dsDECT, either displayed as an overlay

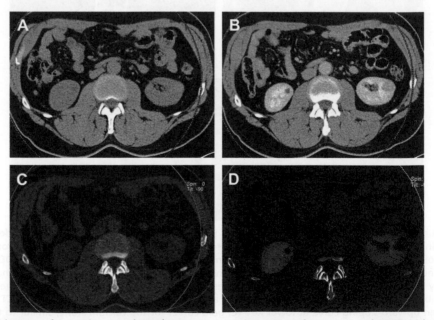

Fig. 4. DECT images of a renal cyst and renal mass. Examination was performed on a dsDECT with tin filtration using 100/140 kVp energies. (A) Unenhanced image: the cyst in the lower pole of the right kidney and mass in the lower pole of the left kidney are difficult to detect. (B) Nephrographic phase: the cyst and enhancing mass are now detectable. (C) VNC image: Similar appearance of the mass, but note the difference in the conspicuity of the cyst. (D) Material-specific iodine image: The image depicts the location of iodine signal. Note the absence of signal in the cyst and homogeneous low-level signal in the renal mass.

image superimposed on the gray-scale CT or as a series showing only the iodine signal, have also been studied as a means to identify an enhancing solid mass. With this method, one does not rely on measured changes in attenuation within a mass to determine enhancement. Rather, direct visualization of iodine signal within the mass differentiates a cyst from solid lesion. As renal cysts do not contain blood vessels centrally, the iodine-specific image sets show a cyst as devoid of iodine signal (see Fig. 4). In contrast, solid renal masses do have vessels within them, and these vessels and the tissue of the mass accumulate iodine after contrast injection. Iodine signal will therefore be identifiable within the center of the mass. Brown and colleagues[77] first described this possible use of DECT in phantom studies. The clinical use of iodine-specific images has since been reported as well.[78]

More recently, Silva and colleagues[79] described the use of quantitative imaging of renal lesions using a ssDECT scanner. They found that the use of VNC and material-specific iodine overlay images significantly improved characterization and reader confidence in differentiating cystic from solid, enhancing renal masses when compared with conventional CT (Fig. 5); however, as a standard window/level has not yet been established for the iodine display, use of spectral CT number curves helped improve reader specificity

after recognizing relatively characteristic "enhancing" and "nonenhancing" curve morphologies (Fig. 6).

In addition to VNC and iodine displays, ssDECT also allows for real-time interaction with CT data on a stand-alone workstation via the construction of computed monochromatic images.[14,72] From a single acquisition, these DECT images can be created representing up to 101 discrete energy levels (ie, 40–140 keV).[14] By taking advantage of iodine's attenuation characteristics, the differential attenuation of renal lesions relative to normal parenchymal tissue can be exploited by examining lower keV images from the computed monochromatic display.

These techniques require further evaluation and validation; however, they have the strong possibility of being clinically capable of differentiating renal cysts from solid masses as well, if not better, than current practices. If this is shown to be the case, the baseline unenhanced CT acquisition can be eliminated, thereby reducing radiation dose to the patient and length of the examinations.

URINARY STONE IN IODINATED SOLUTION (VIRTUAL NONCONTRAST IMAGES)

Unenhanced CT is considered the gold standard for the detection of urinary stones.[46,47] Urinary stones can be obscured by high-attenuation

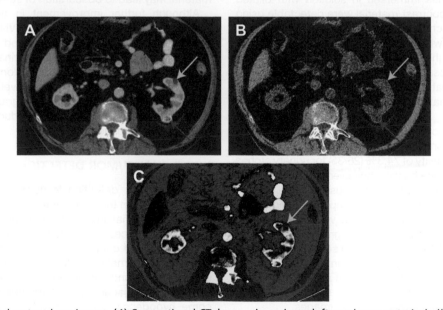

Fig. 5. Renal cyst and carcinoma. (A) Conventional CT shows a hypodense left renal mass anteriorly (blue arrow), which measured 22 HU—indeterminate for renal cyst versus a hypovascular mass. (B) DECT virtual noncontrast image shows that the mass is subtly hypodense (blue arrow) to renal parenchyma. (C) DECT material-specific iodine with color overlay highlights iodine-containing pixels with an orange-yellow hue. Note that the anterior lesion does not contain iodine and is thus avascular, a simple cyst (blue arrow). Compare this with the heterogeneously enhancing left, posterior renal cell carcinoma (A–C, red arrows).

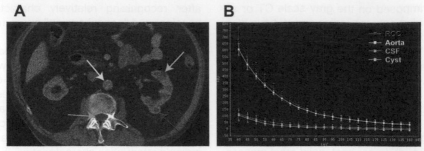

Fig. 6. Renal cyst and carcinoma. (*A*) DECT computed monochromatic image shows no qualitative difference compared with conventional CT (**Fig. 5A**); however, quantitative ROI assessment of the hypodense left renal lesion was 17 HU (*blue arrow*). This is because of inherent decreased susceptibility of the monochromatic display to beam-hardening/pseudoenhancement artifact. (*B*) DECT spectral HU display can be generated from the monochromatic display, depicting the attenuation curve of queried materials. The morphology of the spectral curves can be helpful in differentiating enhancing from avascular lesions, with the former showing a relatively steeper upslope at lower energy values as compared with the latter. Note that the left renal cyst (*A, blue arrow* and *B, blue curve*) has a similar, relatively flat curve as nonenhancing cerebrospinal fluid (*A, peach arrow* and *B, peach curve*), whereas the left renal cell carcinoma (*A, red arrow* and *B, red curve*) has a steep, upward-sloping curve at lower energies, mimicking the enhancing curve morphology in the aorta (*A, yellow arrow* and *B, yellow curve*).

iodinated contrast material in the renal parenchyma or collecting systems on contrast-enhanced CT. Unenhanced CT is not routinely performed for abdominal CT; therefore, renal stones can be missed. On the other hand, unenhanced CT is routinely performed as part of CT urography, given the higher prevalence in the patient population requiring CT urography.[80]

In a phantom study, more than 95% of 2-mm to 4-mm stones immersed in solution with diluted iodinated contrast material were detectable using the VNC technique. The detection rate was limited, however, when stones were immersed in extremely highly concentrated iodine solution. This was the result of failed iodine subtraction when the attenuation value of the iodine solution reached a maximal CT value (3070 HU) on low-kV images.[33]

In a clinical study, virtual noncontrast images created from nephrographic phase CT images had a sensitivity of 74.3% (26/35) for urinary stones on a per-stone basis[81]; however, the stone detection rate did not improve using VNC images compared with the original nephrographic phase CT. In another clinical study, virtual noncontrast images created from pyelographic phase CT images of CT urography had a sensitivity of 65.4% (17/26) for urinary stones on a per-renal-unit basis.[82] Although the detection rate was limited, it was better than the detection rate compared with the original pyelographic phase images.

In a recent study, VNC images created from both nephrographic phase CT and pyelographic phase CT images were evaluated.[83] In this study, the sensitivity of VNC images from nephrographic phase was 77.5% (62/80), whereas that of VNC

images from urographic phase was 73.8% (59/80). The poor detection rate was attributable to the inability to detect 1-mm to 2-mm stones. Oversubtraction of stone signal was a common cause of underdetection of the stones.[82] In addition to the limited ability to detect tiny stones, the stones identified on VNC images often appear smaller than on true unenhanced images.[82,83] Occasionally, undersubtraction of the signal from iodinated contrast material may lead to obscuration of stones.[82]

Although further improvement in the iodine-removal algorithm is necessary, if VNC images reconstructed from contrast-enhanced CT acquisitions eventually accurately detect urinary stones, then routine abdominal DECT detection of unsuspected stones will improve. Alternatively, the true unenhanced CT acquisition in CT urography protocols could be eliminated, thereby reducing radiation dose to the patient.

UROTHELIAL TUMOR DETECTION

Urothelial tumor detection is dependent on the contrast between tumor and the surrounding urine or adjacent normal urothelial wall. Urothelial tumor generally enhances moderately during the parenchymal phase of contrast enhancement, whereas surrounding normal urothelial wall shows minimal enhancement and urine does not enhance.[84] Tumors and adjacent normal urothelial wall become hypodense during the urographic phase, whereas urine becomes opacified.

In a phantom study simulating the pyelographic phase performed with dsDECT, the tumor-to-urine contrast-to-noise ratio increased 35% and lesion conspicuity improved in 67% of lesions

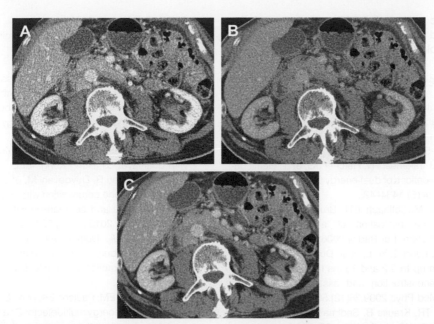

Fig. 7. Urothelial carcinoma in left renal collecting system in a 79-year-old man. (A) Axial CT image obtained in nephrographic phase using DECT 80 kVp and (B) Axial CT image obtained in nephrographic phase using DECT 140 kVp. Note high tumor-to-urine contrast and high image noise on lower-kV image (A) compared with higher kV image (B). (C) Linear blended image (50% from lower-kV image and 50% from higher-kV image). Note tumor-to-urine contrast is between (A) and (B). Improvement of noise level is attributable to summation of 2 images.

using a nonlinear sigmoidal blending technique when the attenuation of iodine in urine was 250 HU. Lesion conspicuity did not improve when the iodine attenuation in urine was higher than 500 HU because the tumor-to-urine contrast was already high.[85] Using this unique DECT technique, tumor conspicuity may improve for examinations when a reduced amount of iodine contrast material is used secondary to renal insufficiency or when only a slow rate of IV injection of iodine contrast material is allowed (Fig. 7).

ADRENAL ADENOMA

Adrenal adenomas are characterized by a large amount of intracytoplasmic fat and typically appear hypoattenuating on standard unenhanced CT, measuring 10 HU or less at unenhanced SECT at 120 kVp, and are referred to as lipid-rich adenomas. In recent studies, DECT has been shown to be useful in characterizing adrenal masses.[86,87]

In a study of adrenal nodules using unenhanced DECT at 80 kVp and 140 kVp, 13 (50%) of 26 adenomas had an attenuation decrease on the 80-kVp images relative to the 140 kVp images, indicative of the presence of intracellular lipid within an adenoma. All 5 metastatic lesions demonstrated relative attenuation increase at 80 kVp.[87] Therefore, a measurable lower attenuation of an adrenal lesion

on 80-kVp images relative to the attenuation of the lesion on the 140-kVp images is a highly specific sign of adrenal adenoma; however, the sensitivity is low because some adenomas, possibly lipid-poor adenomas, had an attenuation increase at 80 kVp.

In a recent study of 39 incidental adrenal nodules (≥1 cm in diameter) using contrast-enhanced DECT obtained at 80 kVp and 140 kVp, sensitivity, specificity, and accuracy in diagnosing lipid-rich adrenal adenomas with VNC images were 91% to 95%, 100%, and 95% to 97%, respectively, when true unenhanced SECT at 120 kVp was used as the reference standard.[86] In this study, a commercially available software was used to generate VNC images after optimization of the parameter settings by attenuation measurements of subcutaneous fat tissue (Fat) and spleen (Tissue) on the VNC and standard unenhanced CT images.[86]

SUMMARY

The recent development of DECT platforms and innovative scanning techniques has provided additional tools for the diagnosis and characterization of renal masses, urolithiasis, and disorders of the uroepithelium. Knowledge of the principal technical aspects of dual-energy scanning and the specific utility of DECT in imaging of the kidneys and urinary tract has become imperative for the radiologist in practice.

REFERENCES

1. Fletcher JG, Takahashi N, Hartman R, et al. Dual-energy and dual-source CT: is there a role in the abdomen and pelvis? Radiol Clin North Am 2009; 47(1):41–57.

2. Vrtiska TJ, Takahashi N, Fletcher JG, et al. Genitourinary applications of dual-energy CT. Am J Roentgenol 2010;194(6):1434–42.

3. Flohr TG, McCollough CH, Bruder H, et al. First performance evaluation of a dual-source CT (DSCT) system. Eur Radiol 2006;16(2):256–68.

4. Flohr TG, Leng S, Yu L, et al. Dual-source spiral CT with pitch up to 3.2 and 75 ms temporal resolution: image reconstruction and assessment of image quality. Med Phys 2009;36(12):5641–53.

5. Johnson TR, Krauss B, Sedlmair M, et al. Material differentiation by dual energy CT: initial experience. Eur Radiol 2007;17(6):1510–17.

6. Primak AN, Giraldo JC, Eusemann CD, et al. Dual-source dual-energy CT with additional tin filtration: dose and image quality evaluation in phantoms and in vivo. Am J Roentgenol 2010;195(5):1164–74.

7. Primak AN, Ramirez Giraldo JC, Liu X, et al. Improved dual-energy material discrimination for dual-source CT by means of additional spectral filtration. Med Phys 2009;36(4):1359–69.

8. Thomas C, Krauss B, Ketelsen D, et al. Differentiation of urinary calculi with dual energy CT: effect of spectral shaping by high energy tin filtration. Invest Radiol 2010;45(7):393–8.

9. Leschka S, Stolzmann P, Baumuller S, et al. Performance of dual-energy CT with tin filter technology for the discrimination of renal cysts and enhancing masses. Acad Radiol 2011;17(4):526–34.

10. Karlo C, Lauber A, Gotti RP, et al. Dual-energy CT with tin filter technology for the discrimination of renal lesion proxies containing blood, protein, and contrast-agent. An experimental phantom study. Eur Radiol 2011;21(2):385–92.

11. Qu M, Ramirez-Giraldo JC, Leng S, et al. Dual-energy dual-source CT with additional spectral filtration can improve the differentiation of non-uric acid renal stones: an ex vivo phantom study. Am J Roentgenol 2011;196(6):1279–87.

12. Wang J, Garg N, Duan X, et al. Quantification of iron in the presence of calcium with dual-energy computed tomography (DECT) in an ex vivo porcine plaque model. Phys Med Biol 2011;56(22):7305–16.

13. Xu D, Langan D, Wu X, et al. Dual energy CT via fast kVp switching spectrum estimation (article no. 72583T). Progress in Biomedical Optics and Imaging - Proceedings of SPIE 2009;7258:72583T.

14. Silva AC, Morse BG, Hara AK, et al. Dual-energy (spectral) CT: applications in abdominal imaging. Radiographics 2011;31(4):1031–46 [discussion: 1047–50].

15. Goodsitt MM, Christodoulou EG, Larson SC. Accuracies of the synthesized monochromatic CT numbers and effective atomic numbers obtained with a rapid kVp switching dual energy CT scanner. Med Phys 2011;38(4):2222–32.

16. Carmi R, Naveh G, Altman A. Material separation with dual-layer CT. Hong Kong: IEEE; 2005.

17. Hidas G, Eliahou R, Duvdevani M, et al. Determination of renal stone composition with dual-energy CT: in vivo analysis and comparison with x-ray diffraction. Radiology 2010;257(2):394–401.

18. Vlassenbroek A. Dual Layer CT. In: Johnson T, Fink C, Schonberg S, et al, editors. Dual Energy CT in Clinical Practice. Berlin (Heidelberg): Springer; 2011. p. 21–34.

19. Boll DT, Merkle EM, Paulson EK, et al. Coronary stent patency: dual-energy multidetector CT assessment in a pilot study with anthropomorphic phantom1. Radiology 2008;247(3):687–95.

20. Boll DT, Merkle EM, Paulson EK, et al. Calcified vascular plaque specimens: assessment with cardiac dual-energy multidetector CT in anthropomorphically moving heart phantom1. Radiology 2008;249(1):119–26.

21. Roessl E, Proksa R. K-edge imaging in x-ray computed tomography using multi-bin photon counting detectors. Phys Med Biol 2007;52:4679.

22. Butler A. Bio-medical X-ray imaging with spectroscopic pixel detectors. Nucl Instrum Methods Phys Res A 2008;591(1):141–6.

23. Schlomka JP, Roessl E, Dorscheid R, et al. Experimental feasibility of multi-energy photon-counting K-edge imaging in pre-clinical computed tomography. Phys Med Biol 2008;53(15):4031.

24. Eiber M, Holzapfel K, Frimberger M, et al. Targeted dual-energy single-source CT for characterisation of urinary calculi: experimental and clinical experience. Eur Radiol 2012;22(1):251–8.

25. Leng S. Renal stone composition differentiation using two consecutive CT scans and a non-rigid registration algorithm. Presented at the 97th Scientific Assembly and Meeting of the Radiological Society of North America. Chicago (IL), November 27 to December 2, 2011.

26. Guimaraes L, Fletcher JG, Harmsen MS, et al. Appropriate Patient Selection at Abdominal Dual energy CT using 80 kV: Relationship Between Patient Size and Image Noise and Image Quality. Radiology 2010;257(3):732–42.

27. Yu L, Primak AN, Liu X, et al. Image quality optimization and evaluation of linearly mixed images in dual-source, dual-energy CT. Med Phys 2009;36(3):1019–24.

28. Holmes DR 3rd, Fletcher JG, Apel A, et al. Evaluation of non-linear blending in dual-energy computed tomography. Eur J Radiol 2008;68(3):409–13.

29. McCollough CH, Schmidt B, Liu X, et al. Dual-Energy Algorithms and Postprocessing Techniques. In: Johnson T, Fink C, Schonberg S, et al, editors. Dual Energy CT in Clinical Practice. Berlin (Heidelberg): Springer; 2011. p. 43–51.

30. Kalender W, Perman W, Vetter J, et al. Evaluation of prototype dual energy computed tomographic apparatus. I. Phantom studies. Med Phys 1986; 13(3):334–9.

31. Alvarez, R, A Macovski, inventors. The Board of Trustees of Leland Stanford Junior University, assignee. X-ray spectral decomposition imaging system. Available at: http://www.patents.com/us-4029963.html. US patent 4029963. July 30, 1976.

32. Liu X, Yu L, Primak AN, et al. Quantitative imaging of element composition and mass fraction using dual-energy CT: three-material decomposition. Med Phys 2009;36(5):1602–9.

33. Takahashi N, Hartman RP, Vrtiska TJ, et al. Dual-energy CT iodine-subtraction virtual unenhanced technique to detect urinary stones in an iodine-filled collecting system: a phantom study. Am J Roentgenol 2008;190(5):1169–73.

34. Hubbell, J. and S. Seltzer. Tables of x-ray mass attenuation coefficients and mass energy-absorption coefficients (version 1.4). Available at: http://physics.nist.gov/xaamdi. Accessed January 7, 2012.

35. Hubbell JH. Review and history of photon cross section calculations. Phys Med Biol 2006;51(13): R245–62.

36. Yu L, Christner JA, Leng S, et al. Virtual monochromatic imaging in dual-source dual-energy CT: radiation dose and image quality. Med Phys 2011;38(12): 6371.

37. Matsumoto K, Jinzaki M, Tanami Y, et al. Virtual monochromatic spectral imaging with fast kilovoltage switching: improved image quality as compared with that obtained with conventional 120-kVp CT. Radiology 2011;259(1):257–62.

38. Yuan R, Shuman WP, Earls JP, et al. Reduced iodine load at CT pulmonary angiography with dual-energy monochromatic imaging: comparison with standard CT pulmonary angiography—a prospective randomized trial. Radiology 2012;262(1):290–7.

39. Venema HW. Virtual monochromatic spectral imaging with fast kilovoltage switching should not be used as standard CT imaging modality. Radiology 2011;260(3):916–7.

40 Leng S, Yu L, Wang J, et al. Noise reduction in spectral CT: reducing dose and breaking the trade-off between image noise and energy bin selection. Med Phys 2011;38(9):4946.

41. Mitcheson HD, Zamenhof RG, Bankoff MS, et al. Determination of the chemical composition of urinary

42. Pearle MS, Calhoun EA, Curhan GC. Urologic diseases in America project: urolithiasis. J Urol 2005;173(3):848–57.

43. Chen MY, Zagoria RJ. Can noncontrast helical computed tomography replace intravenous urography for evaluation of patients with acute urinary tract colic? J Emerg Med 1999;17(2):299–303.

44. Fielding JR, Steele G, Fox LA, et al. Spiral computerized tomography in the evaluation of acute flank pain: a replacement for excretory urography. J Urol 1997;157(6):2071–3.

45. Niall O, Russell J, MacGregor R, et al. A comparison of noncontrast computerized tomography with excretory urography in the assessment of acute flank pain. J Urol 1999;161(2):534–7.

46. Smith RC, Rosenfield AT, Choe KA, et al. Acute flank pain: comparison of non-contrast-enhanced CT and intravenous urography. Radiology 1995; 194(3):789–94.

47. Smith RC, Verga M, Dalrymple N, et al. Acute ureteral obstruction: value of secondary signs of helical unenhanced CT. Am J Roentgenol 1996; 167(5):1109–13.

48. Bellin MF, Renard-Penna R, Conort P, et al. Helical CT evaluation of the chemical composition of urinary tract calculi with a discriminant analysis of CT-attenuation values and density. Eur Radiol 2004; 14(11):2134–40.

49. Demirel A, Suma S. The efficacy of non-contrast helical computed tomography in the prediction of urinary stone composition in vivo. J Int Med Res 2003;31(1):1–5.

50. Hillman BJ, Drach GW, Tracey P, et al. Computed tomographic analysis of renal calculi. Am J Roentgenol 1984;142(3):549–52.

51. Mostafavi MR, Ernst RD, Saltzman B. Accurate determination of chemical composition of urinary calculi by spiral computerized tomography. J Urol 1998;159(3):673–5.

52. Motley G, Dalrymple N, Keesling C, et al. Hounsfield unit density in the determination of urinary stone composition. Urology 2001;58(2):170–3.

53. Nakada SY, Hoff DG, Attai S, et al. Determination of stone composition by noncontrast spiral computed tomography in the clinical setting. Urology 2000; 55(6):816–9.

54. Newhouse JH, Prien EL, Amis ES Jr, et al. Computed tomographic analysis of urinary calculi. Am J Roentgenol 1984;142(3):545–8.

55. Sheir KZ, Mansour O, Madbouly K, et al. Determination of the chemical composition of urinary calculi by noncontrast spiral computerized tomography. Urol Res 2005;33(2):99–104.

56. Zarse CA, McAteer JA, Tann M, et al. Helical computed tomography accurately reports urinary

stone composition using attenuation values: in vitro verification using high-resolution micro-computed tomography calibrated to Fourier transform infrared microspectroscopy. Urology 2004;63(5):828–33.

57. Saigal CS, Joyce G, Timilsina AR. Direct and indirect costs of nephrolithiasis in an employed population: opportunity for disease management? Kidney Int 2005;68(4):1808–14.

58. Coe FL, Keck J, Norton ER. The natural history of calcium urolithiasis. JAMA 1977;238(14):1519–23.

59. Joseph P, Mandal AK, Singh SK, et al. Computerized tomography attenuation value of renal calculus: can it predict successful fragmentation of the calculus by extracorporeal shock wave lithotripsy? A preliminary study. J Urol 2002;167(5):1968–71.

60. Pareek G, Armenakas NA, Fracchia JA. Hounsfield units on computerized tomography predict stone-free rates after extracorporeal shock wave lithotripsy. J Urol 2003;169(5):1679–81.

61. Boll DT, Patil NA, Paulson EK, et al. Renal stone assessment with dual-energy multidetector CT and advanced postprocessing techniques: improved characterization of renal stone composition—pilot study. Radiology 2009;250(3):813–20.

62. Graser A, Johnson TR, Bader M, et al. Dual energy CT characterization of urinary calculi: initial in vitro and clinical experience. Invest Radiol 2008;43(2):112–9.

63. Matlaga BR, Kawamoto S, Fishman E. Dual source computed tomography: a novel technique to determine stone composition. Urology 2008;72(5):1164–8.

64. Primak AN, Fletcher JG, Vrtiska TJ, et al. Noninvasive differentiation of uric acid versus non-uric acid kidney stones using dual-energy CT. Acad Radiol 2007;14(12):1441–7.

65. Stolzmann P, Kozomara M, Chuck N, et al. In vivo identification of uric acid stones with dual-energy CT: diagnostic performance evaluation in patients. Abdom Imaging 2010;35(5):629–35.

66. Stolzmann P, Scheffel H, Rentsch K, et al. Dual-energy computed tomography for the differentiation of uric acid stones: ex vivo performance evaluation. Urol Res 2008;36(3–4):133–8.

67. Thomas C, Patschan O, Ketelsen D, et al. Dual-energy CT for the characterization of urinary calculi: in vitro and in vivo evaluation of a low-dose scanning protocol. Eur Radiol 2009;19(6):1553–9.

68. Manglaviti G, Tresoldi S, Guerrer CS, et al. In vivo evaluation of the chemical composition of urinary stones using dual-energy CT. Am J Roentgenol 2011;197(1):W76–83.

69. Zilberman DE, Ferrandino MN, Preminger GM, et al. In vivo determination of urinary stone composition using dual energy computerized tomography with advanced post-acquisition processing. J Urol 2010;184(6):2354–9.

70. Ascenti G, Siragusa C, Racchiusa S, et al. Stone-targeted dual-energy CT: a new diagnostic approach to urinary calculosis. Am J Roentgenol 2010;195(4):953–8.

71. Schubert G. Stone analysis. Urol Res 2006;34(2):146–50.

72. Silva AC, Robinette AM. Quantitative imaging with single source dual energy CT (ssDECT): potential applications and how we do it. Paper presented at 96th Scientific Assembly and Annual Meeting of the Radiological Society of North America. Chicago (IL), November 27 to December 2, 2011.

73. Israel GM, Bosniak MA. How I do it: evaluating renal masses. Radiology 2005;236(2):441–50.

74. Siegel CL, Fisher AJ, Bennett HF. Interobserver variability in determining enhancement of renal masses on helical CT. Am J Roentgenol 1999;172(5):1207–12.

75. Neville AM, Gupta RT, Miller CM, et al. Detection of renal lesion enhancement with dual-energy multidetector CT. Radiology 2011;259(1):173–83.

76. Graser A, Johnson TR, Hecht EM, et al. Dual-energy CT in patients suspected of having renal masses: can virtual nonenhanced images replace true nonenhanced images? Radiology 2009;252(2):433–40.

77. Brown CL, Hartman RP, Dzyubak OP, et al. Dual-energy CT iodine overlay technique for characterization of renal masses as cyst or solid: a phantom feasibility study. Eur Radiol 2009;19(5):1289–95.

78. Song KD, Kim CK, Park BK, et al. Utility of iodine overlay technique and virtual unenhanced images for the characterization of renal masses by dual-energy CT. Am J Roentgenol 2011;197(6):W1076–82.

79. Silva AC, Bollepalli SD. Differentiating enhancing vs. nonenhancing lesions in the liver and kidney: comparison of single- and dual-energy CT. Paper presented at: 96th Scientific Assembly and Annual Meeting of the Radiological Society of North America. Chicago (IL), November 27 to December 2, 2011.

80. Kawashima A, Glockner JF, King BF Jr. CT urography and MR urography. Radiol Clin North Am 2003;41(5):945–61.

81. Scheffel H, Stolzmann P, Frauenfelder T, et al. Dual-energy contrast-enhanced computed tomography for the detection of urinary stone disease. Invest Radiol 2007;42(12):823–9.

82. Takahashi N, Vrtiska TJ, Kawashima A, et al. Detectability of urinary stones on virtual nonenhanced images generated at pyelographic-phase dual-energy CT. Radiology 2010;256(1):184–90.

83. Moon JW, Park BK, Kim CK, et al. Evaluation of virtual unenhanced CT obtained from dual-energy CT urography for detecting urinary stones. Br J Radiol 2012.

84. Kim JK, Park SY, Ahn HJ, et al. Bladder cancer: analysis of multi-detector row helical CT enhancement pattern and accuracy in tumor detection and perivesical staging. Radiology 2004;231(3):725–31.

85. Takahashi N, Hartman RP, Kawashima A, et al. Dual-energy CT for the detection of tumor in iodine-filled ureter: lesion conspicuity using different blending methods in a phantom study. Presented at the 94th Scientific Assembly and Annual Meeting of the Radiological Society of North America. Chicago (IL), November 30 to December 5, 2008.

86. Gnannt R, Fischer M, Goetti R, et al. Dual-energy CT for characterization of the incidental adrenal mass: preliminary observations. Am J Roentgenol 2012; 198(1):138–44.

87. Gupta RT, Ho LM, Marin D, et al. Dual-energy CT for characterization of adrenal nodules: initial experience. Am J Roentgenol 2010;194(6):1479–83.

Advances in Uroradiologic Imaging in Children

Pooja Renjen, MD[a],*, Richard Bellah, MD[b],
Jeffrey C. Hellinger, MD[c], Kassa Darge, MD, PhD[d]

KEYWORDS

- MR urography • Voiding urosonography • CT angiography
- CT urography

Diagnostic imaging of pediatric urologic disorders is continuously changing as technologic advances are made. Although the backbone of pediatric urologic imaging has been ultrasound (US), voiding cystourethrography (VCUG), and radionuclide scintigraphy, newer and advanced modalities are becoming increasingly important. This article discusses the techniques and clinical applications of three such imaging modalities as they pertain to pediatric urologic disorders: (1) MR urography (MRU); (2) advanced US (harmonic imaging, three-dimensional, and voiding urosonography [VUS]); and (3) CT angiography (CTA).

MRU

MRU is a powerful examination that has the distinct advantage of providing anatomic and functional information in one examination. MRU allows a one-stop-shop evaluation of the renal parenchyma, collecting system, vasculature, bladder, and surrounding structures. MRU has intrinsic high soft tissue contrast resolution and multiplanar three-dimensional reconstruction capabilities, without the use of radiation. Additionally, MRU allows quantification of numerous renal functional parameters

including transit times, an index of glomerular filtration rate (GFR), and differential renal functions (DRF). To date, MRU may serve as the most comprehensive and definitive study in the evaluation of urinary tract obstruction, complex genitourinary anomalies, and infection. The following sections discuss patient preparation, technique, clinical applications, and limitations of MRU as it pertains to the evaluation of pediatric urologic disorders.[1–7]

Patient Preparation

Patient preparation is a crucial part of the successful MRU examination. The examination begins with discussion with the family regarding the purpose and operations of the study. The patient preparation portion of the MRU examination typically takes approximately 1 hour, which includes sedation, hydration, and catheterization. Patients younger than 7 years of age are typically sedated to eliminate patient motion artifact. Although sedation protocols must be adapted according to the experience of each center, at the authors' institution a combination of midazolam, fentanyl, and phenobarbital is typically used. All children undergoing sedation are under continuous close electrocardiogram and pulse oximetry monitoring under the

This article is updated and adapted from Renjen P, Bellah R, Hellinger JC, Darge K. Pediatric urologic advanced imaging: techniques and applications. Urol Clin N Am 2010;37:307–18.

[a] Department of Radiology, Hackensack Radiology Group, Hackensack University Medical Center, Hackensack, NJ 07601, USA
[b] Department of Radiology, The Children's Hospital of Philadelphia, University of Pennsylvania, Philadelphia, PA 19104, USA
[c] Department of Radiology, Stony Brook University Medical Center, Stony Brook, NY 11794, USA
[d] Division of Body Imaging, Department of Radiology, The Children's Hospital of Philadelphia, University of Pennsylvania, Philadelphia, PA 19104, USA
* Corresponding author.
E-mail address: poojarenjen1@gmail.com

Radiol Clin N Am 50 (2012) 207–218
doi:10.1016/j.rcl.2012.02.003
0033-8389/12/$ – see front matter © 2012 Elsevier Inc. All rights reserved.

control of an appropriately trained member of the sedation unit. Older nonsedated children are asked to breathe quietly, or if they are able to cooperate breath-hold imaging is performed.

Provided no contraindications (fluid restriction, congestive heart failure, and so forth) exist, patients are given 20 mL/kg (maximum of 1 L) of normal saline or Ringer solution intravenously over the course of 30 to 60 minutes before the start of imaging. To minimize the need for additional manipulations during the scan, the infusion is stopped before entering the MR scanner room. The administration of intravenous fluid helps to reduce the MR imaging contrast concentration and decrease the potential of T2* effect, making a linear relationship of the gadolinium concentration to the signal intensity possible. It also improves the visualization of the pelvicalyceal system and ureter and optimizes the baseline for subsequent furosemide (Lasix) administration.[8]

A bladder catheter without inflatable balloon is placed to decompress the bladder. In a patient with planned sedation, this is done after sedation. A decompressed bladder is important because it ensures that the contrast washout is not disturbed by full bladder effect or reflux. The catheter may also serve as a urethral marker in cases of possible ureteral ectopy.

The patient is positioned in the MR imaging scanner supine with the arms above the head. Patients with dilated pelvicalyceal system and without contrast in the ipsilateral ureter need to be turned to the prone position for the acquisition of additional delayed sequences.

After the patient is appropriately positioned, before the start of imaging, Lasix is administered intravenously with a dosage of 1 mg/kg up to a maximum dose of 20 mg. The purpose of the Lasix injection is several-fold.[8] Lasix increases urine flow and ensures the urinary tract is distended without increasing GFR. This increased distention of the urinary tract allows improved visualization of nondilated collecting systems. It serves to reduce the gadolinium concentration for the same reasons as discussed under hydration. Lasix results in a more uniform distribution of gadolinium-based contrast, which reduces susceptibility artifacts. It is necessary for the evaluation of the excretory function under diuresis. Finally, Lasix administration shortens the examination time. Contraindications to Lasix administration include anuria, electrolyte imbalance, and hypotension. Patients with sulfonamide allergies may also be allergic to Lasix.[9]

The imaging portion of the examination takes between 30 and 60 minutes, depending on the need of delayed images including after repositioning the patient to the prone position.

Technique

A comprehensive MRU protocol is a two-part imaging technique comprised of precontrast sequences (static MRU) and postcontrast sequences (dynamic or excretory MRU).

Part one: static MRU (precontrast imaging)
Static MRU uses heavily T2-weighted fluid-sensitive sequences in which urine-containing structures are bright (Fig. 1). These T2-weighted images serve to delineate the anatomy of the renal collecting systems and ureters. Unlike the postcontrast excretory MRU images, these T2-weighted images are not dependent on renal function and excretion

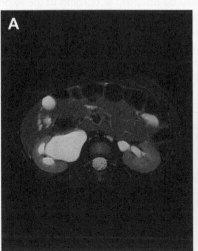
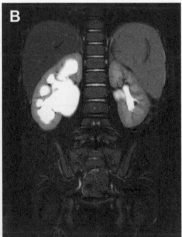
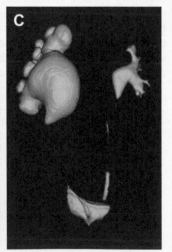

Fig. 1. Ureteropelvic junction (UPJ) obstruction. MRU showing a dilated pelvicalyceal system on the right. Precontrast T2-weighted axial (A) and coronal (B) images and precontrast maximum-intensity projection (C).

of contrast material into the collecting systems to outline the anatomy of the urinary tract. Therefore, the T2-weighted sequences prove to be of greatest value in delineating the anatomy of the collecting system of a poorly or nonfunctioning renal moiety or kidney. These sequences become particularly important in identifying ureteral ectopy (eg, in the case of a patient with constant wetting). Three-dimensional respiratory-triggered T2 sequences can be reconstructed to create maximum intensity projections (MIP) and volume-rendered images of the entire collecting system (see Fig. 1C). Additional high-quality axial T2 sequences are also obtained to provide a high-resolution view of the renal parenchyma.

Part two: dynamic MRU (postcontrast imaging)
Dynamic MRU not only provides anatomic information including that of the vascular system, but it also offers functional information, which is in many ways analogous to a nuclear medicine study (Fig. 2A, B). Intravenous gadolinium is administered and sequential three-dimensional dynamic sequences of the entire urinary tract are acquired. These images can be presented as a MIP and a cine loop. The former provides morphologic information (see Fig. 1C). The dynamic sequences are the basis of the functional calculation, assess renal perfusion, evaluate renal transit and excretion, and allow generation of signal intensity versus time curves. The images are transferred and postprocessed on an external computer using a freely available custom-made software package (www.chop-fmru.com).[10] The software package is used to calculate several functional parameters including calyceal transit time (CTT) and renal transit time (RTT); DRF based on renal parenchymal volume and Patlak number (an index of GFR); and parenchymal volume and Patlak number. Moreover, the software package provides time-signal intensity curves of the renal parenchyma and contrasted part of the pelvicalyceal system corresponding to the renal enhancement and excretion (washout) curves, respectively (Fig. 3).

CTT and RTT refer to the time period between the appearance of contrast in the aorta and just before its appearance in the calyces and proximal ureter, respectively. CTT is the more reliable parameter because RTT can vary according to the volume of the renal pelvis and the morphology of the ureteropelvic junction (UPJ); the RTT value alone may not always differentiate between stasis and obstruction. CTT and RTT should only be interpreted in conjunction with the static and dynamic images. The influence of parenchymal disease on these values should not be underestimated. The cut-off points for normal and abnormal RTT as published in one study do not seem to be universally reliable in classifying UPJ obstruction as compensated and decompensated.[11]

DRF remains the most widely used measure of renal function. With MRU, the DRF is calculated using two distinct methods. The first method is referred to as the "volumetric differential renal function" (vDRF) and is based on the volume of enhancing renal parenchyma, which essentially represents functional renal mass. The vDRF is calculated by measuring the volume of enhancing renal parenchyma at the time point of homogenous renal enhancement before contrast excretion in the calyces as determined by viewing the dynamic series. This method of calculation makes a distinction between functioning enhancing tissue and nonfunctional dysplastic or scarred tissue. This

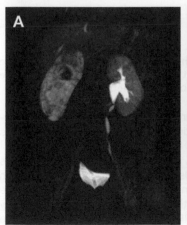
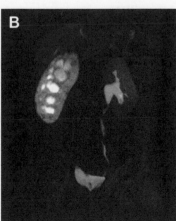
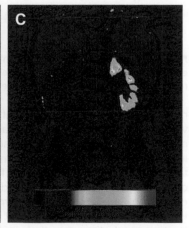

Fig. 2. UPJ obstruction. (*A, B*) MRU postcontrast dynamic series shows delayed dense nephrogram (*A*) and dilated pelvicalyceal system on the right. (*C*) The functional map (Patlak map) reveals significant decrease of function on the right compared with the left. The DRF values were volumetric DRF: R32% and L68%.

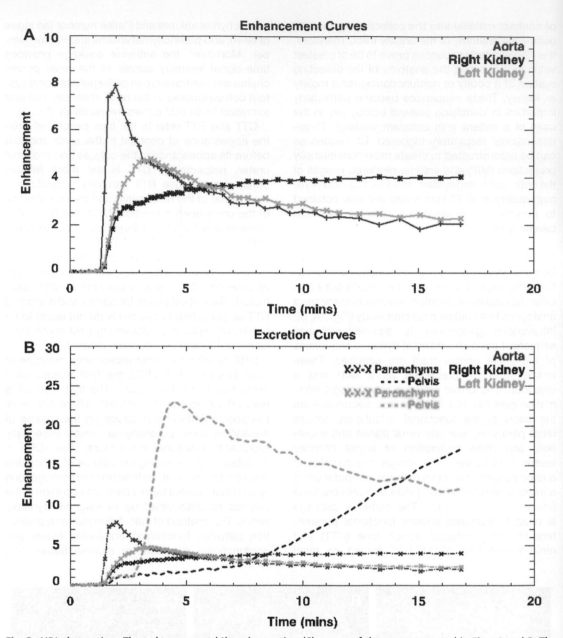

Fig. 3. UPJ obstruction. The enhancement (*A*) and excretion (*B*) curves of the case presented in **Figs. 1** and **2**. The enhancement and excretion curves demonstrate a normal curve on the left but a climbing one on the right. The renal transit time was over 15 minutes on the right compared with 2 minutes on the left.

method also allows for the calculation of the individual contributions from upper and lower pole moieties in duplex kidneys. The second method is referred to as the "Patlak differential renal function" (pDRF), and is an index of GFR. The pDRF is calculated using the Patlak model. The same enhancing parenchyma that determines vDRF is the basis for calculating pDRF, but takes the contrast concentration over time in the aorta into consideration. After the injection of gadolinium, sequential intensity values of the aorta and renal

parenchyma are obtained and subsequently entered automatically in the Patlak equation; this generates the Patlak plot and Patlak numbers.[1] The vDRF is a relatively stable number, whereas the pDRF tends to change with acute changes in GFR. This change in pDRF may reflect a measure of renal function recoverability. Comparatively speaking, vDRF is thought to correlate with the DRF measured by DMSA scintigraphy, whereas pDRF is thought to correlate with MAG3 scintigraphy. When the percentage of the renal parenchyma is taken into consideration with the pDRF, a volumetric pDRF can be calculated.

Comparison with Renal Scintigraphy

MRU has been shown to be superior to renal scintigraphy in many regards.[12] MRU has superior contrast and temporal and spatial resolution and can provide precise anatomic information, which radionuclide studies cannot. MRU has also been shown to be superior to renal scintigraphy in distinguishing between pyelonephritis and scar.[1,13] The functional analysis of MRU also provides more comprehensive functional information.

Limitations

Although MRU is a powerful study with numerous advantages, few limitations do exist. MRU can have relatively long imaging times and is sensitive to motion artifact, which necessitates sedation for young children. This may be considered a minor limitation by some because MRU can provide anatomic and functional information in one examination.

Although to avoid ionizing radiation MRU may be used to follow children with bigger recurrent stone disease, CT remains the gold standard for the detection of small urinary tract calculi, which are not always necessarily resolvable on MR imaging.

The postcontrast dynamic images and interpretation of time signal intensity curves can be used to assess for the possibility of vesicoureteral reflux (VUR). However, MR voiding VCUG is unlikely to replace conventional VCUG because of technical limitations including the inability of sedated patients to completely empty their bladder.

An important limitation of the dynamic postcontrast part of the MRU is that it can be contraindicated in patients with moderate renal insufficiency. As stated, excretory MRU involves the administration of intravenous gadolinium and requires excretion into the collecting systems. Although it was previously thought that gadolinium could be safely administered in patients with renal insufficiency or failure to avoid iodinated contrast material, the disorder nephrogenic systemic fibrosis is now linked to gadolinium administration.[14,15] New recommendations are to make every effort to avoid administering gadolinium-based contrast material in patients with moderate to severe renal insufficiency (GFR <30 mL/min). However, this issue remains a topic of investigation and recommendations may change in the future.

Clinical Applications

MRU can be used in the evaluation of congenital genitourinary anomalies, urinary tract obstruction, infection versus scarring, renal transplantation, hematuria, and surgically altered anatomy. The two most common indications for MRU in the pediatric population include complex congenital anatomic anomalies of the genitourinary tract and hydronephrosis.

Congenital Genitourinary Anomalies

Congenital anomalies of the genitourinary tract are more common than those of any other organ system, with a frequency of between 1:650 and 1:1000. Urinary tract anomalies predispose the child to a variety of complications, including infection, obstruction, wetting, stasis, and stone disease. At present, US is still most often used to provide anatomic information and renal scintigraphy to obtain functional information. MRU has the potential to replace multimodality imaging by providing the three-dimensional anatomic evaluation of the entire urinary tract and the renal functional information that aids in management decisions. For example, in the evaluation of the girl who is "wet all the time," MRU has been shown to be superior to US in the detection of occult upper pole moieties and in demonstrating ureteral ectopy.[3,16,17] In this instance, excretory function of the kidney is not a limiting factor in diagnosing an ectopic ureter because the static-fluid MRU images are sufficient. This is also true for the detection of dysplastic ectopic kidneys that are very difficult to see with other imaging modalities. MRU can also clarify the anatomy and complications related to complex urinary tract anomalies, such as crossed fused renal ectopia and horseshoe kidney.

Hydronephrosis and Obstruction

Hydronephrosis is the most common abnormality seen in the kidney on prenatal and postnatal imaging. UPJ obstruction is the most common cause of hydronephrosis in childhood. Although in neonates UPJ obstruction is most often caused by intrinsic narrowing of the proximal ureter, in older children this is often caused by a crossing vessel causing extrinsic compression and kinking of the ureter. Prognosis and need for surgical intervention is best predicted on basis of renal function.

MRU can provide the anatomic and functional information necessary to guide management.[18,19] Obstruction is suggested morphologically by dilation of the renal pelvis and narrowing of the ureter (see **Fig.** 2A, B). MRU can depict the site of ureteral narrowing, assess for a possible crossing vessel, and evaluate for possible obstructing urothelial mass. Obstruction is suggested functionally by nonexcretion or delayed excretion of contrast material.

Dynamic MRU can also be used to assess the success of pyeloplasty. Prepyeloplasty parameters, vDRF, pDRF, and RTT can be compared with those obtained postpyeloplasty to ascertain the effect of surgery.[20]

Pyelonephritis Versus Scar

MRU can demonstrate pyelonephritis but may also distinguish acute pyelonephritis from renal scarring, which is a distinct advantage compared with renal scintigraphy.[1,3,13] MRU has also been shown to be more sensitive in detecting renal scarring compared with US, a finding of clinical importance when deciding if a Deflux procedure should be performed.[21] The normal renal cortex demonstrates homogenous low signal intensity on T2-weighted images. Acute pyelonephritis appears as areas of abnormal T2 signal hyperintensity in the renal cortex and also demonstrates a striated or patchy nephrogram on postcontrast imaging similar to that seen with CT. Unlike acute pyelonephritis, renal scarring appears as focal areas of parenchymal volume loss with deformity of the renal contour, with or without associated deformity of the underlying calyx.

Renal Transplant

Renal transplant complications can be categorized as prerenal (vascular); renal (intrinsic parenchymal disease); and postrenal (obstruction). MRU has the ability to evaluate and distinguish among these complications in a single comprehensive examination. Because gadolinium is administered for the dynamic portion of the MRU, MR angiography can also be performed during the first pass of contrast material through the aorta and renal arteries. As such, evaluation for possible renal artery stenosis can be made. Additionally, delayed images allow assessment for patency of the renal veins. Intrinsic parenchymal disease can be suggested on the T2-weighted images if increased cortical T2 signal and loss of corticomedullary differentiation are seen. The T2-weighted sequences can also be used to depict hydronephrosis, ureteral stenosis or kinks, lymphoceles, and urinomas. The dynamic MRU can provide functional information of the transplant kidney, such as GFR. Decreased transplant function may provide an earlier clue to acute or chronic rejection and potentially reduce the need for biopsy.[4]

Hematuria

MRU can evaluate for possible renal parenchymal lesions, vascular lesions, and urothelial abnormalities as an etiology for hematuria. Additionally, MRU may be used to follow children with big recurrent stone disease to avoid ionizing radiation.[4,5] Urinary tract calculi appear as filling defects in the collecting systems on the static-fluid urography images and excretory MRU images. Secondary signs of stone disease, such as perirenal edema, renal enlargement, and urothelial thickening, can be demonstrated.

ADVANCED ULTRASONOGRAPHY
Harmonic Imaging

Harmonic imaging is a technical method that has proved to be useful in urosonography based on nonlinear properties of US that provide clearer and sharper US images than fundamental US.[22–24] Harmonic imaging constructs images based on higher frequencies than conventional US, and also reduces US artifacts. Harmonic imaging improves border recognition and tissue differentiation, particularly of fluid-filled structures (Fig. 4). Additionally, it

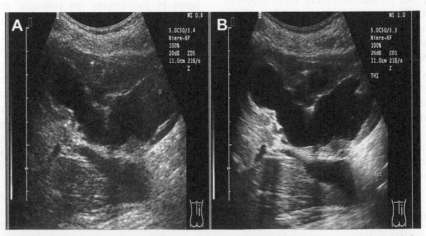

Fig. 4. Conventional US (A) and harmonic US (B) of a hydronephrotic kidney. The US image with harmonic image is clearer without artifacts and the different structures are better delineated.

improves the conspicuity of even a small amount of echo-enhancing agents.[25] It has been shown to improve the detection of renal stones, renal parenchymal lesions, and the overall US scan of the urinary tract in children.[26,27] However, the improved border recognition may create artifacts that have to be recognized; specifically, harmonic imaging exaggerates the normal corticomedullary differentiation and may falsely mimic nephrocalcinosis.

Three-Dimensional US

Three-dimensional US combines conventional two-dimensional US with position information to provide a three-dimensional data set. Three-dimensional US has numerous advantages.[23,24,28] First, three-dimensional US can create multiplanar views, similar to MR imaging and CT. This multiplanar capability provides greater anatomic information. For example, it may help in distinguishing a renal cyst from a calyceal diverticulum. Three-dimensional US also allows for better evaluation of surfaces and curved structures and, as such, may better delineate the collecting system of a complex duplex kidney, or a dilated, hydronephrotic kidney. Three-dimensional US has been shown to have increased accuracy in the calculation of renal parenchymal volumes and, thereby, improve standardization of renal measurements, particularly of hydronephrotic and scarred kidneys. It also provides more exact bladder volume measurement.

VUS Technique, Clinical Application, and Limitations

VUS is a relatively new modality in the detection of VUR in children. Although VCUG and radionuclide cystography (RNC) are currently the two methods most commonly used to evaluate for VUR, recent developments of commercially available echo-enhancing agents have significantly improved the sonographic detection of fluid movement within the urinary tract (Fig. 5). The most commonly used echo-enhancing agent is Levovist (Bayer-Schering, Berlin, Germany), which is composed of 99.9% microcrystalline galactose particles and 0.1% palmitic acid. This introduces stabilized microbubbles, which allow improved visualization of fluid movement. More recently a newer generation of US contrast agent (SonoVue; Bracco, Milan, Italy) with distinctly more practical advantages than Levovist is being used.[29–31] These US contrast agents have made VUS a reliable alternative to VCUG and RNC with the distinct advantage of avoiding ionizing radiation and, at the same time, increasing the detection rate of VUR. Given that radiation exposures continue to be a concern in the pediatric population, strong consideration to performing VUS over conventional methods may be given. In the following sections, the patient preparation, technique, and clinical applications and limitations of VUS are discussed.[29,30,32,33]

Overall, the VUS examination consists of scanning the patient before, during, and after the

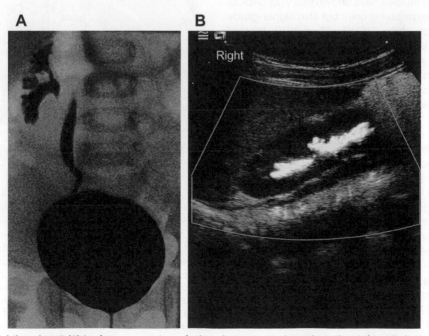

Fig. 5. VCUG (A) and VUS (B) in the same patient during the same study session. The right-sided grade II reflux is equally well demonstrated with both modalities.

intravesical administration of US contrast agent, and during voiding. First, the patient is placed in the supine position on the examination table for a baseline US examination of the urinary tract. Subsequently, a bladder catheter is inserted under aseptic conditions and urine is allowed to drain. The bladder is then slowly filled with a warmed saline solution under physiologic pressure until the predicted bladder volume is reached ([age + 2] × 30) or the patient feels an urge to void. The saline infusion is warmed to minimize patient discomfort. The US contrast agent is intravesically administered during the early filling phase. The kidneys, ureter, and bladder are then imaged to assess for possible VUR, which is diagnosed by the presence of echogenic microbubbles in either the ureters or the renal pelves. The patient is then asked to void around the catheter and additional sonographic images of the kidneys, ureters, and bladder are obtained during voiding. Although most patients are able to void in the supine, prone, or decubitus position, if the child is older a potty or urine bottle may be offered to the child and the child may be scanned from the back while seated or standing. If desired, cyclic filling may also be performed with the procedure repeated under the same conditions using the same filling volume and the same catheter, which needs to be left in place after the first cycle.

VUS can be used in work-up of urinary tract infections, follow-up of known VUR, and in the evaluation of reflux in renal transplant patients. Comparative studies have shown that VUS depicts not only more refluxing units but also higher-grade refluxes than does VCUG. Most VUR labeled grade I on VCUG actually are grade II or higher on VUS. A reflux grading system similar to the one used in VCUG is used in VUS, as follows: grade I, microbubbles reaching the ureter only; grade II, microbubbles reaching the nondilated renal pelvis; grade III, microbubbles reaching the moderately dilated pyelocalyceal system; grade IV, microbubbles reaching the significantly dilated pyelocalyceal system; and grade V, microbubbles reaching the significantly dilated pyelocalyceal system with loss of the normal renal pelvic contour and with a dilated, tortuous ureter.

The main limitation of VUS is the evaluation of the urethra, although this may be less of a consideration in female patients. This limitation may potentially be overcome by incorporating transperineal US with the examination. Like RNC, VUS is an excellent technique for screening patients and for follow-up of known VUR in patients of both sexes.

A second minor limitation is that the examination is longer than VCUG. Specifically, the examination may take up to 30 minutes to perform including catheterization, whereas a VCUG may only take approximately 15 minutes. However, the examination time may be decreased with the use of harmonic imaging or newer contrast-specific modalities, and if a baseline US does not need to be performed. The 10% increase in reflux detection rate combined with the absence of radiation compensates for the longer duration of the study.

CT

State-of-the-art CT technology offers two advanced imaging protocols for pediatric urological applications: 3D CT angiography (CTA) (Fig. 6), and 3D CT urography (CTU) (Fig. 7). For both, workstation image post-processing is essential. CTA and CTU require precise synchronization between contrast medium delivery and the scan acquisition. With CTA, synchronization is to the arterial or venous phase, while for CTU, synchronization is to the delayed excretory renal phase. Although inherently dependent upon radiation and iodinated contrast medium, CTA and CTU can be performed safely in pediatric patients using low radiation and contrast medium dose strategies.

Technical Considerations

Current state-of-the-art scanners with 64- to 320-channel multidetector-row CT (MDCT) technology,

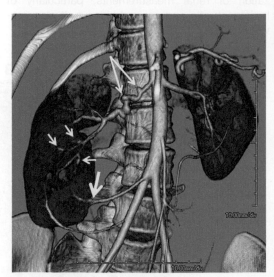

Fig. 6. A 14-year-old girl with neurofibromatosis type 1 and progressively worsening hypertension underwent renal CTA. Coronal volume-rendered image shows three right and single left renal arteries. Advanced extraparenchymal (postostial, *long arrows*) and intraparenchymal (second to third order, *short arrows*) beading and irregularity involve the main right renal artery distribution. Note intraparenchymal collateral flow from the first accessory right renal artery (*thick arrow*). No disease was identified in the left renal arteries.

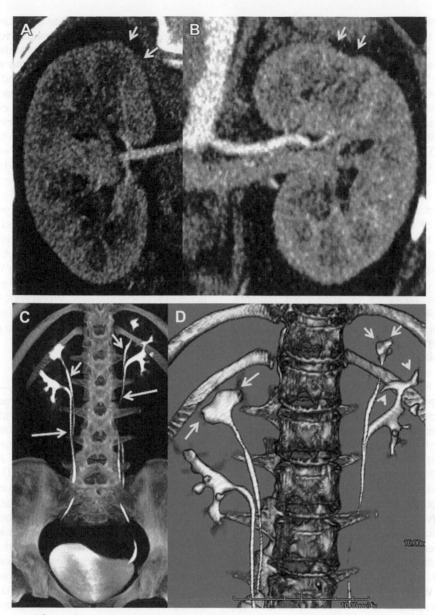

Fig. 7. CTA was performed in a 16-year-old girl with hypertension. Single bilateral renal arteries were patent; however, preliminary review of the renal parenchyma demonstrated right (A) and left (B) upper pole mild focal cortical thinning (arrows) prompting a delayed urographic acquisition. CT urography revealed bilateral duplex configurations (C, MIP image; arrows) with calyceal blunting involving the bilateral upper pole moieties (D, volume rendering; arrows), consistent with reflux nephropathy. Mild calyceal blunting was also noted to involve the superior portion of the left lower pole moiety (D, arrowheads).

can generate isotropic (0.5- to 0.75-mm thick images) and high-resolution (1.25- to 1.5-mm thick images) volumetric datasets. In most instances, however, a high-resolution acquisition provides sufficient detail for accurate CTA and CTU diagnoses and subsequent treatment planning. In selecting this mode, patients are exposed to less radiation as submillimeter collimation is not required. Additional basic strategies and acquisition parameters to control radiation exposure include restricting coverage to the anatomy of interest and using the lowest possible voltage (kilovolt [peak] kV[p]) and amperage (milliampere). Coverage, voltage, and amperage all have direct relationships with the amount of patient radiation exposure. The minimum coverage for assessment of the native renal vasculature is from the upper abdomen to the upper pelvis. This coverage accounts for possible anomalous renal arteries, which may arise from as high as the supraceliac aorta down to the iliac arteries. If the examination is to assess prerenal or postrenal transplant vasculature, coverage is limited to the pelvis and lower abdomen. Regarding CTU coverage, the scan volume includes the abdomen and pelvis, from the suprarenal regions through to the bladder. Voltage options for most vendors include 80, 100, 120, and 140 kV(p). 80 kV(p) is recommended until 50 kg, 100 kV(p) from 50 to 90 kg, and 120 kV(p) greater than 90 kg. Amperage is typically prescribed using an automated dose algorithm. This delivers a variable range of amperage over the length of the coverage, based on prescan determined body density and a targeted threshold value for acceptable noise.

In our experience using a 64-channel MDCT scanner for abdominal CTA and abdominal–pelvis CTU in the neonates to adolescent patients, average radiation exposures are approximately 1-2mSv.[34] This radiation dose is equivalent to that of approximately 50-100 chest radiographs.[35] Sub-millisievert exposure can be achieved using 64-channel scanners by decreasing the amperage while using 80 or 100kVp. However, the tradeoff is higher image noise and decreased image quality. Adjunct, advanced strategies to reduce image noise and maintain high image quality include iterative reconstruction and 3D workstation structural preservation techniques.[36,37] 128-320 channel systems offer the potential for routine sub-mSv exposure with less compromise in image quality. Iterative reconstruction and 3D workstation structural preservation techniques also apply to these advanced scanners.

When a renal CTA or CTU is performed on a 64-channel scanner, the scan time ranges between 1.5 and 4 seconds, depending on the scan coverage. When taking into consideration the technical preparations for the scan, the average room time is approximately 10 to 15 minutes. To optimize image quality and minimize respiratory and patient motion artifact, sedation or anesthesia may be required, leading to additional room time. Depending upon the coverage, 128- to 320-channel scanners can generate subsecond scan times for submillimeter abdominal and abdominal–pelvis CT examinations, inherently minimizing the potential for motion artifacts. This technology may obviate the need for sedation or anesthesia in pediatric patients undergoing renal CTA and CTU, which may enhance patient safety and workflow efficiency.

Three-dimensional CTA and three-dimensional CTU are best reviewed on a server-based thin client or independent thick client workstation using a combination of multiplanar and curved planar reconstructions, three-dimensional volume rendering, and MIPs. Alternatively, static postprocessed images are generated on the workstation and transferred to a Picture Archive and Communications System for subsequent review along with the original axial and reconstructed coronal and sagittal images. Thin client workstations offer the advantage of being able to review studies and perform advanced analysis for treatment planning from any location. Select images can be captured and transmitted electronically for communication with other physicians. Virtual group conferences for treatment planning are possible, with remote sharing of the workstation screen and interactive two- and three-dimensional display options. The most recent thin client technology streams data over the Internet from a server with a World Wide Web–based interface that does not require additional executable software. World Wide Web–client workstation technology is available on select hand-held and tablet devices, which has the potential to further enhance patient care.

Clinical Considerations

Pediatric CTA and CTU are considered only after US and MR imaging have been attempted without satisfactory answer to the clinical question(s), or in cases where CT is considered superior for the specific clinical imaging objectives. Appropriate primary indications for CTA and CTU, based on the advantages of CT technology, include the presence of metallic hardware and implantable devices; the requirement for higher spatial resolution; and the need for rapid scan time, such as in emergent imaging or in the high sedation and anesthesia risk patient. If MR imaging or US is nondiagnostic or negative and there remain clinical requirements for additional imaging, CTA and CTU should be considered before conventional catheter angiograms and intravenous pyelograms, respectively.

After there is a decision to proceed forward with CT, it is imperative to confirm the patient has normal renal function and does not have an allergy to iodinated contrast. It should also be determined if sedation or anesthesia is required. It is recommended to counsel the family and patient on the risks, benefits, and precautionary radiation protective measures for CT, including use of low radiation dose strategies. Examinations for neonates, infants, and toddlers should be scheduled with consideration to feeding schedules, because most imaging departments have 2- to 4-hour food restrictions before a contrast-enhanced CT. On the day of the examination, a suitable size peripheral vein is accessed for optimized contrast delivery. This is often in the hand for the neonate or infant and the forearm or antecubital fossa for toddler, young child, or adolescent. In a neonate, a 24-gauge intravenous catheter is placed, whereas in an infant, a 22- or 24-gauge is used. Beyond this age, a 20- or 22-gauge is recommended.

CTA applications for the pediatric urology patient include evaluation of suspected or known renovascular hypertension (see Fig. 6); crossing renal hilar vessels (in the setting of UPJ obstruction); renal aneurysms (commonly syndromic related); small vessel vasculitis; renal venous occlusive disease (ie, tumor invasion); vascular malformations (in the setting of hematuria); and traumatic renovascular injury. An additional indication is preoperative vascular mapping as may be required prior to resection of vascular renal and adrenal tumors. Diagnostic quality pediatric renal CT arteriograms are those that are motion free, achieving robust enhancement of extraparenchymal renal arteries through to at least the third- to fourth-order intraparenchymal segments, with the goal of depicting the subcapsular fourth- to fifth-order arteries. This is particularly important in the setting of renovascular hypertension secondary to fibromuscular dysplasia, because it is not uncommon to have isolated intraparenchymal arterial disease. As with conventional angiography, assessment addresses the number, caliber, contour, course, and patency of native and anomalous renal arteries and veins. Although arterial flow is not directly evaluated, global and regional enhancement patterns provide indirect measures of flow and parenchymal perfusion; global and regional kidney size and cortical thickness serve as means to assess renal function and potential sequelae from vascular or alternatively, nonvascular pathology.

CTU applications include the evaluation of suspected or known congenital anomalies, obstructive uropathy, traumatic nephroureteral injury, reflux nephropathy (see Fig. 7), and papillary necrosis. Acquisitions may be performed as a single dedicated urographic 8- to 10-minute delay acquisition or as a second series after a routine CT or CTA acquisition. In the authors' experience, given the dominant role for MRU in the diagnosis and surveillance of pediatric renal parenchymal and nephroureteral disease, CTU is most commonly performed after the first-pass phase of the CT arteriogram. In this instance, if preliminary review of the CTA images reveals parenchymal abnormalities, with or without vascular abnormalities, the monitoring physician determines whether an 8- or 10-minute delayed urographic series is warranted to elucidate the cause for the patient's symptoms (see Fig. 7). Diagnostic-quality CT urograms are those that are motion free, achieving

dense enhancement of the upper and lower collecting systems and the bladder, while maintaining enhancement in the renal parenchyma. As with MRU or conventional intravenous pyelograms, evaluation addresses the number, caliber, contour, course, and patency of native and anomalous upper and lower collecting systems. Renal pelvis, infundibular, and calyceal abnormalities are assessed with regards to feeding arteries and draining veins and regional parenchymal abnormalities. Normal ipsilateral and contralateral segments are used as internal normative references, applying flexible visualization techniques. While urographic flow is not directly evaluated, delayed renal parenchymal enhancement patterns can provide an indirect measure of urinary flow. As with the vascular phase, global and regional kidney size and cortical thickness serve as means to assess nephron function.

REFERENCES

1. Grattan-Smith JD, Jones RA. MR urography in children. Pediatr Radiol 2006;36:1119–32.
2. Grattan-Smith JD, Little SB, Jones RA. MR urography in children: how we do it. Pediatr Radiol 2008; 38(Suppl 1):S3–17.
3. Cerwinka WH, Grattan-Smith JD, Kirsch AJ. Magnetic resonance urography in pediatric urology. J Pediatr Urol 2008;4:74–83.
4. Kalb B, Votaw JR, Salman K, et al. Magnetic resonance nephrourography: current and developing techniques. Radiol Clin North Am 2008;46:11–24.
5. Leyendecker JR, Barnes CE, Zagoria RJ. MR Urography: techniques and clinical applications. Radiographics 2008;28:23–48.
6. Darge K, Anupindi SA, Jaramillo D. MR imaging of the abdomen and pelvis in infants, children, and adolescents. Radiology 2011;261(1):12–29.
7. Darge K, Grattan-Smith JD, Riccabona M. Pediatric uroradiology: state of the art. Pediatr Radiol 2011; 41(1):82–91.
8. Grattan-Smith JD, Perez-Bayfield MR, Jones RA, et al. MR imaging of kidneys: functional evaluation using F-15 perfusion imaging. Pediatr Radiol 2003; 33:293–304.
9. Healy R, Jankowski TA. Which diuretics are safe and effective for patients with a sulfa allergy? J Fam Pract 2007;56:488–90.
10. Khrichenko D, Darge K. Functional analysis in MR urography - made simple. Pediatr Radiol 2010; 40(2):182–99.
11. Grattan-Smith JD, Little SB, Jones RA. MR urography evaluation of obstructive uropathy. Pediatr Radiol 2008;38(Suppl 1):S49–69.
12. Perez-Brayfield MR, Kirsch AJ, Jones RA, et al. A prospective study comparing ultrasound, nuclear

scintigraphy and dynamic contrast enhanced magnetic resonance imaging in the evaluation of hydronephrosis. J Urol 2003;170:1330–4.

13. Kavanagh EC, Ryan S, Awan A, et al. Can MRI replace DMSA in the detection of renal parenchymal defects in children with urinary tract infections? Pediatr Radiol 2005;35:275–81.

14. Grobner T. Gadolinium: a specific trigger for the development of nephrogenic fibrosing dermopathy and nephrogenic systemic fibrosis? Nephrol Dial Transplant 2006;21:1104–8.

15. Thomsen HS, Morcos SK, Dawson P. Is there a causal relation between the administration of gadolinium based contrast media and the development of nephrogenic systemic fibrosis (NSF)? Clin Radiol 2006;61:905–6.

16. Avni FE, Nicaise N, Hall M, et al. The role of MR imaging for the assessment of complicated duplex kidneys in children: preliminary report. Pediatr Radiol 2001;31:215–23.

17. Staatz G, Rohrmann D, Nolte-Ernsting CC, et al. Magnetic resonance urography in children: evaluation of suspected ureteral ectopia in duplex systems. J Urol 2001;166:2346–50.

18. Rorhrschneider WK, Haufe S, Wiesel M, et al. Functional and morphologic evaluation of congenital urinary tract dilatation by using combined static-dynamic MR urography: findings in kidneys with a single collecting system. Radiology 2002;224:683–94.

19. Jones RA, Easley K, Little SB, et al. Dynamic contrast-enhanced MR urography in the evaluation of pediatric hydronephrosis. Part I. Functional assessment. AJR Am J Roentgenol 2005;185:1598–607.

20. Kirsch AJ, McMann LP, Jones RA, et al. Magnetic resonance urography for evaluating outcomes after pediatric pyeloplasty. J Urol 2006;176:1755–61.

21. Rodriguez LV, Spielman D, Herfkens RJ, et al. Magnetic resonance imaging for the evaluation of hydronephrosis, reflux, and renal scarring in children. J Urol 2001;166:1023–7.

22. Tranquart F, Grenier N, Eder V, et al. Clinical use of ultrasound tissue harmonic imaging. Ultrasound Med Biol 1999;25:889–94.

23. Riccabona M. Modern pediatric ultrasound: potential applications and clinical significance. A review. Clin Imaging 2006;30:77–86.

24. Riccabona M. Potential of modern sonographic techniques in pediatric uroradiology. Eur J Radiol 2002;43:110–21.

25. Darge K, Zeiger B, Rohrschneider W, et al. Contrast-enhanced harmonic imaging for the diagnosis of vesicoureteral reflux in pediatric patients. AJR Am J Roentgenol 2001;177:1411–5.

26. Kim B, Lim HK, Choi MH, et al. Detection of parenchymal abnormalities in acute pyelonephritis by pulse inversion harmonic imaging with or without microbubble ultrasonographic contrast agent: correation with computed tomography. J Ultrasound Med 2001;20:5–14.

27. Bartnam U, Darge K. Harmonic versus conventional ultrasound imaging of the urinary tract in children. Pediatr Radiol 2005;35:655–60.

28. Riccabona M, Fritz G, Ring E. Potential applications of three-dimensional ultrasound in the pediatric urinary tract: pictorial demonstration based on preliminary results. Eur Radiol 2003;13:2680–7.

29. Darge K. Voiding urosonography with ultrasound contrast agents for the diagnosis of vesicoureteral reflux in children. I. Procedure. Pediatr Radiol 2008;38:40–53.

30. Darge K. Voiding urosonography with US contrast agents for the diagnosis of vesicoureteric reflux in children. II. Comparison with radiological examinations. Pediatr Radiol 2008;38:54–63.

31. Robrecht J, Darge K. In-vitro comparison of a 1st and 2nd generation US contrast agent for reflux diagnosis. Rofo 2007;179:818–25 [in German].

32. Giordano M, Marzolla R, Puteo F, et al. Voiding urosonography as first step in diagnosis of vesicoureteral reflux in children: a clinical experience. Pediatr Radiol 2007;37(7):674–7.

33. Darge K, Troeger D, Duetting T, et al. Reflux in young patients: comparison of voiding US of the bladder and retrovesical space with echo enhancement versus voiding cystourethrography for diagnosis. Radiology 1999;210:201–7.

34. Hellinger JC, Pena A, Poon M, et al. Pediatric CT angiography: Imaging the cardiovascular system gently. Radiol Clin North 2010;48(2):439–67.

35. Brody AS, Frush DP, Huda W, et al. Radiation risk to children from computed tomography. Pediatrics 2007;120:677–82.

36. Prakash P, Kalra MK, Kambadakone AK, et al. Reducing abdominal CT radiation dose with adaptive statistical iterative reconstruction technique. Invest Radiol 2010;45:202–10.

37. Hellinger JC, Jacobs S, Salazar P, et al. Image quality improvement using a 3D edge-sensitive noise reduction filter in low dose pediatric retrospective ECG-gated cardiac CT angiography (CCTA). J Cardiovasc Comput Tomogr 2011;5(4S):S6–7.

Adrenal Imaging: A Comprehensive Review

Myles Taffel, MD[a,*], Shawn Haji-Momenian, MD[b],
Paul Nikolaidis, MD[c], Frank H. Miller, MD[c]

KEYWORDS

- Adrenal neoplasm
- Adrenal adenoma
- Adrenal characterization

ARTICLE OBJECTIVES

1. Review the characteristic imaging features of common adrenal masses.
2. Learn the recommended algorithm for the workup of an incidental adrenal mass.
3. Develop an understanding of emerging technologies in the evaluation of adrenal masses.

With the proliferation of medical imaging, physicians are increasingly facing the diagnostic challenges that are associated with the discovery of an unsuspected mass on radiologic imaging. Among the most common "incidentalomas" are lesions discovered in the adrenal gland. Adrenal lesions are seen in approximately 4% of abdominal CTs performed for various reasons.[1] The prevalence of these lesions increases to 10% in the elderly.[1]

With an increasing number of adrenal lesions being identified, radiologists must have a sound understanding of imaging characteristics and their implications. When an adrenal lesion is encountered, two questions must be answered: is the lesion functional, and is the lesion malignant. Despite being typically asymptomatic on presentation, the endocrinology literature recommends that patients undergo a clinical assessment that includes a hormonal workup to evaluate for subclinical Cushing syndrome, pheochromocytoma, or hyperaldosteronism. This evaluation includes a 1-mg dexamethasone suppression test, plasma or urine metanephrines, and a ratio of plasma aldosterone concentration to plasma renin activity.[2]

Improvements in imaging techniques often allow a definitive diagnosis of benignity, and can obviate any additional workup. In indeterminate lesions, the radiologist should guide intervention when treatment is warranted and differentiates them from the "leave alone" mass. With this in mind, the American College of Radiology developed recommendations for the management of incidental findings (**Fig. 1**). The committee consensus was published as a White Paper to provide guidance.[3] These guidelines promote greater consistency in recognizing, reporting, and managing adrenal lesions. The anticipated benefits of these guidelines included reducing patient risk from unnecessary examinations, limiting costs of management, and providing guidance to radiologists concerned about litigation risk.

BENIGN LESIONS

Adrenal Adenomas

The adrenal cortex contains increased amounts of intracytoplasmic fat (cholesterol, fatty acids, neutral fat), which acts as a precursor for hormone production. Approximately 70% of adrenal adenomas are lipid-rich and contain significant amounts of intracytoplasmic fat. Unfortunately, up to 30% are lipid-poor adenomas and do not

[a] Department of Radiology, George Washington University Medical Center, Washington, DC, USA
[b] Association of Alexandria Radiologists, Alexandria, VA, USA
[c] Department of Radiology, Northwestern University, Feinberg School of Medicine, 676 North Saint Clair, Suite 800, Chicago, IL 60611, USA
* Corresponding author.
E-mail address: taffelm@gmail.com

Radiol Clin N Am 50 (2012) 219–243
doi:10.1016/j.rcl.2012.02.009
0033-8389/12/$ – see front matter © 2012 Elsevier Inc. All rights reserved.

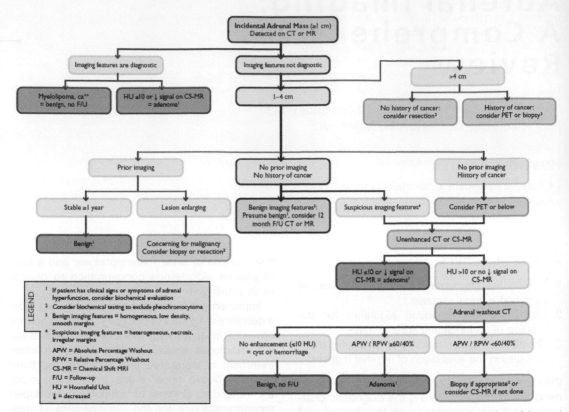

Fig. 1. American College of Radiology White Paper algorithm for management of incidental adrenal lesions. (*From* Berland LL, Silverman SG, Gore RM, et al. Managing incidental findings on abdominal CT: White Paper of the American College of Radiology Incidental Findings Committee. J Am Coll Radiol 2010;7(10):764. Copyright © 2010 American College of Radiology; with permission.)

contain substantial amounts of lipids, making them difficult to distinguish from other adrenal masses. Adenomas are often smaller than 3 cm, homogeneous, and have well-defined margins; however, these morphologic features overlap with malignant lesions, limiting their diagnostic usefulness. Achieving a high level of specificity is imperative in diagnosing an adenoma to prevent the incorrect classification of a malignant lesion. Without this high specificity, patients with cancer who have incorrectly classified metastases may be precluded from undergoing curative treatment.[4]

Although often asymptomatic, some adenomas secrete hormones independent of adrenocorticotropic hormone stimulation or the renin–angiotensin system. Approximately 5.3% of patients with incidentally discovered adrenal lesions have autonomous cortisol secretion.[5] Some patients may present with obvious signs of Cushing syndrome or hyperaldosteronism; however, sequelae of mildly elevated cortisol levels may not be as apparent in others. When autonomous cortisol secretion is seen in patients without the typical symptomatology of Cushing syndrome,

the condition is defined as subclinical Cushing syndrome. These patients are at risk for the adverse effects of long-term elevated cortisol levels, including hypertension, obesity, diabetes, and osteoporosis. To identify patients with this subtle condition accurately, an overnight dexamethasone suppression test is recommended as one of the tests for patients with incidentally discovered adrenal lesions.

Most incidentally discovered adrenal lesions are lipid-rich adenomas. Song and colleagues[6] studied 973 patients with 1049 incidental adrenal masses discovered on CT, none of whom had a history of malignancy. One-year follow-up imaging or at least a 2-year clinical follow-up was performed for each patient. Adenomas accounted for 75% of all lesions, with 78% of these lesions being lipid-rich.

Some discrepancies exist between the radiology and the endocrinology literature regarding follow-up imaging of incidentally found, hormonally inactive benign adenomas. Despite little data to support their recommendation, the National Institutes of Health State-of-the-Science statement asserts that a repeat CT at 6 to 12 months is reasonable.[7] Multiple clinical guidance publications by Young and colleagues[8–10] suggest additional imaging be considered at 24 months. This recommendation is in contrast to the Appropriateness Criteria published by the American College of Radiology.[11] If the lesion has diagnostic features of a benign neoplasm, no data support strict serial follow-up imaging.[11]

Adenomas have been characterized using the presence of intracytoplasmic fat for almost 2 decades. Using densitometry on unenhanced CT, Lee and colleagues[12] were the first to effectively differentiate many adrenal adenomas from non-adenomatous lesions. Densitometry is performed by placing a region of interest over the lesion that encompasses one-half to two-thirds of the adrenal lesion surface area. This large region of interest prevents measurement inaccuracies that are secondary to sampling error and noise. With specificity as a high priority, Lee and colleagues[12] showed that a Hounsfield unit (HU) threshold of 0 allowed an adenoma to be diagnosed at a specificity of 100%, but the sensitivity was low at 47%. Multiple studies have been performed to assess HU values and their relative sensitivities and specificities in the diagnosis of adrenal adenomas. A meta-analysis by Boland and colleagues[4] found that if the threshold HU value was raised to 10, a very small false-negative rate was able to be maintained (specificity of 98%) with significant improvements in sensitivity (71%). Therefore, a cutoff of less than 10 HU is generally used to diagnose an adenoma, a technique endorsed by the American College of Radiology appropriateness criteria.[11]

The relative abundance of intracellular lipid in adenomas is also the basis of the signal loss seen on MR chemical shift imaging (CSI). CSI takes advantage of the different resonant frequencies of fat and water protons. Because of the longer chemical side chains present in fat, the hydrogen protons precess at a lower frequency than those in water. For in-phase (IP) imaging, the echo time is selected to align the fat and water proton signals to be additive (exact echo time is dependent on field strength). In opposed-phase (OP) imaging, the echo time is selected so the fat and water signals are opposed 180°. This 180° opposition causes signal cancellation, resulting in a drop in signal if both water and fat protons are within the same voxel. Masses with either fat or water components in a single voxel, but not both, will not display signal cancellation. Korobkin and colleagues[13] showed that an inverse relationship exists between the percentage of lipid-rich cortical cells in adrenal adenomas and the relative change in signal intensity on CSI. On the OP sequences, almost a complete signal intensity loss is seen when equal concentrations of fat and water are present in most voxels. Conversely, if the proton ratio of lipid-to-water is low, the signal intensity on the OP sequences is essentially unchanged and the lesion remains indeterminate. This same study showed a similar inverse relationship between the percentage of intracytoplasmic fat in an adrenal adenoma and its CT attenuation values.[13] With CSI, the sensitivities and specificities of differentiating adenomas range from 81% to 100% and 94% to 100%, respectively.[14]

Current imaging protocols allow the acquisition of the IP and OP sequences simultaneously in a single breath hold. All slices are obtained in the same anatomic position and no hardware or sequence-related variability exists between the acquisitions, which is a problem with older acquisition techniques. Many radiologists assess the loss of signal visually, and this may be sufficient with a significant decrease in signal. If only visual inspection is used to assess for a loss of signal, the radiologist must use the same contrast window and level when viewing the IP and OP sequences so that differences in image contrast do not influence perceived signal differences. Caution is advised in lesions with more equivocal loss of signal. Postprocessing subtraction techniques (reconstructed after subtracting the OP images from the IP images) can enhance qualitative evaluation. This technique increases visual conspicuity and obviates window/level concerns. Savci and colleagues[15] retrospectively reviewed 35 patients with 42 adrenal masses who underwent CSI. The two radiologists reviewing

Table 1
Quantitative analysis for chemical shift MRI

Parameter	Formula	Value Indicating Adenoma
Adrenal-to-spleen chemical shift ratio	(Lesion SI_{OP}/Spleen SI_{OP})/(Lesion SI_{IP}/Spleen SI_{IP})	<0.71
Adrenal SI index	$(SI_{IP}-SI_{OP})/SI_{IP} \times 100\%$	>16.5%

Abbreviations: IP, in-phase sequence; OP, opposed-phase sequence; SI, signal intensity.

the subtracted images observed high qualitative specificity using this technique.

Despite the relative ease and efficiency of qualitative analysis, increased accuracy may be seen when quantitative measures are used.[16,17] Multiple methods can be used to perform these quantitative calculations using internal references. Because the liver can have fatty infiltration, the spleen is generally the optimal internal reference organ. The CSI signal loss is measured quantitatively using the adrenal-to-spleen chemical shift ratio or the adrenal sensitivity index. The adrenal-to-spleen chemical shift ratio (ASR) is calculated by dividing the lesion-to-spleen signal intensity (SI) ratio on OP sequences by the ratio on the IP sequences (Lesion SI_{OP}/Spleen SI_{OP})/(Lesion SI_{IP}/Spleen SI_{IP}) (Table 1). McNicholas and colleagues found that all adrenal adenomas had an ASR of 70 or less.[18,19] The adrenal SI index is calculated using ([IP–OP]/IP) × 100.[16] Fujiyoshi and colleagues[20] assessed these quantitative methods in a study of 102 adrenal tumors in 88 patients. The parameters were also compared with lesion-to-muscle and lesion-to-liver ratios. In this study, the adrenal SI index was the most reliable, with 100% accuracy when the SI index was between 11.2% and 16.5%. No adenomas in their series had an SI index of less than 16.5%. Although the adrenal-to-spleen ratio was the

second most accurate parameter, considerable overlap was seen between adenomas and metastatic tumors when an ASR of less than 71 was used. Other organs are less accurate when used as internal references. The liver should not be used because of the frequent incidence of hepatic steatosis, which also results in signal loss on the OP sequences from the presence of intracytoplasmic fat. Muscle is not typically used because it is also subject to fatty infiltration.

As nonenhanced CT and CSI are both based on detection of intracellular lipid, debate exists over which modality is superior for characterizing incidentally discovered adrenal lesions. Outwater and colleagues[21] showed a high correlation between CT attenuation values and CSI ratios. Both techniques resulted in indeterminate characterization of a similar subset of benign lesions. One study by Haider and colleagues[22] specifically evaluated the performance of CSI on lesions with an HU value between 10 and 30. Within these parameters, CSI showed 89% sensitivity (17 of 19 lesions) and 100% specificity (11 of 11 lesions) for adenoma characterization. These findings suggest that CSI can characterize some adenomas that do not meet unenhanced CT criteria (Fig. 2).

Because up to 30% of adrenal adenomas are lipid-poor, both noncontrast CT and CSI are limited in evaluation of these lesions. Fortunately,

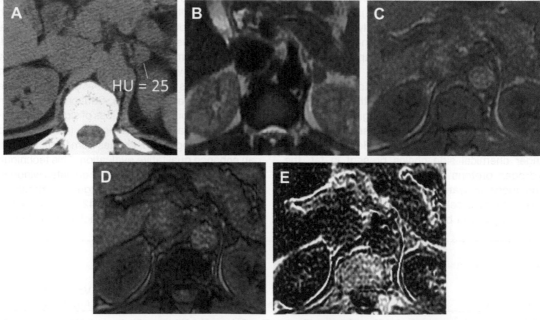

Fig. 2. MRI evaluation of a hyperattenuating adrenal mass (10–30 HU). CSI can characterize some lipid-rich adenomas that do not meet unenhanced CT criteria. (A) An incidental left adrenal mass was identified on an unenhanced CT, with attenuation greater than 10 HU. (B) Corresponding T2-weighted image again shows the left adrenal mass. (C, D) On gradient-echo CSI, a drop in signal intensity is seen on the OP (D) compared with the IP (C). (E) This signal loss is confirmed with CSI subtraction (IP minus OP).

several authors showed that delayed CT enhancement parameters allow characterization of both lipid-poor and lipid-rich adenomas.[23–25] Adenomas de-enhance faster than nonadenomatous lesions. The high vascular density and permeability associated with disorganized angiogenesis in malignancy is believed to lead to prolonged contrast accumulation in malignant adrenal lesions. An absolute attenuation measurement on delayed scans has not been found to be reliable.[26]

The washout percentage calculation provides a reproducible method to assess contrast de-enhancement when characterizing adrenal lesions. Two methods are available to calculate percent washout: absolute percentage washout (APW), which incorporates a precontrast attenuation value, and relative percentage washout (RPW) (Table 2, Fig. 3). The APW is derived from the formula ([enhanced HU–delayed HU]/[enhanced HU–noncontrast HU]) × 100. The RPW is derived from ([enhanced HU–delayed HU]/enhanced HU) × 100. Incorporation of the noncontrast HU value results is in a more accurate determination of washout; therefore, APW should be calculated when possible. RPW is typically performed when an astute technologist identifies an adrenal mass on a contrast-enhanced examination while the patient is on the table. The precontrast HU value should supersede the washout characteristics if the value indicates benignity.[27] Any lesion with an intrinsic noncontrast HU value of 43 or more should be viewed with a high suspicion for malignancy regardless of the washout characteristics.[27]

Caoili and colleagues[26] found that lipid-poor adenomas showed 15-minute delayed washout characteristics similar to lipid-rich adenomas, and significantly less than nonadenomas. An APW threshold of 60% was set for lipid-poor adenomas, resulting in 95% specificity and 89% sensitivity. An RPW threshold of 40% resulted in 93% specificity and 83% sensitivity. In an effort to expedite examinations and increase scanner throughput, some practices use a 10-minute delay. Because there is less time for de-enhancement to occur, lower thresholds for RPW and APW are expected. Using an APW value of 52%, Blake and colleagues[27] reported a specificity and sensitivity of 100% and 98%, respectively. Using a 10-minute delay to assess 122 adrenal masses, an RPW value of 37.5 or higher yielded a specificity of 100% and sensitivity of 98%.[27] This study included both lipid-rich and lipid-poor adenomas, which helps explain the increased sensitivity and specificity compared with the Caoili study, which assessed only lipid-poor adenomas. A similar more recent study with a larger cohort of 323 adrenal lesions did not show this high level of sensitivity when using the 10-minute delayed scan.[28] This study's APW threshold of 60% for lipid-poor adenomas resulted in a 93.3% specificity and 38.8% sensitivity. Using the RPW threshold of 37.5%, the sensitivity of lipid poor adenomas was a paltry 30.6%. These findings suggest that a 5-minute shorter delay significantly decreases the sensitivity of the examination, limiting the clinical value. As a result, most radiologists currently use a 15-minute delay when quantifying washout.

In the absence of a history of malignancy, an incidentally discovered adrenal lesion statistically likely represents an adenoma. If no prior examinations are available to document stability, further characterization of the lesion should be performed with CS-MRI or noncontrast CT; we prefer CS-MRI, because it is slightly more accurate than noncontrast CT and does not expose the patient to radiation. If these examinations do not diagnose a lipid-rich adenoma, an adrenal washout examination with a 15-minute delay should be performed. Currently, no data support lesion follow-up imaging if it is clearly characterized as an adenoma.[11]

Myelolipoma

Myelolipoma is a benign tumor composed primarily of fatty tissue with scattered hematopoietic elements that resemble bone marrow histologically. These lesions are hormonally inactive and

Table 2
Percent washout for delayed-contrast CT examinations

		Washout Value Percentage	
Percent Washout	Formula	Adenoma Characterization Using 15 min Delay	Adenoma Characterization Using 10 min Delay[a]
APW	(E–D)/(E–U) × 100	>60%	>52.5%
RPW	(E–D)/E × 100	>40%	>37.5%

Abbreviations: APW, absolute percentage washout; D, delayed HU value; E, enhanced HU value; H, Hounsfield unit; RPW, relative percentage washout; U, unenhanced HU value.
[a] Use controversial because of questionable sensitivity of examination.[28]

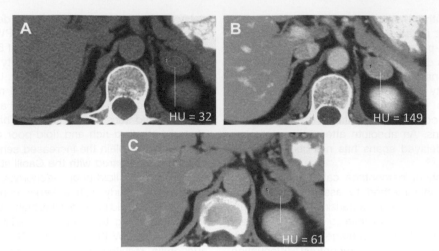

Fig. 3. Incidental left adrenal mass in a 56-year-old woman. (*A–C*) The mass measures 32 HU on noncontrast CT (*A*), 149 HU in the portal venous phase (*B*), and 61 HU in the 15-minute delayed phase (*C*). The absolute washout of this lesion is 75%, consistent with an adenoma.

most often are found incidentally. In the study by Song and colleagues,[6] myelolipoma was the second most common lesion of the adrenal gland, accounting for 6% of incidentally discovered lesions. This finding was higher than previous pathologic series, in which myelolipomas accounted for 2.6% of primary adrenal lesions.[29] Symptoms may arise secondary to mass effect or rarely hemorrhage.[30] No malignant potential has been shown. Although surgical intervention is often advised for adrenal masses larger than 4 to 6 cm because of the correlation of tumor size to malignancy risk, asymptomatic myelolipomas should be excluded from this doctrine, because these benign lesions can often exceed 6 cm.[31]

The imaging diagnosis of myelolipomas is based on the presence of macroscopic fat. On CT, the lesion contains macroscopic fat (HU≤30) with interspersed, denser myeloid tissue. MRI characteristics include T1-hyperintense signal that suppresses with frequency selective fat saturation (**Fig. 4**). Similar to renal angiomyolipomas, the presence of the india ink (chemical shift) artifact at the myelolipoma–adrenal interface or within an adrenal mass on OP images should indicate a myelolipoma.[32] Multiplanar evaluation is also important to confirm that the fatty mass is adrenal in origin, and not an exophytic renal angiomyolipoma or retroperitoneal liposarcoma.

Myelolipomas can contain various amount of fat (**Fig. 5**). In a review of 74 cases from the Armed

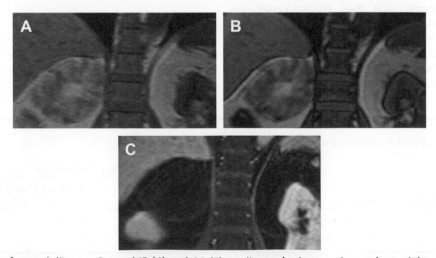

Fig. 4. MRI of a myelolipoma. Coronal IP (*A*) and OP (*B*) gradient-echo images show a large right adrenal mass with hyperintense signal. Coronal frequency selective fat-saturated gadolinium-enhanced T1 image shows loss of signal in the mass (*C*). The predominance of macroscopic fat is consistent with a myelolipoma.

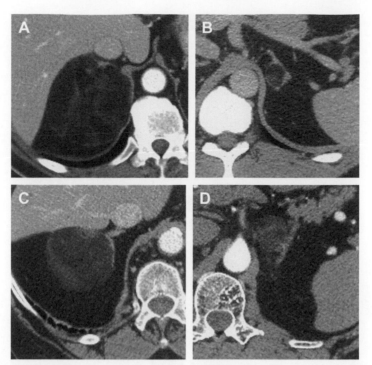

Fig. 5. Four examples of myelolipoma showing varying appearances of this neoplasm (*A–D*). These tumors can have varying proportions of macroscopic fat and myeloid elements.

Forces Institute of Pathology, 80% of myelolipoma cases were scored as being composed of at least 50% fat, with 32% having more than 90% fat.[33] Calcifications, usually small, were identified in 24% of cases. A pseudo-capsule consisting of a thin rim of residual adrenal cortex was often identified. In 18 of the cases that were archived as myelolipoma, reexamination suggested myelolipomatous elements within other pathologic conditions.[33] In this series, the vast majority were large non-functioning adenomas. The median fat content of these 18 lesions was very low (<10%). Calcification, often extensive, was found in 11 of these cases.

Multiple case reports have described focal macroscopic fat in other tumors, making small quantities of macroscopic fat not completely specific for myelolipoma. In addition to adenomas (Fig. 6), a recent retrospective study of 41 adrenocortical carcinomas suggested that 10% contained foci of macroscopic fat.[34] In contrast to renal angiomyolipomas, small amounts of macroscopic fat should be considered characteristic, but not diagnostic of myelolipomas. Other imaging features (margins, invasion, heterogeneity, etc.) should be considered to exclude a rare fat-containing malignancy. Otal and colleagues[18] reported that lesions with composition of greater than 50% macroscopic fat can be managed as a myelolipoma.

Adrenal Hemorrhage

Adrenal hemorrhage occurs secondary to traumatic and nontraumatic etiologies. In a large series from one center, adrenal hemorrhage was noted in 1.9% (51 of 2692 patients) of trauma patients who underwent CT, and was associated with higher injury severity scores and higher mortality.[35] The right adrenal gland is more prone to hemorrhage than the left; 20% of adrenal hematomas are bilateral. In the pediatric population, adrenal hemorrhage can also be seen with nonaccidental trauma.[36,37] Nontraumatic causes of adrenal hemorrhage include coagulopathy, stress (eg, surgery, sepsis, hypotension), venous hypertension (from adrenal vein or inferior vena cava thrombosis[38]), and hemorrhagic neoplasms (Box 1).

The clinical manifestations of adrenal hemorrhage vary depending on the amount of blood loss. Patients may report upper abdominal, flank, or back pain, with signs of blood loss. Addison's disease is a rare sequela of bilateral adrenal hemorrhage.[39,40]

A high-attenuation adrenal mass on CT is typical for adrenal hemorrhage. Hematomas appear as round or oval masses. Stranding of the periadrenal fat may be present, with possible extension into the perinephric space. Acute to subacute hematomas show hyperdense attenuation (50–90 HU).[41] Hematomas decrease in size and attenuation over

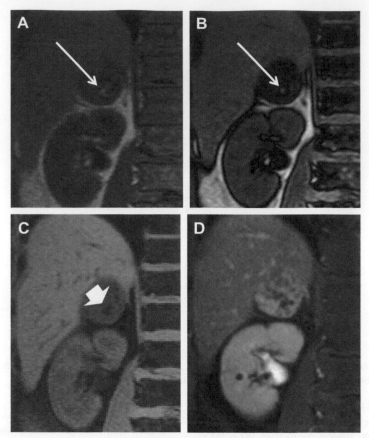

Fig. 6. Adenoma with macroscopic fat. Coronal IP (*A*) and OP (*B*) gradient-echo images show a 5-cm mass that shows loss of signal on the OP, compatible with intracellular fat. A focus of T1 hyperintense signal is seen in this mass (*arrows*) that loses signal (*arrowhead*) on the coronal T1 fat-saturated image (*C*), consistent with macroscopic fat. The lesion shows heterogeneous enhancement after gadolinium administration (*D*), a nonspecific finding. Because of its size, the lesion was resected. Pathology showed an adrenal adenoma with a component of macroscopic fat. Although the presence of macroscopic fat is characteristic of myelolipoma, it is not always diagnostic.

time, and most will completely resolve. An adrenal hematoma may calcify after 1 year. A chronic organized hematoma with hypodense fluid attenuation and a thin peripheral rim is called a pseudocyst.

Using MRI, the acute stage (<7 days) of a hematoma appears isointense to slightly hypointense on T1 sequences, and markedly hypointense on T2 sequences. In the subacute stage (1–7 weeks), hematomas appear hyperintense on T1 fat-saturated sequences and T2 sequences (Fig. 7); high T1 signal appears at the periphery of the hematoma and fills in centrally over several weeks. Heterogeneous signal may be present in the setting of a multiloculated hematoma with blood products in various stages of oxidation. In the chronic stage (after 7 weeks), a hypointense rim is present on T1 and T2 sequences secondary to hemosiderin deposition. The rim demonstrates "blooming" on gradient echo sequences. MRI

can also evaluate for possible renal vein or inferior vena cava thrombosis.

In patients without risk factors for nontraumatic adrenal hemorrhage, further imaging is necessary to exclude an underlying hemorrhagic neoplasm. Adrenal pseudocysts, myelolipomas, pheochromocytomas, adrenocortical adenomas and carcinomas, and metastases can all present with hemorrhage. Contrast-enhanced CT or MRI is performed to evaluate for any enhancing solid component of the hematoma (Fig. 8); subtraction imaging may be necessary. In questionable cases, follow-up imaging can be performed to confirm the decreasing size and eventual resolution of a benign hematoma, and exclude an underlying mass.

Adrenal Cysts

Cysts of the adrenal gland are extremely rare. Fortunately, the imaging features are typically

Box 1
Causes of adrenal hemorrhage

Traumatic
- Pediatric: nonaccidental trauma

Nontraumatic
- Bleeding diathesis and coagulopathy
  - Anticoagulation
  - Antiphospholipid syndrome
  - Disseminated intravascular coagulopathy
- Venous hypertension
  - Inferior vena cava thrombosis
  - Renal vein thrombosis
- Stress
  - Sepsis
  - Surgery
  - Burns
  - Hypotension
  - Pregnancy
  - Cardiovascular disease
  - Exogenous steroids
  - Neonatal
    - Difficult labor/delivery
    - Asphyxia/hypoxia
    - Extracorporeal membrane oxygenation
- Hemorrhagic tumor
  - Myelolipoma
  - Pheochromocytoma
  - Adrenocortical carcinoma
  - Metastases
  - Adrenal adenoma
  - Pseudocyst
  - Hemangioma

diagnostic, because they show typical CT and MR features of cystic lesions. The size of these cysts can range from a few millimeters to 20 cm. Wall calcification is commonly identified on CT. In a small series by Rozenblit and colleagues,[42] 51% of the cystic lesions had wall calcification (19 of 37 cases). Typical rim-like calcification was seen in a significant (n = 15) number of the cases.

The three subtypes of adrenal cysts are endothelial cysts, pseudocysts, and parasitic cysts. Endothelial cysts are the most common subtype. Also known as a simple cyst, they constitute approximately 45% of adrenal cysts.[43] Simple cysts have fluid characteristics ($\leq$20 HU and/or high T2 signal) with thin walls that show no enhancement.

Pseudocysts constitute the second most common subtype (39%).[43] Pseudocysts are caused by a prior episode of hemorrhage or infarct; the cyst wall is composed of fibrous tissue. Although low-density, the pseudocyst can be more complex and may present with thicker walls, internal septations, and calcifications (**Fig. 9**). MRI is the best modality for characterization because of its increased sensitivity in detecting hemorrhagic elements and superior septation characterization.[44]

Parasitic infections account for 7% of adrenal cysts. They are most commonly secondary to echinococcal infection. The imaging appearance can vary from simple cyst to complex multicystic mass, depending on the stage of the disease.

CT and MRI detect cystic lesions with a high level of sensitivity, and the multiplanar capability also allows differentiation from cysts arising from adjacent organs (kidneys, liver, pancreas). With increasing complexity of the cyst, suspicion should rise that the lesion could represent a cystic malignancy, including metastases and pheochromocytoma. In these cases, additional clinical workup and follow-up should be recommended.

ADRENAL METASTASIS

The likelihood of an incidental adrenal lesion representing a metastasis in the absence of a history of malignancy is exceedingly low. In a study of 1049 incidental lesions in patients with no history of cancer, no malignant lesions were identified.[6] With a history of malignancy, the likelihood of an adrenal mass representing metastatic disease is much higher. The adrenal gland is the fourth most common site of metastatic disease after lung, liver, and bone. In patients with known extra-adrenal cancer, 50% to 75% of adrenal masses represent metastases.[45–47] The primary malignancy associated with adrenal metastases is most often lung, breast, thyroid, colon, or melanoma.[48,49] Although cancer of an unknown primary can occasionally involve the adrenal gland, metastatic cancer presenting as an isolated adrenal mass is extremely uncommon. In a review of 1639 patients with suspected carcinoma of unknown primary from MD Anderson Cancer Center, 95 (5.8%) had adrenal gland involvement at presentation.[50] Only 4 of these patients had isolated adrenal metastases, all of which were larger than 6 cm.

Adrenal metastases present as round soft tissue masses or a diffusely enlarged gland, and tend to

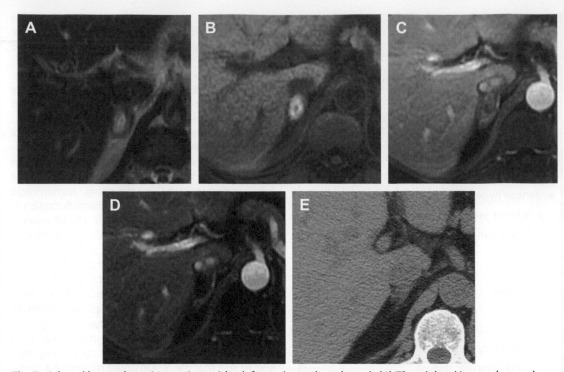

Fig. 7. Adrenal hemorrhage in a patient with a left renal mass (not shown). (*A*) T2-weighted image shows a hyperintense lesion in the right adrenal gland. (*B*) T1 fat-saturated precontrast image also shows hyperintense signal in the lesion, compatible with hemorrhage. This lesion is again noted on the post–gadolinium-enhanced image (*C*). Qualitative evaluation for enhancement is suboptimal because of the underlying high T1 signal. (*D*) Postcontrast subtraction image confirms that the lesion does not enhance. Additional history revealed recent trauma, and a diagnosis of adrenal hematoma was rendered. The patient proceeded to a partial nephrectomy for the renal mass. (*E*) Routine postsurgical follow-up CT showed near-complete resolution of the hematoma.

be larger, heterogeneous, and less well defined. Metastases have an unenhanced CT value of greater than 10 HU and a SII greater than 16.5% on CS-MRI (**Fig. 10**). These parameters are optimized to maximize specificity for the diagnosis of adenoma while maintaining clinically acceptable sensitivity. Although the specificity for diagnosing adenomas with MRI is high, it is not

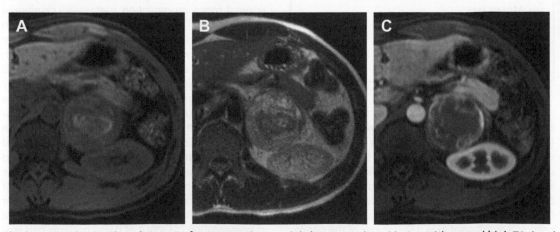

Fig. 8. Hemorrhagic adrenal mass. T1 fat-saturated image (*A*) shows an adrenal lesion with central high T1 signal compatible with hemorrhage. T2-weighted image (*B*) shows an intermediate T2 signal rind of soft tissue surrounding the hematoma, which has arterial hyperenhancement on the T1 post–gadolinium-enhanced image (*C*). This finding is compatible with a hemorrhagic neoplasm; biochemical evaluation and surgical resection confirmed a pheochromocytoma.

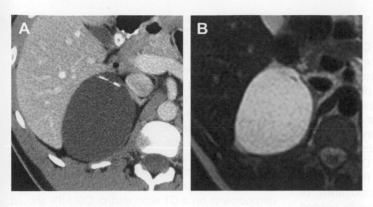

Fig. 9. Adrenal cyst. (*A*) A contrast-enhanced CT image shows a large mass with fluid attenuation and a partially calcified septation. (*B*) T2-weighted image on a 1-year follow-up MRI shows hyperintense fluid signal. The septation is partially visualized as a thin linear hypointense structure.

100%. Rarely, metastases from primary malignancies containing intracytoplasmic fat, such as clear cell renal cell carcinoma and hepatocellular carcinoma, result in a false-positive diagnosis of adenomas because they lose signal on OP imaging. In patients with these primary malignancies, an adrenal mass containing microscopic fat may require additional imaging (washout CT,

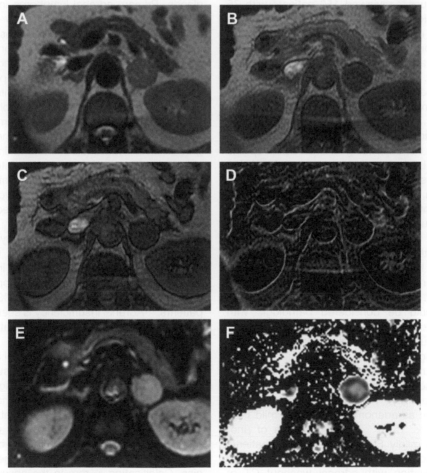

Fig. 10. Isolated left adrenal metastasis in a patient with right upper lobe lung carcinoma. (*A*) T2-weighted image shows a left adrenal mass. IP (*B*) and OP (*C*) gradient-echo images do not show any loss of signal in this mass. Subtraction image (*D*), IP minus OP, confirms no loss of signal in this mass. The mass shows a high signal on the b400 diffusion-weighted image (*E*) and low signal on the apparent diffusion coefficient map (*F*), consistent with restricted diffusion.

18F-fluorodeoxyglucose [FDG] PET) or short-term follow-up.

The proliferation of ^{18}F-FDG PET-CT in staging malignancy adds an additional tool for lesion characterization. In addition to the densitometric characteristics provided by the CT portion, PET detects the increased metabolic activity of malignant masses. The 5-mm resolution of PET is sufficient for evaluation of the small adrenal glands. Despite their vascularity and metabolic activity, normal adrenal glands do not show FDG activity.[51]

A recent meta-analysis by Boland and colleagues[52] examined the diagnostic utility of FDG PET across 15 studies. Their results yielded specificity, sensitivity, and accuracy of 91%, 97, and 98%, respectively. These calculations may be underestimations, because most PET scans are now performed on hybrid PET-CT scanners. The correlative unenhanced CT images add further specificity in cases of lipid-rich adenomas. Metser and colleagues[53] reviewed 150 patients with 75 adrenal lesions that received PET-CT. Using a standard uptake value (SUV) criterion of less than 3.1 alone, the sensitivity and specificity for diagnosing an adenoma were 98.5% and 93%, respectively. When a lesion met either criteria of SUV less than 3.1 or HU value less than 10, the sensitivity and specificity rose to 100% and 98%, respectively. This difference in specificity was clinically significant. Unfortunately, using absolute SUVs (and corresponding standardized uptake ratios) can be inconsistent because of differing body habitus, variability in time between injection and imaging, fluctuations in plasma glucose levels, and different reconstruction algorithms. Boland and colleagues[54] performed a qualitative analysis using liver activity as the reference. When combining the qualitative PET data with unenhanced CT, the sensitivity and specificity of diagnosing benignity were 99% and 100%, respectively. FDG adrenal uptake exceeding liver uptake should be considered pathologic with a high suspicion for malignancy. A lesion with little or no FDG uptake can confidently be characterized as benign.

Although most malignant lesions are markedly FDG-avid, some metastases may show only mild metabolic activity. Furthermore, some benign lesions, such as adenomas, can show mild FDG uptake (up to 15%).[55] In the absence of prior imaging, all mildly FDG-avid lesions in patients with a history of malignancy should undergo further evaluation with adrenal washout CT or biopsy. The results of this extensive workup can have dramatic implications on management, because the presence of an adrenal metastasis may preclude the patient from definitive surgery.

Collision Tumor

Collision tumors are defined as the coexistence of two adjacent but histologically distinct tumors with no significant tissue admixture.[56] The adjacent lesions can both be benign (adenoma and myelolipoma) or one may be malignant (adenoma and metastasis). Although extremely rare, the occurrence of metastatic collision tumors is not surprising given the relative high prevalence of adrenal adenomas and the propensity of malignancy to metastasize to the adrenal gland. With a history of malignancy, the presence of two tumor components on a CT scan and/or CS-MRI should raise suspicion (**Fig. 11**). PET-CT may be helpful for further evaluation and biopsy guidance.

Adrenal Lymphoma

Occasionally, lymphoma can involve the adrenal glands. Primary adrenal lymphoma involves only the adrenal gland and is extremely rare. Singh and colleagues[57] reported four cases (0.83%) from a series of 241 patients with non–Hodgkin's lymphoma (NHL). Zhou and colleagues[58] performed a retrospective review of 32 patients with adrenal lymphoma. Of these patients, six were diagnosed with primary adrenal lymphoma, three of whom had bilateral disease. The mean size of these lesions was 10 cm. Although they generally grow in an infiltrative manner and maintain a triangular adreniform appearance, the heterogeneous enhancement and presence of necrotic or cystic components can make them difficult to distinguish from adrenocortical carcinoma, pheochromocytoma, or metastases.[59]

Secondary adrenal involvement is typically seen with NHL. A review of 173 patients with diffuse NHL found that 4% had adrenal involvement, 43% of which was bilateral.[60] On autopsy, adrenal involvement can be seen in up to 25% of afflicted patients.[57] Adrenal insufficiency is seen in approximately two-thirds of patients with bilateral adrenal involvement.[57]

In early secondary disease, adrenal involvement may not be apparent or may only result in diffuse adrenal enlargement with no change in gland configuration. More nodular enlargement is noted in progressive disease.[61] Extensive retroperitoneal tumor may engulf the entire gland. On CT, the masses generally appear homogeneous and the washout characteristics resemble other malignancies. Calcification is rare in the absence of prior therapy.[62] The MR characteristics are nonspecific and similar to metastases. Typically, the T1 signal intensity is lower than that of liver and the T2 signal is heterogeneously hyperintense. They typically

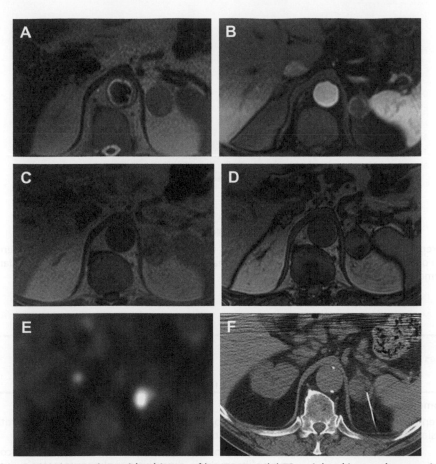

Fig. 11. Collision tumor in a patient with a history of lung cancer. (*A*) T2-weighted image shows an intermediate signal left adrenal mass with heterogeneous enhancement on T1 post–gadolinium-enhanced image (*B*). IP (*C*) and OP (*D*) gradient-echo images show small areas of signal loss on the OP, compatible with intracellular lipid related to the adenomatous component of the mass. However, most of the lesion does not show signal loss on the OP, and a collision tumor was suspected given the history of lung cancer. FDG PET image (*E*) shows marked FDG activity medially within the mass, and CT-guided biopsy (*F*) confirmed coexisting metastatic lung carcinoma in this collision tumor.

show only mild to moderate homogeneous (or mildly heterogeneous) enhancement after gadolinium.[58]

Like most lymphomas elsewhere, adrenal lymphoma involvement shows FDG activity. After successful treatment, decreased FDG avidity is seen in adrenal lesions and other metastatic foci,[53] and the involved adrenal glands will often return to their original size and configuration (Fig. 12).

Adrenal Pheochromocytoma

Pheochromocytomas are tumors composed of chromaffin cells, the predominant cells of the adrenal medulla. Extra-adrenal pheochromocytomas are found along the sympathetic chain, can occur anywhere from the skull base to the pelvis, and are referred to as paragangliomas.

Pheochromocytomas have been called the "10% tumor," because approximately 10% occur bilaterally, 10% are extra-adrenal, 10% occur in children, and 10% are malignant. Local invasion and metastatic spread are the only reliable criteria for malignant disease. Pheochromocytomas can also be seen with various syndromes, including multiple endocrine neoplasia (MEN) syndrome types IIa[63] and IIb,[64] neurofibromatosis type 1, von Hippel-Lindau syndrome, tuberous sclerosis, Sturge-Weber syndrome, nonsyndromic familial pheochromocytoma, and Carney triad (Table 3).

Most commonly encountered during the fourth through sixth decades of life, pheochromocytomas classically present with new or recently exacerbated, refractory paroxysmal hypertension. Patients may also have palpitations, headaches, diaphoresis, and flushing. The diagnosis of pheochromocytoma is often made clinically; 90% of patients have elevated 24-hour urinary metanephrines or vanillylmandelic acid levels.

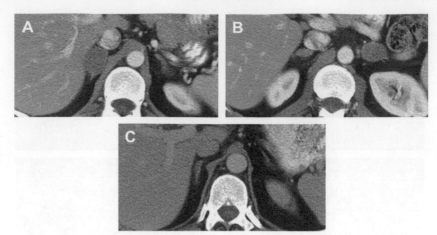

Fig. 12. Adrenal lymphoma. (*A*, *B*) Contrast-enhanced CT images show bilateral soft tissue adrenal masses in patient with diffuse large B-cell lymphoma. (*C*) After treatment with chemotherapy, the adrenal glands returned to their normal configuration.

Table 3
Syndromes associated with adrenal neoplasms

	Constellation of Findings and Associated Tumors
Pheochromocytomas	
Multiple endocrine neoplasia (MEN) IIa	Medullary thyroid carcinoma, pheochromocytoma, parathyroid hyperplasia/adenoma
MEN IIb	Medullary thyroid carcinoma, pheochromocytoma, mucosal neurofibromatosis, digestive ganglioneuromatosis
Neurofibromatosis type 1	Multiple neurofibromas, optic gliomas, café-au-lait spots, Lisch nodules, rarely pheochromocytoma
Von Hippel-Lindau syndrome	Central nervous system hemangioblastomas, renal and pancreatic cysts, renal cell carcinoma, pancreatic cystadenocarcinoma and islet cell tumor, pheochromocytoma, epididymal cystadenomas
Tuberous sclerosis	Central nervous system cortical and subependymal tubers, giant cell astrocytoma, angiomyolipoma, lymphangioleiomyomatosis, cardiac rhabdomyoma, adenoma sebaceum, rarely pheochromocytoma
Sturge-Weber syndrome	Port wine nevus, leptomeningeal angiomas, rarely pheochromocytomas
Carney triad	Gastric leiomyosarcoma, pulmonary chondroma, and extra-adrenal pheochromocytomas
Adrenocortical carcinoma	
MEN type I	Pituitary prolactinoma, parathyroid hyperplasia, pancreatic (islet cell) tumors, rarely adrenocortical carcinoma
Li-Fraumeni cancer syndrome	Risk of several cancers, including sarcomas, leukemia, breast, brain, lung cancers, adrenocortical carcinoma
Carney complex	Cardiac and cutaneous myxomas, Sertoli cell tumors, thyroid adenomas, primary pigmented nodular adrenocortical disease (bilateral adrenocortical hyperplasia), hyperpigmented skin, rarely adrenocortical carcinoma
Beckwith Wiedemann	Prenatal and postnatal overgrowth, organomegaly (macroglossia, hepatosplenomegaly), omphalocele, Wilms tumor, rarely adrenocortical carcinoma

Pheochromocytomas are typically larger than adenomas, and smaller than adrenocortical carcinomas. In a series of 51 adrenal masses consisting of adenomas, pheochromocytomas, and adrenocortical carcinomas, Szolar and colleagues[65] reported mean sizes of 2.2, 5.1, and 9.8 cm, respectively. Nonfunctioning pheochromocytomas typically present at a larger size than their functioning counterparts.[66] Smaller pheochromocytomas have homogeneous soft tissue attenuation on CT. Larger pheochromocytomas can have heterogeneous attenuation from internal hemorrhage, cystic[67] and myxoid[68] degeneration, and necrosis. Calcification can be seen in 10% of pheochromocytomas. Ramsay and colleagues[69] also reported lipid degeneration in pheochromocytomas resulting in the presence of intracellular fat. Blake and colleagues[70] reported two cases of pheochromocytomas with attenuation values less than 10 HU. They also suggested that these lesions might show loss of signal on CSI (although these cases did not undergo MRI). Cases such as these could result in a false-positive diagnosis of adenoma, and are the reason that attenuation and chemical shift features are not 100% specific for adenomas. Pheochromocytomas can also have small quantities of macroscopic fat[71]; a finding that is not completely specific for myelolipoma.

On MRI, pheochromocytomas show low T1 signal and are classically described as having high T2 signal (Fig. 13). Early studies suggested that the uniform high T2 signal of these lesions could distinguish them from other adrenal neoplasms.[72,73] Subsequent studies have shown the variability of the T2 signal in pheochromocytomas, and the overlap in T2 signal features of pheochromocytomas and other adrenal masses. Up to 30% of pheochromocytomas can show low T2 signal[74,75]; heterogeneous signal is secondary to hemorrhagic (Fig. 8), cystic, or myxoid degeneration (Fig. 14). MRI is also helpful in cases of extra-adrenal pheochromocytomas, in which the high T2 signal may be more conspicuous on fat-suppressed sequences. MR spectroscopy has also been used to identify unique spectral resonance based on the presence of catecholamine and catecholamine metabolites in pheochromocytomas.[76]

Compared with adenomas, pheochromocytomas avidly enhance and typically show some contrast retention on delayed scans. Szolar and colleagues[65] reported mean APW and RPW of pheochromocytomas to be less than those of adenomas, and relatively similar to those of adrenocortical carcinomas and metastases. This study used only a 10-minute delay for washout. Using a 15-minute delay, Park and colleagues[77] reported that 5 of 31 (16%) pheochromocytomas showed greater than 60% washout on delayed-contrast enhanced CT, mimicking an adenoma. There are additional case reports of pheochromocytomas with washout characteristics that have met adenoma criteria.[70,78,79] Although washout characteristics may be complimentary, the diagnosis of pheochromocytoma should be based primarily on other imaging findings and clinical parameters.

Metaiodobenzylguanidine (MIBG) is an analog of guanethidine and norepinephrine, and is taken up by adrenergic tissue. Iodine-131 (I-131)– or I-123–labeled MIBG scintigraphy detects adrenergic tumors, including pheochromocytomas, paragangliomas, and neuroblastomas. I-123 results in a lower radiation dose to the patient, whereas

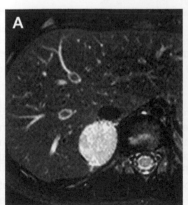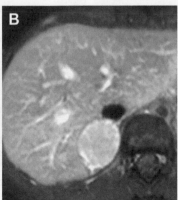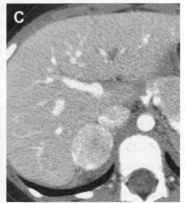

Fig. 13. Classic appearance of a pheochromocytoma. (A) T2-weighted image shows the classically reported high T2 signal of a pheochromocytoma (light bulb sign). T1 post–gadolinium-enhanced image (B) and arterial phase of a contrast-enhanced CT (C) show the hypervascular nature of these neoplasms. (Courtesy of Rami Sartawi, MD, Nashville, TN.)

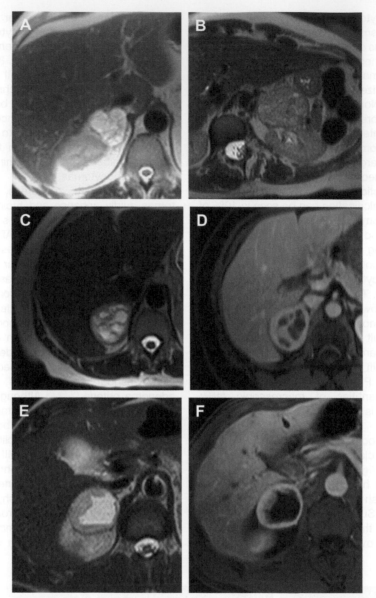

Fig. 14. Various imaging appearances of pheochromocytomas. Although some pheochromocytomas can show uniform high T2 signal (*A*), they can also show variable or uniformly intermediate T2 signal (*B*). Pheochromocytomas can also have varying degrees of cystic degeneration best seen on T2-weighted images (*C, E*). The hypervascularity of the surrounding rind of soft tissue in the arterial phase (*D, F*) can help distinguish them from other adrenal malignancies.

I-131 allows for delayed imaging and greater washout of background activity. MIBG scintigraphy is performed when pheochromocytomas cannot be localized with CT or MRI. Larger pheochromocytomas and paragangliomas have an increased risk of metastases, which may be better detected with scintigraphy. MIBG has a reported sensitivity of 82%[80] and specificity of greater than 95%[81] for pheochromocytomas. An advantage of scintigraphy includes imaging of the entire body on a single scan. Disadvantages include

lower spatial resolution and a 1- to 3-day study time requirement. MIBG single photon emission computed tomography/CT has also been shown to improve diagnostic certainty in equivocal cases.[82] FDG PET shows increased tracer activity in pheochromocytomas,[83,84] but this finding is not specific. PET is also helpful in MIBG-negative pheochromocytomas.[85]

Historically, patients with suspected pheochromocytoma were premedicated with adrenergic blockers before CT imaging with ionic iodinated contrast, based on reports of hypertensive crises.[86] However, subsequent studies with nonionic contrast material did not show a correlation,[87,88] and premedication is no longer performed.[89] If percutaneous biopsy is indicated for a suspected pheochromocytoma, it should be performed in consultation with endocrine and anesthesia services in the setting of hemodynamic monitoring and endocrine blockade.

Adrenocortical Carcinoma

Adrenocortical carcinoma (ACC) is an aggressive tumor arising from the adrenal cortex. It occurs in approximately 1 to 2 cases per 1 million.[90] ACC has a bimodal age distribution, occurring in the first and fourth/fifth decades. Patients can present with fever, weight loss, a palpable mass, and abdominal pain. Hypertension is also common in functioning ACCs. Although most ACCs are sporadic, they can be associated with Li-Fraumeni syndrome, Carney complex, Beckwith-Wiedemann syndrome, familial adenomatous polyposis coli, and MEN type 1 (see Table 3).

ACCs are functional in approximately 60% of cases,[91] although this occurs more commonly in children (approximately 85%)[92,93] than in adults (15%–30%).[94] Functional ACCs manifest as Cushing syndrome, feminization, virilization, or hyperaldosterism. Nonfunctioning ACCs present later, and approximately 21% to 34% of cases present with metastatic disease.[94,95] ACC is staged based on the TNM classification scheme, which separates the tumors based on size of less than or greater than 5 cm, local invasion, and metastases to local lymph nodes and distant sites.[95] ACC metastasizes most commonly to the liver, with other sites including lung and bone.

Surgical guidelines suggest resection of solid adrenal masses larger than 6 cm because most of these lesions are malignant. Most ACCs are larger than 6 cm on initial presentation, which partly guides this principle. Ng and Libertino[93] reported a mean diameter of 9.8 cm (4–25 cm range) in a meta-analysis of 602 cases of ACC. Fishman and colleagues[96] reported ACC diameters of 3 to 25 cm, with the rate of hormone activity inversely related to size. Although ACCs show soft tissue attenuation, masses greater than 6 cm often have heterogeneous attenuation secondary to central necrosis and internal hemorrhage (Fig. 15). Calcification can be seen in up to 30% of ACCs. Rarely, macroscopic fat can be seen with ACCs.[94] Irregular tumor margins and invasion of adjacent structures may also be present.

On contrast enhanced CT, there is typically heterogeneous enhancement of these tumors secondary to areas of central necrosis. Some ACCs show a thin capsule-like rim of enhancement.[96] Schlund and colleagues[97] also described peripheral mural-based nodular enhancement in seven of eight ACCs. Compared with adenomas, ACCs retain some contrast and show less absolute and relative washout.[65,98] Since case reports exist of ACCs with washout characteristics similar to adenomas,[34,99] tumor size greater than 4 cm and heterogeneous enhancement are the most reliable indicators of an malignant adrenal mass.[100]

On MRI, ACCs are typically heterogeneous in signal because of the presence of hemorrhage and necrosis.[101] On T1-weighted sequences, these tumors are isointense to hypointense to liver, with high T1 signal in areas of hemorrhage (Fig. 16). ACCs can also contain intracytoplasmic lipid, which is attributed to the presence of cortisol and other fatty precursors in hormonally active tissue,[102] which could result in signal loss on opposed-phase images.[97,103] Generally, ACCs with fat can be distinguished from adenomas based on their heterogeneous appearance and

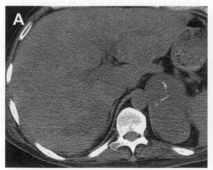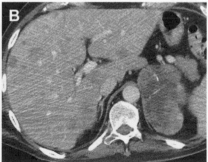

Fig. 15. Adrenocortical carcinoma. (A) Unenhanced CT image shows a large left adrenal mass with foci of calcification. (B) The mass enhances heterogeneously on the portal venous phase, and hypodense liver metastases are identified. Adrenocortical carcinomas typically present as large adrenal masses, and often with metastatic disease.

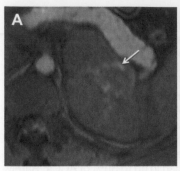 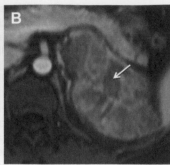

Fig. 16. Adrenocortical carcinoma. (A) T1 fat-saturated image shows a large left mass with foci of high T1 signal (arrow), compatible with internal hemorrhage. (B) Areas of nonenhancing necrosis are seen on the T1 post–gadolinium-enhanced image.

size. ACC has a propensity to invade veins. The presence of an adrenal mass with renal vein or inferior vena cava invasion is highly suggestive of ACC.[104] MRI has been shown to be superior to CT for evaluating inferior venal cava invasion (Fig. 17).[105,106]

FDG PET can also identify malignant adrenal masses, given their increased metabolic activity. The advantage of FDG PET is its ability to detect distant metastases of ACC, which are seen in one-third of patients on presentation.[107] Becherer and colleagues[108] prospectively evaluated a series of 10 patients with ACC and reported that FDG PET identified additional lesions (in the lung, abdomen, and skeleton). These findings affected tumor staging in three of patients, and changed therapeutic management in two.

The definitive treatment of ACC is en bloc resection. Tumor debulking is performed when complete resection is not possible. Although typically performed in nonsurgical candidates, ACCs can also be treated with radiofrequency ablation. Treatment with adrenolytic drug mitotane is used as both primary and adjuvant therapy.[107] Radiotherapy is performed in patients with risk for local recurrence, advanced locoregional disease, or incomplete resection.

OTHER MISCELLANEOUS LESIONS OF THE ADRENAL GLAND

Neuroblastoma

Although neuroblastoma is the third most common malignant tumor seen in children, it is rare in the adult population. Neuroblastomas most often arise in the adrenal glands, but can occur anywhere along the sympathetic chain. Soft tissue adrenal masses are seen, which are often calcified.[109] Neuroblastoma often presents with disseminated disease, with similar imaging findings of metastatic disease or lymphoma.

Ganglioneuroma

Ganglioneuromas are benign neoplasms composed of Schwann cells and ganglion cells that arise from the sympathetic ganglia; 20% to 30% arise in the adrenal medulla. These lesions do not secrete hormones, and are incidental findings. Ganglioneuromas show soft tissue attenuation, variable size, and homogenous or mildly heterogeneous enhancement.[110] On MRI, these lesions are low in T1 signal and can have heterogeneous hyperintense T2 signal.[74]

Hemangioma

Hemangiomas of the adrenal gland are extremely rare. These lesions have soft tissue attenuation on CT, hyperintense signal of T2-weighted MRI sequences, and show peripheral nodular enhancement that persists on delayed phase.[18,111] Like hemangiomas in other locations, these lesions can contain calcification from phleboliths or prior hemorrhage.

Infection

Tuberculosis, histoplasmosis, and other granulomatous diseases can occur in the adrenal gland, often with bilateral involvement. Imaging features are nonspecific, and may include soft tissue masses, cystic changes, and calcification[112]; the diagnosis is established through clinical history and biopsy.

EMERGING TECHNOLOGIES

Diffusion-weighted imaging (DWI) is an exciting new MRI technique that evaluates thermally induced Brownian motion in cellular tissues.[113] With increased cellularity of tissues (as seen in malignancy), a proportional increase occurs in water molecule diffusion restriction. After the acquisition of at least two b-values, an apparent diffusion coefficient (ADC) map can be calculated that reflects the unique diffusion properties of the tissue. ADC mapping can be used as an imaging biomarker for tissue characterization and cancer detection, and to assess response to treatment.[114] This technique holds the most value in patients who are unable to receive contrast.

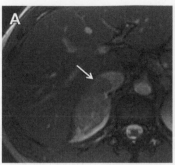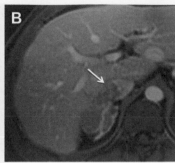

Fig. 17. Adrenocortical carcinoma with inferior vena cava invasion. Steady-state free precession (*A*) and post–gadolinium-enhanced (*B*) images show a right adrenocortical carcinoma extending into the inferior vena cava (*arrows*).

Unfortunately, no standard DWI protocol exists. The sequences are acquired using free breathing, respiratory triggering, or breath-hold techniques. Furthermore, no consensus exists on the number and maximum b-values that should be required. These variables lead to inconsistencies across various magnets and institutions. Nevertheless, diffusion has proven useful in differentiating benign and malignant lesions in other anatomic areas.[115,116] Many institutions have incorporated diffusion-weighted sequences into their standard imaging protocols without significantly adding to overall acquisition time.

Although many malignant adrenal masses show restriction (Fig. 10), adenomas can also restrict. Initial studies using ADC values to characterize adrenal lesions were disappointing. Tsushima and colleagues[115] analyzed 43 tumors and found no difference in ADC value between adenomas and metastases. Similarly, Miller and colleagues[117] reviewed 160 adrenal lesions and found no significant difference between the ADC values of benign and malignant adrenal lesions. More recent studies suggest that use of ADC values in lesions with an indeterminate SI index on CSI may be helpful. Sandrasegaran and colleagues[118] evaluated lesions with indeterminate SI index and found that all lesions with an ADC value greater than 1.5×10^{-3} mm^2/s were benign. Although the specificity was 100%, only 4 of 26 lesions met these criteria. Nine of 11 lesions (82%) with an ADC value less than 1.0×10^{-3} mm^2/s were malignant. Using a 3T MRI, Song and colleagues[119] reviewed 51 hyperattenuating lesions (>10 HU) on unenhanced CT. This study suggested that benignity could be diagnosed with 85.7% specificity when a lesion showed an ADC value greater than 1.04×10^{-3} mm^2/s.

The promise of DWI for adrenal characterization is that it obviates the necessity of contrast administration and does not expose the patient to radiation. Unfortunately, initial studies show significant overlap between the ADC values of benign and malignant lesions, raising doubts about its use. Although it may prove to be an adjunct to CSI in characterization, larger cohort studies with more standardized DWI protocols are necessary to fully evaluate the true value of DWI.

An exciting new technology that is entering clinical practice is dual-energy CT (DECT). When DECT is used, two images are acquired at a given location with two different energies (80 and 140 kVp).[120] On postcontrast DECTs, virtual unenhanced images can be reconstructed through subtracting the iodine content with a three-material decomposition technique. In Song's study of 1049 adrenal lesions,[119] 38% of the lesions required additional imaging after the initial CT, often postcontrasted examinations.[6] Therefore, the generation of virtual noncontrast images from contrasted DECT acquisitions has exciting implications for lipid-rich adenoma characterization in patients who have only received a postcontrast examination.

Gupta and colleagues[121] performed a prospective study evaluating 31 adrenal lesions in 17 patients with noncontrast DECT. The mean change in attenuation was calculated between 80 and 140 kVp. An attenuation decrease was seen at 80 kVp in 50% of the adenomas. At 80 kVp, all of the metastatic lesions showed an increase in attenuation. The sensitivity, specificity, and positive predictive value in the diagnosis of adenoma were 50%, 100%, and 100%, respectively. As expected, the low sensitivity was believed to be caused by the prevalence of lipid-poor adenomas.

Gnannt and colleagues[122] performed a retrospective review to evaluate the accuracy of the virtual unenhanced images. They reviewed 140 patients referred for DECT for follow-up of endovascular aortic aneurysm repair. All patients received a precontrast examination in addition to a dual-energy examination in the portal venous

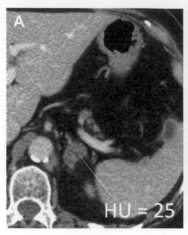
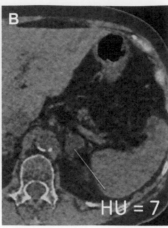

Fig. 18. Dual-energy CT evaluation of an adrenal mass. (*A*) A left adrenal mass was identified on a dual-energy CT urogram performed to evaluate for hematuria. Attenuation of the lesion was 25 HU. (*B*) A virtual noncontrast CT image of the left adrenal mass shows a Hounsfield value of 7. Although larger studies are needed to validate this presumption, this is believed to represent a benign adenoma. (*Courtesy of David Levi, MD, Galloway, NJ.*)

Table 4
Summary of adrenal masses

	Incidence	CT/MR Features	Other Considerations
Benign, with diagnostic imaging features			
Adenoma	Very common, 50%–80%	Smaller (1–4 cm) More homogeneous NC CT <10 HU APW >60% RPW >40% SII >16.5% ASR <71	Exclude a rare collision tumor, fatty metastasis
Myelolipoma	5%–10%	Variable size, often large Macroscopic fat	If small amounts of fat, consider ACC or adenoma
Hematoma	~1%	↑Attenuation ↑T1 signal on T1 FS Blooming on GRE	Exclude a hemorrhagic neoplasm
Cyst	~1%	Fluid attenuation/signal Thin fine wall ± Wall calcification	Exclude a cystic neoplasm
Malignant, with nonspecific imaging features			
Metastasis	Uncommon in absence of history of malignancy	Larger mass Extra-adrenal metastases typically present	
Adrenocortical carcinoma	<5%	Usually >4–5 cm Heterogeneous: Ca+, necrotic, hemorrhagic	Evaluate for renal vein/ IVC invasion, metastasis
Pheochromocytoma	<5%	Intermediate size mass Classically ↑ T2 signal, can be variable ± Cystic component	+ Urine metanephrine, VMA
Lymphoma	Primary rare, metastatic more common	Solid homogeneous Ca+ post-treatment	

Abbreviations: ACC, adrenocortical carcinoma; APW, absolute percent washout; ASR, adrenal-to-spleen chemical shift ratio; Ca+, calcification; GRE, Gradient echo sequence; IVC, inferior vena cava; NC CT, non-contrast computed tomography; RPW, relative percentage washout; SI index, adrenal signal intensity index; T1 FS, T1 fat saturated sequence; VMA, vanillylmandelic acid.

phase. In these patients, 51 incidental adrenal masses were detected in 42 patients. They reported good accuracy of the virtual unenhanced HU values when compared with the values on the noncontrast CTs (**Fig. 18**). When evaluating lesions greater than 1 cm, the specificity for characterizing a lesion as likely benign was 100% (the gold standard was an HU value <10 on the unenhanced scan). The smaller lesions were difficult to characterize because of increased image noise seen on the virtual noncontrast images.

Although these small studies are promising, evaluation of adrenal lesions using DECT requires further validation before widespread clinical use. The HU unit characterization on conventional noncontrast CT was developed using 120 kVp settings, and exact values on DECT have not yet been established.[123] Similarly, additional studies are needed to determine exact HU value thresholds for virtual noncontrasted sequences to characterize benignity.

SUMMARY

With the explosion of cross-sectional imaging, an increasing number of adrenal lesions are encountered unexpectedly. These "adrenal incidentalomas" have created a public health challenge. Both benign and malignant lesions can be present in the adrenal gland with variable imaging characteristics (**Table 4**). Although clinicians should conduct hormonal testing, CT, MRI, and PET can evaluate whether a lesion is benign or malignant with a high level of specificity. DWI and DECT are new technologies that may add more accuracy to noninvasive adrenal lesion diagnosis. Radiologists must have a strong understanding of principles and techniques of adrenal imaging to guide appropriate evaluation and management.

REFERENCES

1. Kloos RT, Gross MD, Francis IR, et al. Incidentally discovered adrenal masses. Endocr Rev 1995; 16(4):460–84.
2. Zeiger MA, Siegelman SS, Hamrahian AH. Medical and surgical evaluation and treatment of adrenal incidentalomas. J Clin Endocrinol Metab 2011; 96(7):2004–15.
3. Berland LL, Silverman SG, Gore RM, et al. Managing incidental findings on abdominal CT: white paper of the ACR incidental findings committee. J Am Coll Radiol 2010;7(10):754–73.
4. Boland GW, Lee MJ, Gazelle GS, et al. Characterization of adrenal masses using unenhanced CT: an analysis of the CT literature. AJR Am J Roentgenol 1998;171(1):201–4.
5. Young WF Jr. The incidentally discovered adrenal mass. N Engl J Med 2007;356(6):601–10.
6. Song JH, Chaudhry FS, Mayo-Smith WW. The incidental adrenal mass on CT: prevalence of adrenal disease in 1,049 consecutive adrenal masses in patients with no known malignancy. Am J Roentgenol 2008;190(5):1163–8.
7. Grumbach MM, Biller BM, Braunstein GD, et al. Management of the clinically inapparent adrenal mass ("incidentaloma"). Ann Intern Med 2003;138: 424–9.
8. Young WF. The adrenal incidentiloma. In: Basow DS, editor. UpToDate. Waltham (MA); 2012.
9. Young WF. Management approaches to adrenal incidentalomas. A view from Rochester, Minnesota. Endocrinol Metab Clin North Am 2000;29(1):159–85, x.
10. Management of the clinically inapparent adrenal mass (incidentaloma). U.S. Department of Health & Human Services, National Institutes of Health Web site. Available at: http://consensus.nih.gov/ 2002/2002AdrenalIncidentalomasos021html.htm. Accessed February 11, 2012.
11. Choyke PL. ACR Committee on Appropriateness Criteria. ACR Appropriateness Criteria on incidentally discovered adrenal mass. J Am Coll Radiol 2006;3(7):498–504.
12. Lee MJ, Hahn PF, Papanicolaou N, et al. Benign and malignant adrenal masses: CT distinction with attenuation coefficients, size, and observer analysis. Radiology 1991;179(2):415–8.
13. Korobkin M, Giordano TJ, Brodeur FJ, et al. Adrenal adenomas: relationship between histologic lipid and CT and MR findings. Radiology 1996; 200(3):743–7.
14. Boland GW, Blake MA, Hahn PF, et al. Incidental adrenal lesions: principles, techniques, and algorithms for imaging characterization. Radiology 2008;249(3):756–75.
15. Savci G, Yazici Z, Sahin N, et al. Value of chemical shift subtraction MRI in characterization of adrenal masses. AJR Am J Roentgenol 2006; 186(1):130–5.
16. Mayo-Smith W, Lee M, McNicholas M, et al. Characterization of adrenal masses. Am J Roentgenol 1995;165(1):91.
17. Israel GM, Korobkin M, Wang C, et al. Comparison of unenhanced CT and chemical shift MRI in evaluating lipid-rich adrenal adenomas. AJR Am J Roentgenol 2004;183(1):215–9.
18. Otal P, Escourrou G, Mazerolles C, et al. Imaging features of uncommon adrenal masses with histopathologic correlation. Radiographics 1999;19(3): 569–81.
19. McNicholas MM, Lee MJ, Mayo-Smith WW, et al. An imaging algorithm for the differential diagnosis of adrenal adenomas and metastases. AJR Am J Roentgenol 1995;165(6):1453–9.

20. Fujiyoshi F, Nakajo M, Fukukura Y, et al. Characterization of adrenal tumors by chemical shift fast low-angle shot MR imaging: comparison of four methods of quantitative evaluation. Am J Roentgenol 2003;180(6):1649.

21. Outwater E, Siegelman E, Huang A, et al. Adrenal masses: correlation between CT attenuation value and chemical shift ratio at MR imaging with in-phase and opposed-phase sequences. Radiology 1996;200(3):749.

22. Haider MA, Ghai S, Jhaveri K, et al. Chemical shift MR imaging of hyperattenuating (>10 HU) adrenal masses: does it still have a role? Radiology 2004; 231(3):711–6.

23. Szolar DH, Kammerhuber F. Quantitative CT evaluation of adrenal gland masses: a step forward in the differentiation between adenomas and nonadenomas? Radiology 1997;202(2):517–21.

24. Boland GW, Hahn PF, Peña C, et al. Adrenal masses: characterization with delayed contrast-enhanced CT. Radiology 1997;202(3):693–6.

25. Korobkin M, Brodeur FJ, Francis IR, et al. CT time-attenuation washout curves of adrenal adenomas and nonadenomas. AJR Am J Roentgenol 1998; 170(3):747–52.

26. Caoili EM, Korobkin M, Francis IR, et al. Delayed enhanced CT of lipid-poor adrenal adenomas. AJR Am J Roentgenol 2000;175(5):1411–5.

27. Blake MA, Kalra MK, Sweeney AT, et al. Distinguishing benign from malignant adrenal masses: multi-detector row CT protocol with 10-minute delay. Radiology 2006;238(2):578–85.

28. Sangwaiya MJ, Boland GWL, Cronin CG, et al. Incidental adrenal lesions: accuracy of characterization with contrast-enhanced washout multidetector CT–10-minute delayed imaging protocol revisited in a large patient cohort. Radiology 2010;256(2): 504–10.

29. Lam KY, Lo CY. Adrenal lipomatous tumours: a 30 year clinicopathological experience at a single institution. J Clin Pathol 2001;54(9):707–12.

30. Patel VG, Babalola OA, Fortson JK, et al. Adrenal myelolipoma: report of a case and review of the literature. Am Surg 2006;72(7):649–54.

31. Meyer A, Behrend M. Presentation and therapy of myelolipoma. Int J Urol 2005;12(3):239–43.

32. Israel GM, Hindman N, Hecht E, et al. The use of opposed-phase chemical shift MRI in the diagnosis of renal angiomyolipomas. AJR Am J Roentgenol 2005;184(6):1868–72.

33. Kenney PJ, Wagner BJ, Rao P, et al. Myelolipoma: CT and pathologic features. Radiology 1998; 208(1):87–95.

34. Zhang HM, Perrier ND, Grubbs EG, et al. CT features and quantification of the characteristics of adrenocortical carcinomas on unenhanced and contrast-enhanced studies. Clin Radiol 2012;67(1):38–46.

35. Rana AI, Kenney PJ, Lockhart ME, et al. Adrenal gland hematomas in trauma patients. Radiology 2004;230(3):669–75.

36. Nimkin K, Teeger S, Wallach MT, et al. Adrenal hemorrhage in abused children: imaging and post-mortem findings. AJR Am J Roentgenol 1994; 162(3):661–3.

37. Westra SJ, Zaninovic AC, Hall TR, et al. Imaging of the adrenal gland in children. Radiographics 1994; 14(6):1323–40.

38. Hinrichs CR, Singer A, Maldjian P, et al. Inferior vena cava thrombosis: a mechanism of posttraumatic adrenal hemorrhage. AJR Am J Roentgenol 2001;177(2):357–8.

39. Xarli VP, Steele AA, Davis PJ, et al. Adrenal hemorrhage in the adult. Medicine (Baltimore) 1978; 57(3):211–21.

40. Ten S, New M, Maclaren N. Clinical review 130: Addison's disease 2001. J Clin Endocrinol Metab 2001;86(7):2909–22.

41. Dunnick NR. Hanson lecture. Adrenal imaging: current status. AJR Am J Roentgenol 1990; 154(5):927–36.

42. Rozenblit A, Morehouse HT, Amis ES. Cystic adrenal lesions: CT features. Radiology 1996; 201(2):541–8.

43. Foster D. Adrenal cysts: review of literature and report of case. Arch Surg 1966;92(1):131–43.

44. Guo YK, Yang ZG, Li Y, et al. Uncommon adrenal masses: CT and MRI features with histopathologic correlation. Eur J Radiol 2007;62(3):359–70.

45. Lenert JT, Barnett CC, Kudelka AP, et al. Evaluation and surgical resection of adrenal masses in patients with a history of extra-adrenal malignancy. Surgery 2001;130(6):1060–7.

46. Gillams A, Roberts C, Shaw P, et al. The value of CT scanning and percutaneous fine needle aspiration of adrenal masses in biopsy-proven lung cancer. Clin Radiol 1992;46(1):18–22.

47. Belldegrun A, Hussain S, Seltzer S. Incidentally discovered mass of the adrenal gland. Surg Gynecol Obstet 1986;163(3):203–8.

48. Korobkin M. Overview of adrenal imaging/adrenal CT. Urol Radiol 1989;11(4):221–6.

49. Abrams HL, Spiro R, Goldstein N. Metastases in carcinoma; analysis of 1000 autopsied cases. Cancer 1950;3(1):74–85.

50. Lee JE, Evans DB, Hickey RC, et al. Unknown primary cancer presenting as an adrenal mass: frequency and implications for diagnostic evaluation of adrenal incidentalomas. Surgery 1998; 124(6):1115–22.

51. Blake MA, Cronin CG, Boland GW. Adrenal imaging. AJR Am J Roentgenol 2010;194(6):1450–60.

52. Boland GW, Dwamena BA, Sangwaiya MJ, et al. Characterization of adrenal masses by using FDG PET: a systematic review and meta-analysis of

diagnostic test performance. Radiology 2011; 259(1):117–26.

53. Metser U, Miller E, Lerman H, et al. 18F-FDG PET/CT in the evaluation of adrenal masses. J Nucl Med 2006;47(1):32–7.

54. Boland GW, Blake MA, Holalkere NS, et al. PET/CT for the characterization of adrenal masses in patients with cancer: qualitative versus quantitative accuracy in 150 consecutive patients. Am J Roentgenol 2009;192(4):956–62.

55. Vikram R, Yeung HD, Macapinlac HA, et al. Utility of PET/CT in differentiating benign from malignant adrenal nodules in patients with cancer. Am J Roentgenol 2008;191(5):1545–51.

56. Schwartz LH, Macari M, Huvos AG, et al. Collision tumors of the adrenal gland: demonstration and characterization at MR imaging. Radiology 1996; 201(3):757–60.

57. Singh D, Kumar L, Sharma A, et al. Adrenal involvement in Non-Hodgkin's lymphoma: four cases and review of literature. Leuk Lymphoma 2004;45(4): 789–94.

58. Zhou L, Peng W, Wang C, et al. Primary adrenal lymphoma: radiological; pathological, clinical correlation. Eur J Radiol 2012;81(3):401–5.

59. Kato H, Itami J, Shiina T, et al. MR imaging of primary adrenal lymphoma. Clin Imaging 1996; 20(2):126–8.

60. Palling MR, Williamson BR. Adrenal involvement in non-Hodgkin lymphoma. AJR Am J Roentgenol 1983;141(2):303–5.

61. Hussain HK, Korobkin M. MR imaging of the adrenal glands. Magn Reson Imaging Clin N Am 2004;12(3):515–44, vii.

62. Sohaib SA, Reznek RH. Adrenal imaging. BJU Int 2000;86(Suppl 1):95–110.

63. Cho KJ, Freier DT, McCormick TL, et al. Adrenal medullary disease in multiple endocrine neoplasia type II. AJR Am J Roentgenol 1980;134(1):23–9.

64. Demos TC, Blonder J, Schey WL, et al. Multiple endocrine neoplasia (MEN) syndrome type IIB: gastrointestinal manifestations. AJR Am J Roentgenol 1983;140(1):73–8.

65. Szolar DH, Korobkin M, Reittner P, et al. Adrenocortical carcinomas and adrenal pheochromocytomas: mass and enhancement loss evaluation at delayed contrast-enhanced CT. Radiology 2005; 234(2):479–85.

66. Newhouse JH, Heffess CS, Wagner BJ, et al. Large degenerated adrenal adenomas: radiologic-pathologic correlation. Radiology 1999;210(2): 385–91.

67. Andreoni C, Krebs RK, Bruna PC, et al. Cystic phaeochromocytoma is a distinctive subgroup with special clinical, imaging and histological features that might mislead the diagnosis. BJU Int 2008;101(3):345–50.

68. Park BK, Kim CK, Kwon GY, et al. Re-evaluation of pheochromocytomas on delayed contrast-enhanced CT: washout enhancement and other imaging features. Eur Radiol 2007;17(11):2804–9.

69. Ramsay JA, Asa SL, van Nostrand AW, et al. Lipid degeneration in pheochromocytomas mimicking adrenal cortical tumors. Am J Surg Pathol 1987; 11(6):480–6.

70. Blake MA, Krishnamoorthy SK, Boland GW, et al. Low-density pheochromocytoma on CT: a mimicker of adrenal adenoma. AJR Am J Roentgenol 2003; 181(6):1663–8.

71. Blake MA, Kalra MK, Maher MM, et al. Pheochromocytoma: an imaging chameleon. Radiographics 2004;24(Suppl 1):S87–99.

72. Quint LE, Glazer GM, Francis IR, et al. Pheochromocytoma and paraganglioma: comparison of MR imaging with CT and I-131 MIBG scintigraphy. Radiology 1987;165(1):89–93.

73. van Gils AP, Falke TH, van Erkel AR, et al. MR imaging and MIBG scintigraphy of pheochromocytomas and extraadrenal functioning paragangliomas. Radiographics 1991;11(1):37–57.

74. Rha SE, Byun JY, Jung SE, et al. Neurogenic tumors in the abdomen: tumor types and imaging characteristics. Radiographics 2003;23(1): 29–43.

75. Francis IR, Korobkin M. Pheochromocytoma. Radiol Clin North Am 1996;34(6):1101–12.

76. Kim S, Salibi N, Hardie AD, et al. Characterization of adrenal pheochromocytoma using respiratory-triggered proton MR spectroscopy: initial experience. Am J Roentgenol 2009;192(2):450–4.

77. Park BK, Kim B, Ko K, et al. Adrenal masses falsely diagnosed as adenomas on unenhanced and delayed contrast-enhanced computed tomography: pathological correlation. Eur Radiol 2006;16(3): 642–7.

78. Yoon JK, Remer EM, Herts BR. Incidental pheochromocytoma mimicking adrenal adenoma because of rapid contrast enhancement loss. Am J Roentgenol 2006;187(5):1309–11.

79. Caoili EM, Korobkin M, Francis IR, et al. Adrenal masses: characterization with combined unenhanced and delayed enhanced CT. Radiology 2002;222(3):629–33.

80. Wiseman GA, Pacak K, O'Dorisio MS, et al. Usefulness of 123I-MIBG scintigraphy in the evaluation of patients with known or suspected primary or metastatic pheochromocytoma or paraganglioma: results from a prospective multicenter trial. J Nucl Med 2009;50(9):1448–54.

81. Tenenbaum F, Lumbroso J, Schlumberger M, et al. Comparison of radiolabeled octreotide and meta-iodobenzylguanidine (MIBG) scintigraphy in malignant pheochromocytoma. J Nucl Med 1995;36(1): 1–6.

82. Rozovsky K, Koplewitz BZ, Krausz Y, et al. Added value of SPECT/CT for correlation of MIBG scintigraphy and diagnostic CT in neuroblastoma and pheochromocytoma. Am J Roentgenol 2008; 190(4):1085–90.

83. Shulkin BL, Thompson NW, Shapiro B, et al. Pheochromocytomas: imaging with 2-[fluorine-18]fluoro-2-deoxy-D-glucose PET. Radiology 1999;212(1): 35–41.

84. Ilias I, Yu J, Carrasquillo JA, et al. Superiority of 6-[18F]-fluorodopamine positron emission tomography versus [131I]-metaiodobenzylguanidine scintigraphy in the localization of metastatic pheochromocytoma. J Clin Endocrinol Metab 2003;88(9):4083–7.

85. Arnold D, Villemagne V, Civelek A. FDG-PET: a sensitive tool for the localization of MIBG negative pelvic pheochromocytomas. The …. 1998.

86. Raisanen J, Shapiro B, Glazer GM, et al. Plasma catecholamines in pheochromocytoma: effect of urographic contrast media. AJR Am J Roentgenol 1984;143(1):43–6.

87. Bessell-Browne R, O'Malley ME. CT of pheochromocytoma and paraganglioma: risk of adverse events with i.v. administration of nonionic contrast material. Am J Roentgenol 2007;188(4):970–4.

88. Hurley ME, Herts BR, Remer EM, et al. Three-dimensional volume-rendered helical CT before laparoscopic adrenalectomy. Radiology 2003; 229(2):581–6.

89. Johnson P, Horton K. Adrenal mass imaging with multidetector CT: pathologic conditions, pearls, and pitfalls. Radiographics 2009;29(5):1333–51.

90. Hedican SP, Marshall FF. Adrenocortical carcinoma with intracaval extension. J Urol 1997; 158(6):2056–61.

91. Wooten MD, King DK. Adrenal cortical carcinoma. Epidemiology and treatment with mitotane and a review of the literature. Cancer 1993;72(11): 3145–55.

92. Wajchenberg BL, Albergaria Pereira MA, Medonca BB, et al. Adrenocortical carcinoma: clinical and laboratory observations. Cancer 2000; 88(4):711–36.

93. Ng L, Libertino JM. Adrenocortical carcinoma: diagnosis, evaluation and treatment. J Urol 2003; 169(1):5–11.

94. Bharwani N, Rockall AG, Sahdev A, et al. Adrenocortical carcinoma: the range of appearances on CT and MRI. Am J Roentgenol 2011;196(6):W706–14.

95. Lloyd R, De Lellis R, Heitz P. Lloyd: World Health Organization Classification of. - Google Scholar. International Agency for Research on Cancer … 2004.

96. Fishman EK, Deutch BM, Hartman DS, et al. Primary adrenocortical carcinoma: CT evaluation with clinical correlation. AJR Am J Roentgenol 1987;148(3):531–5.

97. Schlund J, Kenney P, Brown E. Adrenocortical carcinoma: MR imaging appearance with current techniques. Journal of Magnetic…. 1995.

98. Slattery JM, Blake MA, Kalra MK, et al. Adrenocortical carcinoma: contrast washout characteristics on CT. Am J Roentgenol 2006;187(1):W21–4.

99. Simhan J, Canter D, Teper E, et al. Adrenocortical carcinoma masquerading as a benign adenoma on computed tomography washout study. Urology 2012;79(2):e19–20.

100. Hussain S, Belldegrun A, Seltzer SE, et al. Differentiation of malignant from benign adrenal masses: predictive indices on computed tomography. AJR Am J Roentgenol 1985;144(1):61–5.

101. Elsayes KM, Mukundan G, Narra VR, et al. Adrenal Masses: MR imaging features with pathologic correlation1. Radiographics 2004;24(Suppl 1): S73–86.

102. Mackay B, el-Naggar A, Ordonez NG. Ultrastructure of adrenal cortical carcinoma. Ultrastruct Pathol 1994;18(1–2):181–90.

103. Ferrozzi F, Bova D. CT and MR demonstration of fat within an adrenal cortical carcinoma. Abdom Imaging 1995;20(3):272–4.

104. Mezhir JJ, Song J, Piano G, et al. Adrenocortical carcinoma invading the inferior vena cava: case report and literature review. Endocr Pract 2008;14(6):721–5.

105. Hricak H, Amparo E, Fisher M, et al. Abdominal venous system: assessment using MR. Radiology 1985;156(2):415–22.

106. Soler R, Rodríguez E, López MF, et al. MR imaging in inferior vena cava thrombosis. Eur J Radiol 1995; 19(2):101–7.

107. Luton JP, Cerdas S, Billaud L, et al. Clinical features of adrenocortical carcinoma, prognostic factors, and the effect of mitotane therapy. N Engl J Med 1990;322(17):1195–201.

108. Becherer A, Vierhapper H, Pötzi C, et al. FDG-PET in adrenocortical carcinoma. Cancer Biother Radiopharm 2001;16(4):289–95.

109. David R, Lamki N, Fan S, et al. The many faces of neuroblastoma. Radiographics 1989;9(5):859–82.

110. Radin R, David CL, Goldfarb H, et al. Adrenal and extra-adrenal retroperitoneal ganglioneuroma: imaging findings in 13 adults. Radiology 1997; 202(3):703–7.

111. Krebs TL, Wagner BJ. MR imaging of the adrenal gland: radiologic-pathologic correlation. Radiographics 1998;18(6):1425–40.

112. Wilson DA, Muchmore HG, Tisdal RG, et al. Histoplasmosis of the adrenal glands studied by CT. Radiology 1984;150(3):779–83.

113. Gass A, Niendorf T, Hirsch JG. Acute and chronic changes of the apparent diffusion coefficient in neurological disorders–biophysical mechanisms and possible underlying histopathology. J Neurol Sci 2001;186(Suppl 1):S15–23.

114. Malayeri AA, Khouli El RH, Zaheer A, et al. Principles and applications of diffusion-weighted imaging in cancer detection, staging, and treatment follow-up. Radiographics 2011;31(6):1773–91.

115. Tsushima Y, Takahashi-Taketomi A, Endo K. Diagnostic utility of diffusion-weighted MR imaging and apparent diffusion coefficient value for the diagnosis of adrenal tumors. J Magn Reson Imaging 2009;29(1):112–7.

116. Chandarana H, Taouli B. Diffusion and perfusion imaging of the liver. Eur J Radiol 2010;76(3):348–58.

117. Miller FH, Wang Y, McCarthy RJ, et al. Utility of diffusion-weighted MRI in characterization of adrenal lesions. Am J Roentgenol 2010;194(2):W179–85.

118. Sandrasegaran K, Patel AA, Ramaswamy R, et al. Characterization of adrenal masses with diffusion-weighted imaging. Am J Roentgenol 2011;197(1):132–8.

119. Song J, Zhang C, Liu Q, et al. Utility of chemical shift and diffusion-weighted imaging in characterization of hyperattenuating adrenal lesions at 3.0T. Eur J Radiol 2011. [Epub ahead of print].

120. Silva AC, Morse BG, Hara AK, et al. Dual-energy (spectral) CT: applications in abdominal imaging. Radiographics 2011;31(4):1031–46.

121. Gupta RT, Ho LM, Marin D, et al. Dual-energy CT for characterization of adrenal nodules: initial experience. Am J Roentgenol 2010;194(6):1479–83.

122. Gnannt R, Fischer M, Goetti R, et al. Dual-energy CT for characterization of the incidental adrenal mass: preliminary observations. Am J Roentgenol 2012;198(1):138–44.

123. Yeh BM, Shepherd JA, Wang ZJ, et al. Dual-energy and low-kVp CT in the abdomen. Am J Roentgenol 2009;193(1):47–54.

Common and Less-Common Renal Masses and Masslike Conditions

Ranu Taneja, MD[a], Puneet Bhargava, MD[b],*,
Carlos Cuevas, MD[c], Manjiri K. Dighe, MD[c]

KEYWORDS

- Renal mass • Incidental renal mass • Genitourinary imaging
- Kidney disease • Renal disease

Approximately 50% of middle-aged adults have an incidental renal lesion.[1] The most common incidental renal lesion is a cyst,[1] and the prototypical solid lesion seen is renal cell carcinoma (RCC). Imaging appearance of renal masses other than RCC and cysts are elucidated in this review.

Renal lesions can be divided into neoplastic and non-neoplastic lesions. Neoplastic renal masses include RCC; transitional cell carcinoma; oncocytoma; angiomyolipoma (AML); mesenchymal tumors, such as liposarcomas; lymphoma; leukemia; plasmacytoma; metastases; and rare tumors, such as medullary cell carcinoma, metanephric adenoma, renal solitary fibrous tumor, and primitive neuroectodermal tumor (PNET). Non-neoplastic renal lesions include parapelvic cysts, acute focal pyelonephritis, xanthogranulomatous pyelonephritis, renal parenchymal scar, intrarenal splenules, hematoma, and renal infarcts.

Renal lesions can also be subdivided into exophytic and infiltrative based on their appearance and growth pattern. Exophytic lesions enlarge by additive expansion and deform the renal contour, producing a bulge along the renal contour. These lesions are well appreciated on contrast-enhanced imaging as compressing the renal parenchyma and distorting the collecting system. They may possess a pseudocapsule of compressed renal parenchyma. Infiltrative lesions, on the other hand, use the renal interstitium to grow. These lesions cause nephromegaly without distorting the reniform shape. They are difficult to appreciate on unenhanced imaging but usually well seen on contrast-enhanced imaging.[2,3]

NON-NEOPLASTIC LESIONS
Parapelvic Cysts

Parapelvic cysts are not true renal cysts but may be lymphatic in origin or develop from embryologic rests.[4] These cysts do not communicate with the collecting system and, therefore, do not fill with contrast material during excretory urography or contrast-enhanced computed tomography (CT)/magnetic resonance (MR) imaging. They are commonly seen as hypoattenuating parapelvic and cortical lesions consistent with cysts. On ultrasound (US) these are seen as anechoic lesions with increased through transmission. However, because the parapelvic cysts are located in the renal pelvis, they may be mistaken for hydronephrosis (Fig. 1).[4] The absence of central communication in the renal pelvis should

[a] Department of Radiology, Changi General Hospital, 2 Simei Street 3, Singapore 529889
[b] Department of Radiology, VA Puget Sound Health Care System, University of Washington, Mail Box 358280, S-114/Radiology, 1660 South Columbian Way, Seattle, WA 98108-1597, USA
[c] Department of Radiology, University of Washington Medical Center, Box 356510, 1959 Northeast Pacific Street, Seattle, WA 98195-7117, USA
* Corresponding author.
E-mail address: bhargp@uw.edu

Radiol Clin N Am 50 (2012) 245–257
doi:10.1016/j.rcl.2012.02.006
0033-8389/12/$ – see front matter Published by Elsevier Inc.

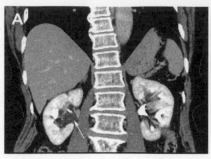
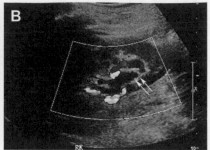

Fig. 1. Parapelvic cysts. Coronal reformat (*A*) from the delayed phase of a CT intravenous urogram shows fluid-filled hypodense areas within the renal pelvis that do not fill with contrast consistent with parapelvic cysts (*arrow*). Color Doppler US (*B*) shows fluid-filled anechoic areas in the renal pelvis, which can be mistaken for hydronephrosis (*double arrow*).

suggest the diagnosis of parapelvic cysts over hydronephrosis.

Acute Pyelonephritis

Urinary tract infection typically originates in the urinary bladder; when it migrates to the kidney or is seeded there hematogenously, a tubulointerstitial inflammatory reaction ensues, involving the renal pelvis and parenchyma. The condition is characterized as pyelonephritis. Imaging is usually not warranted in uncomplicated pyelonephritis. When imaging is warranted because of nonresponsiveness to treatment or complications, CT is the modality of choice for evaluating acute bacterial nephritis. It provides comprehensive anatomic and physiologic information that accurately characterizes both intrarenal and extrarenal pathologic conditions. Unenhanced CT is excellent for identifying urinary tract gas, calculi, hemorrhage, renal enlargement, and obstruction. After the administration of contrast material, acute bacterial nephritis most commonly manifests as one or

more wedge-shaped areas or streaky zones of lesser enhancement that extend from the papilla to the renal cortex, reflecting underlying pathophysiology of tubular obstruction caused by inflammatory debris within the lumen, interstitial edema, and vasospasm, which decreases the flow of contrast through the tubule. This condition results in delayed and persistent enhancement of the involved tubules. CT is also the best modality for fully evaluating the secondary signs of renal inflammatory disease and its complications, which include focal or global enlargement of the kidney, perinephric stranding, thickening of Gerota fascia, and abscess formation (**Fig. 2**).[5-8]

US findings in pyelonephritis include hydronephrosis, renal enlargement, loss of renal sinus fat caused by edema, changes in echogenicity caused by edema (hypoechoic) or hemorrhage (hyperechoic), loss of corticomedullary differentiation, abscess formation, and areas of hypoperfusion (visible with power Doppler interrogation). However, US is limited in the definitive differentiation of calcification from intraparenchymal or

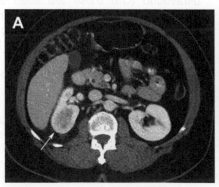
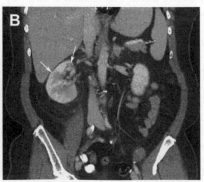

Fig. 2. Focal pyelonephritis. Axial postcontrast (*A*) image shows a rounded, masslike, hypodense lesion in the right kidney (*arrow*). Coronal reformat (*B*) shows this structure to have a striated appearance typical of pyelonephritis (*arrows*) and mild perinephric stranding involving the right kidney. In the clinical context of urinary tract infection, fever and flank pain, this is consistent with acute pyelonephritis.

collecting system gas (manifested respectively as clean shadowing and dirty shadowing with echoes and reverberations), identification of perinephric extension of infection, and visualization of small microabscesses that are common in early acute infections.[9,10]

When confined to a single lobe, focal pyelonephritis can mimic a focal renal mass. Sonographically, it appears as either a hypoechoic or hyperechoic lesion in the renal cortex and mimics a mass. The focal abnormality typically extends from the renal medulla to the renal capsule and shows decreased perfusion on color-flow Doppler imaging.[11] CT shows a focal wedge-shaped or rounded area of low attenuation without a well-defined surrounding wall, typically without an overlying bulge on the renal surface, which helps to distinguish it from RCC. The clinical history of flank pain, fever/chills, and pyuria is often present and aids in establishing the diagnosis. Renal cortical scintigraphy, using 99mTc-labeled glucoheptonate or dimercaptosuccinic acid, shows a focal cortical defect in the kidney.[12] Striations may also be observed in the nephrogram.[11,13]

Soft tissue stranding in the perinephric fat may give the appearance of renal malignancy. In particular, it may be difficult to distinguish this appearance from infiltrative neoplasms, such as medullary renal carcinoma. Clinical history of flank pain, fever with chills, and pyuria should be helpful in establishing the diagnosis of pyelonephritis. Also, pyelonephritis is more likely to occur in patients with diabetes and in those who are immunocompromised.[11]

Xanthogranulomatous Pyelonephritis

Xanthogranulomatous pyelonephritis (XGP) is a rare inflammatory condition usually secondary to chronic obstruction caused by nephrolithiasis and resulting in infection and irreversible destruction of the renal parenchyma. XGP is associated with a staghorn calculus in approximately 70% of cases. Patients with diabetes are particularly predisposed to the formation of XGP. XGP may rarely present with the classic urographic triad of unilaterally decreased or absent renal excretion, staghorn calculus, and diffuse renal enlargement.[7,11] XGP may present in a diffuse or focal pattern. Focal or segmental XGP is seen in a smaller number of patients (approximately 10%) and is more likely to mimic RCC on imaging.[14] Establishing a definite preoperative diagnosis only by imaging in both focal and diffuse forms of XGP is difficult. Sonographically, XGP may appear as single or multiple hypoechoic areas in the parenchyma of an enlarged kidney, with central echogenic foci representing calculi. Sonographic findings are nonspecific but can nevertheless suggest a diagnosis of XGP.[13] Although not confirmatory, CT evaluation can be considered helpful in the presence of features, such as abscess replacing the renal parenchyma, with low-attenuation areas (lipid-rich xanthogranulomatous tissue) and calcification in the mass.[11,15] If calculi are not present, focal XGP with a low-attenuation area in the renal parenchyma may suggest a diagnosis of renal tumor.

Autoimmune Pancreatitis

Lymphoplasmacytic renal focal lesions can be found in up to 35% of patients with autoimmune pancreatitis.[16] These masses are usually multiple, bilateral, wedge shaped, hypovascular, and do not alter the renal contour (**Fig. 3**).[16–18] Differential diagnosis includes lymphoma, metastasis, ischemia, and pyelonephritis. The key for the diagnosis is the presence of characteristic findings in the pancreas, including the presence of a peripancreatic halo and a smooth, rounded contour of the enlarged pancreas. Lymphoplasmacytic masses in the lungs, biliary ducts, or retroperitoneum may also be present.[17,19,20] The diagnosis can be confirmed with elevated serum immunoglobulin G4 measurements or biopsy.[19] Most of these lesions show complete or partial response to corticosteroid treatment.[16]

Renal Pseudotumor/Scar

Severely scarred renal parenchyma secondary to infectious processes, such as pyelonephritis or renal infarcts, may also present as a potential pseudotumor on imaging. Regions of preserved parenchyma may seem masslike on sonography or even in the nephrographic phase of CT and MR imaging. Appropriate corticomedullary differentiation in the early phases of enhancement on CT or MR imaging may be required to exclude a mass.[11]

Splenule

Ectopic splenic tissue can occur in congenital or acquired forms. The congenital form, called accessory spleen, occurs in 10% of the population. In distinction, the term splenosis refers to the acquired form, produced by seeding of splenic tissue, generally after trauma or splenectomy. First described by Buchbinder and Lipkoff[21] in 1939, splenosis has been reported to occur in 26% to 67% of patients after trauma associated with splenic rupture or after splenectomy.[22,23] It is most frequently encountered in the serous surface of the small intestine, followed by the greater

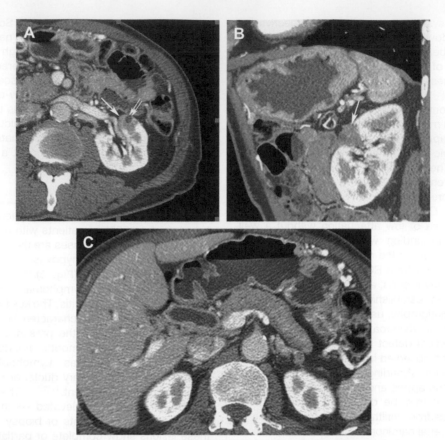

Fig. 3. Autoimmune pancreatitis. Axial (*A*) and sagittal (*B*) contrast-enhanced CT obtained during corticomedullary-phase show a hypovascular, wedge-shaped mass (*arrow*) in the left kidney with preservation of the normal renal contour. The mass is encasing a small renal cyst (*double arrow*). Axial (*C*) contrast-enhanced CT in the same patient shows a low density rim surrounding and edematous appearing pancreas consistent with autoimmune pancreatitis. After 1 month of corticosteroid treatment, there was almost complete resolution of the lesions and the renal cyst was unchanged.

omentum, parietal peritoneum, large intestine, diaphragm undersurface, and thorax in cases of associated diaphragmatic injury.[24] The usual mechanism of seeding of splenic tissue is by local dissemination from disruption of the splenic capsule. Heterotopic perirenal splenic tissue may arise in the subcapsular region, separate from the adjacent renal parenchyma, as a developmental anomaly or secondary to prior trauma or splenectomy.[22]

On CT or gadolinium-enhanced MR imaging, it appears as a solid enhancing mass that may seem to arise from the kidney. Sometimes, it can be difficult to distinguish if the lesion is on the surface of the kidney rather than arising from the renal parenchyma and growing exophytically. Conventional imaging methods (US, CT) might lead to a false diagnosis of tumor (**Fig. 4**). The key to the diagnosis of this entity is to suspect it based on the previous history of trauma, splenectomy, or the presence of additional splenules. If a multiphasic

CT study is available, comparing enhancement patterns and the attenuation values with that of the spleen is useful. Similarly, MR signal intensities of accessory splenic tissue follow that of the spleen across all sequences. The tests with the greatest reported specificity for the diagnosis of both normal and ectopic splenic tissue are 99mTc-sulfur colloid liver-spleen scintigraphy, 99mTc-labeled heat-damaged erythrocytes spleen scintigraphy, and ferumoxide-enhanced MR imaging, which show uptake by the splenic tissue and help make a more-definitive diagnosis. With increased awareness of accessory splenic tissue in various locations, especially in the regions surrounding the spleen, and ever-improving imaging capability, radiologists should be aware of this entity to avoid unnecessary biopsy or surgery.[11,25,26]

Infarct

In the appropriate clinical setting, a wedge-shaped hypodensity in the kidney on CT or MR imaging is

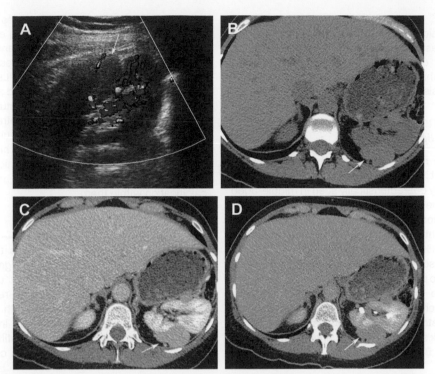

Fig. 4. Splenule. Color Doppler US image (*A*) shows an avascular isoechoic lesion along the peripheral aspect of the left kidney (*arrow*). Multiphase CT performed shows mild enhancement of the mass (*arrow*) with contrast administration: (*B*) noncontrast, (*C*) nephrographic phase, and (*D*) pyelographic phase. Given the history of a prior splenectomy, a splenule was suspected. Biopsy of this lesion was performed at the request of the clinical service and confirmed a splenule.

suspicious for a renal infarct. A thin, dense rim of enhancement is often seen around the kidney during the nephrographic phase, corresponding to a viable rim of cortex, likely caused by collateral circulation from the renal capsule. It is considered that this nephrographic rim sign is diagnostic of total renal infarction or cortical necrosis (**Fig. 5**).[27] Although most of the cases are straightforward for the diagnosis of renal infarction, cases with tumefactive lesions and global infarctions without the well-known cortical rim sign may be difficult to distinguish from renal masses. Suzer and

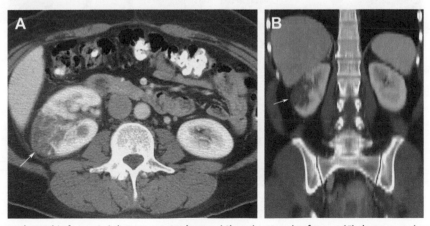

Fig. 5. Segmental renal infarct. Axial postcontrast image (*A*) and coronal reformat (*B*) show a wedge-shaped area of hypodensity in the right kidney (*arrow*). A cortical rim sign was not present. Because the patient presented with pain and did not have any clinical features to suggest pyelonephritis, this was thought to be caused by segmental renal infarction.

colleagues[28] described a flip-flop enhancement pattern, which the investigators think is caused by extravasation of contrast from ischemic destruction of glomerular membrane in delayed contrast-enhanced CT images, and this solidifies the diagnosis of renal infarction.

NEOPLASTIC LESIONS
Angiomyolipoma

AML is the most common benign mesenchymal neoplasm. It is the prototypical fat-containing lesion in the kidney characteristically seen in middle-aged women. These tumors are benign tumors containing angiomatous, myomatous, and lipomatous tissue. Eighty percent of AMLs are sporadic, whereas 20% are associated with tuberous sclerosis (autosomal dominant phakomatosis). The latter tend to be larger at presentation. Sonographic appearance of an AML is mostly echogenic caused by either fat or hemorrhage. Macroscopic fat demonstrates negative Hounsfield values on CT and dark signal on MR sequences with fat saturation (Fig. 6). Risk of bleeding in AML increases when the size of the mass increases to greater than 4 cm because of the lack of an elastic layer within the angiomatous component and the presence of intralesional aneurysms greater than 5 mm.[29] Approximately 4.5% of AMLs may not show identifiable macroscopic fat and are indistinguishable from RCC on imaging studies alone (Fig. 7). Studies indicate that in contradistinction to RCCs, AMLs with minimal fat show uniform, prolonged contrast enhancement and a higher signal intensity index on double-echo, chemical shift MR imaging.[30,31] Rarely, AMLs may have necrosis and calcification within them.

Transitional Cell Carcinoma

Transitional cell carcinoma (TCC) is the second most-common primary renal malignancy, accounting for approximately 10% of upper tract tumors.[32] Although not an unusual renal lesion, specific imaging features are worth reviewing. Renal TCC most frequently arises in the renal pelvis, and spreads outwards, infiltrating the renal parenchyma but preserving its contour. On

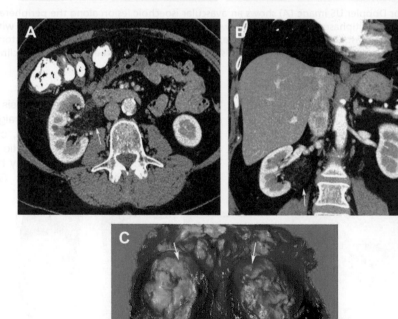

Fig. 6. Angiomyolipoma. Axial postcontrast CT (A) and coronal reformat (B) images show a fat-containing mass in the renal hilum (arrow). Gross specimen (C) from a right nephrectomy show the large, fat-containing mass (arrows) in the renal sinus with extension into the upper pole of the kidney. This mass was confirmed to be an angiomyolipoma on histopathology.

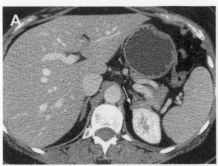
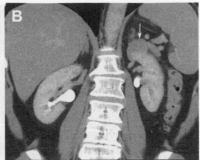

Fig. 7. Lipid-poor angiomyolipoma. Axial postcontrast (*A*) and coronal reformat (*B*) from a delayed-phase CT shows a homogenous mildly enhancing mass (*arrow*) in the upper pole of the left kidney. The mass showed an increase in size from the prior study and concern for an RCC was raised. The mass was excised, and histopathology revealed a lipid poor angiomyolipoma.

unenhanced studies, the intraluminal portion of the tumor often shows increased attenuation relative to urine. After contrast administration, the mass typically enhances, although to a lesser degree than normal renal parenchyma and characteristically less than conventional RCC (Fig. 8).[32] The central location of these tumors makes their identification in the corticomedullary phase nearly impossible, underscoring the importance of nephrographic phase imaging.[3]

Oncocytoma

Oncocytoma is a benign renal cell neoplasm that accounts for approximately 5% of all adult primary renal epithelial neoplasms. The peak age of incidence is in the seventh decade; men are more likely to be affected than women. Most tumors occur sporadically in asymptomatic patients. They typically appear as solitary, well-demarcated, unencapsulated, fairly homogeneous renal cortical tumors. Multiple, bilateral tumors are known to occur. A characteristic central stellate

fibrotic scar (more often seen with large tumors) is seen in up to 33% of tumors. Hemorrhage may be found in up to 20% of cases. A spoke-wheel pattern of feeding arteries associated with a homogeneous nephrogram is a characteristic finding on catheter angiography.[33] However, oncocytomas cannot be distinguished from RCCs by imaging findings alone (Fig. 9). In addition, oncocytomas may be associated with RCCs either as hybrid tumors (pathologic features of both oncocytomas and chromophobe or other RCC subtypes) or as collision tumors.[34] Thus, despite advances in histopathologic techniques (including immunocytochemistry and cytogenetics), a partial nephrectomy is typically required for accurate characterization.[35]

Medullary Carcinoma

Medullary carcinomas are rare tumors, accounting for less than 1% of all tumors. It is thought to arise from the calyceal epithelium in or near the renal papilla, from which it grows in an infiltrative pattern. It occurs in relatively young males aged

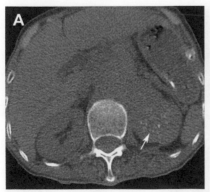
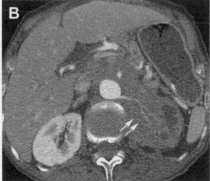

Fig. 8. Transitional cell carcinoma. Axial precontrast CT (*A*) shows calcifications (*arrow*) in the left kidney. Postcontrast axial CT image (*B*) shows an infiltrative mass in the poorly functioning left kidney centered on the left renal pelvis (*double arrow*). Urine cytology was positive for urothelial carcinoma.

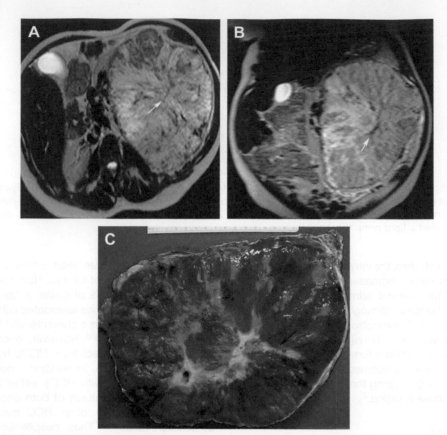

Fig. 9. Oncocytoma. Axial T2-weighted image (*A*) and coronal T2-weighted image (*B*) shows a large T2 hyperintense left renal mass displacing but not infiltrating surrounding structures with a central scar (*arrow*). The patient's glomerular filtration rate (GFR) was not able to receive intravenous contrast because of a low GFR. Histopathology revealed an oncocytoma on resection. Gross photograph (*C*) of left kidney replaced by oncocytoma, with classic mahogany brown parenchyma and central tan-white stellate scar (*black arrow*).

between 11 and 40 years and is found almost exclusively in patients with sickle cell trait.[36] They are aggressive, infiltrating tumors with a high propensity for local invasion and early metastatic disease. Radiologically, medullary carcinoma appears as an ill-defined, heterogeneously enhancing mass centered on the renal medulla without deforming the renal contour (**Fig. 10**).[37]

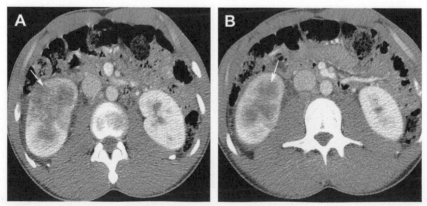

Fig. 10. Medullary carcinoma. Axial postcontrast CT images (*A, B*) show a heterogeneously, hypoenhancing ill-defined mass (*arrow*) in the right kidney. This mass was consistent with medullary carcinoma on resection.

Solitary Fibrous Tumor

Solitary fibrous tumors (SFT) are rare fibrous tumors arising from serosal surfaces of organs, most commonly pleura. They can be benign or malignant and are frequently asymptomatic. They present as large exophytic masses that can be confused with RCC.[38] Tissue diagnosis is usually necessary. The cross-sectional imaging findings of renal solitary fibrous tumors are attributable to the combination of variable cellularity, dense collagen content, and focal hemangiopericytomatous vascular pattern. More than 50% of the renal SFTs have occurred in patients older than 40 years (from 33–76 years, with an average age of 52 years). The male-to-female ratio seems to be almost equal (1.0:1.5).[39]

On CT images, renal solitary fibrous tumor appears as a well-circumscribed lobulated soft-tissue mass in the region of the renal sinus or capsule.[39] The tumors typically show relatively homogeneous enhancement despite the large size of the mass (Fig. 11). Necrosis, hemorrhage, and calcifications are rare. At MR imaging, solitary fibrous tumors are isointense to the renal cortex on T1-weighted images. On T2-weighted MR images, alternate areas of extremely low signal intensity and moderately high signal intensity are distributed in a radial configuration. A heterogeneous spoke-wheel pattern of enhancement has been observed in some cases.[40] Surgical removal is the treatment of choice. Most solitary fibrous tumors are benign; however, 10% to 15% of extrapleural solitary fibrous tumors show malignant behavior in the form of recurrence or metastatic disease.[41]

Metastases

Frequency of metastasis to the kidney varies between 7% and 13% in patients with a preexisting primary tumor.[42] Common primaries are bronchogenic carcinomas, colorectal cancer, and breast cancer.[43] They present more commonly as exophytic lesions and less often as an infiltrative lesions (Fig. 12). Because of the possibility of a synchronous primary RCC, tissue diagnosis is still necessary.

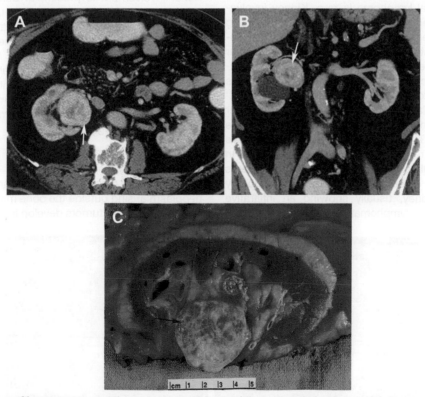

Fig. 11. Solitary fibrous tumor. Axial postcontrast CT image (A) and coronal reformat (B) shows an enhancing mass (arrow) in the right renal pelvis. This mass was suspicious for an RCC and, hence, patient underwent surgery. Histopathology revealed a solitary fibrous tumor. Gross photograph (C) of right kidney shows a well-circumscribed, mass confined to the renal hilum (black arrow). The mass did not involve the renal parenchyma.

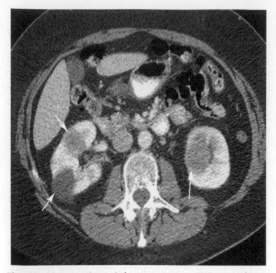

Fig. 12. Metastasis. Axial postcontrast CT image shows bilateral hypoenhancing renal masses (*arrows*). Given a history of breast cancer and the interval development of the lesions compared with the prior study, these lesions were thought to be secondary to metastases.

Lymphoma

Primary renal lymphoma is rare. Kidney involvement by lymphoma typically occurs in the setting of widespread disease and usually with non-Hodgkin histologic types. Lymphoma may enter the kidney hematogenously or through sinus, perinephric, or capsular lymphatics. Several patterns of renal involvement have been described.[44,45] Multiple bilateral renal masses, with either a mass-forming or infiltrative growth pattern, are seen in 50% to 60% of patients. Most have associated retroperitoneal lymphadenopathy. In up to 25% of patients, renal lymphoma represents contiguous spread from adjacent adenopathy into the kidney, usually showing an infiltrative pattern. Diffuse lymphomatous infiltration producing

smooth generalized renal enlargement occurs in approximately 20% of patients and it is almost always bilateral. Renal lymphoma as a solitary mass is the least common pattern of involvement, which is seen in fewer than 10% of patients.[44,45]

At CT, renal lymphoma is a soft tissue attenuation mass that enhances homogeneously but less intensely than normal renal parenchyma after contrast material administration.[44–46] Nephrographic-phase CT imaging is essential because lymphomatous deposits in the kidney may be small and medullary in location, making them inconspicuous on corticomedullary-phase images (**Fig. 13**).

On MR, renal lymphoma appears as a hypointense signal on T1-weighted MR images and is slightly hypointense or isointense relative to normal renal cortex on T2-weighted images. After the intravenous administration of gadolinium-based contrast material, lymphomatous deposits enhance less than the surrounding normal parenchyma, although some lesions can demonstrate progressive enhancement on delayed images.[45]

Leukemia

Renal involvement is present at autopsy in approximately 65% of patients with leukemia. The involvement tends to be infiltrative rather than exophytic. Moderate nephromegaly is the most-common finding reported in multiple studies.[44,47–50] Focal parenchymal abnormalities were also seen in renal leukemia, with the study by Hilmes[51] describing focal involvement in 42% of cases. Acute lymphoblastic leukemia accounts for most cases (**Fig. 14**).

Plasmacytoma

Extramedullary plasmacytoma is a rare malignant neoplasm arising outside the bone marrow. Eighty percent to 90% of tumors develop in the head and

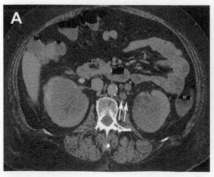
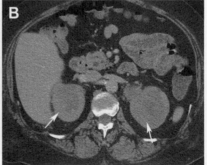

Fig. 13. Lymphoma. Axial postcontrast CT images (*A*, *B*) show bilateral hypoattenuating infiltrative masses (*arrows*) in the kidneys and associated lymphadenopathy (*double arrow*). Because the patient had a history of lymphoma and other areas of recurrence, it was considered that these were caused by renal lymphoma.

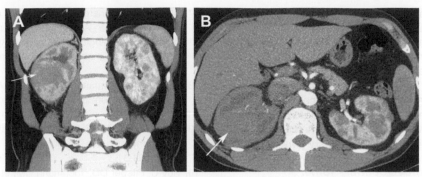

Fig. 14. Leukemia. Coronal reformat (*A*) and axial postcontrast (*B*) CT images show a hypoattenuating mass (*arrow*) in the interpolar region of the right kidney with multiple other similar smaller masses in the left kidney. Biopsy confirmed the diagnosis of myeloid leukemia infiltration in the right kidney.

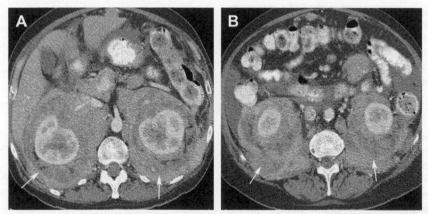

Fig. 15. Plasmacytoma. Axial postcontrast CT images (*A, B*) show heterogeneously enhancing masses (*arrows*) in the perinephric space. Because of the history of multiple myeloma and the perinephric extension, this was suggestive of extramedullary plasmacytoma.

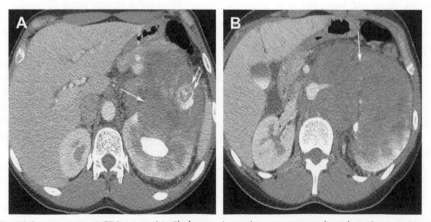

Fig. 16. PNET. Axial postcontrast CT images (*A, B*) show a large heterogeneously enhancing retroperitoneal mass encasing the vessels and invading the left kidney (*arrow*). This mass was confirmed on excision to represent a PNET. Note areas of calcification within this mass (*double arrow*).

neck area and compose up to 1% of the tumors of the head and neck region.[52] Patients with renal plasmacytoma have a history of multiple myeloma or plasmacytoma involving other organs. Primary extramedullary neoplasms of B cells are rare and account for only 5%. Renal involvement has been reported in up to 17% of cases of multiple myeloma. Imaging features similar to other infiltrative tumors with preservation of the reniform shape and tissue diagnosis is necessary (**Fig. 15**).[53]

Primary Neuroectodermal Tumor

These neoplasms are uncommon and represent undifferentiated peripheral small cell neoplasms. They are highly aggressive and considered to have a poor prognosis.[54] Outside the central nervous system, they can involve the chest wall, paraspinal areas, and rarely organs, such as the kidney. Imaging appearance is that of a minimally enhancing large mass with multiple septumlike structures, peripheral hemorrhage, venous thrombosis, accompanied by distant metastases in a young adult.[55] Tissue diagnosis is necessary to make this diagnosis (**Fig. 16**).

SUMMARY

Renal masses are frequently incidental findings. These findings can be exophytic or infiltrative. Imaging is invaluable in characterizing the lesions and is confirmatory in some benign lesions. RCC remains the primary diagnostic consideration, and the assessment of imaging pattern in the right clinical context can improve diagnostic accuracy for these uncommon and unusual renal neoplasms.

REFERENCES

1. Silverman SG, Israel GM, Herts BR, et al. Management of the incidental renal mass. Radiology 2008; 249:16–31.
2. Hartman DS, Davidson AJ, Davis CJ, et al. Infiltrative renal lesions: CT-sonographic-pathologic correlation. AJR Am J Roentgenol 1988;150:1061–4.
3. Dyer R, DiSantis DJ, McClennan BL. Simplified imaging approach for evaluation of the solid renal mass in adults. Radiology 2008;247:331–43.
4. Hidalgo H, Dunnick NR, Rosenberg ER, et al. Parapelvic cysts: appearance on CT and sonography. AJR Am J Roentgenol 1982;138:667–71.
5. Harrison RB, Shaffer HA. The roentgenographic findings in acute pyelonephritis. JAMA 1979;241: 1718–20.
6. Goldman SM, Fishman EK. Upper urinary tract infection: the current role of CT, ultrasound, and MRI. Semin Ultrasound CT MR 1991;12:335–60.
7. Pickhardt PJ, Lonergan GJ, Davis CJ, et al. From the archives of the AFIP. Infiltrative renal lesions: radiologic-pathologic correlation. Armed Forces Institute of Pathology. Radiographics 2000;20: 215–43.
8. Soulen MC, Fishman EK, Goldman SM, et al. Bacterial renal infection: role of CT. Radiology 1989;171: 703–7.
9. Allen HA, Walsh JW, Brewer WH, et al. Sonography of emphysematous pyelonephritis. J Ultrasound Med 1984;3:533–7.
10. Roy C, Pfleger DD, Tuchmann CM, et al. Emphysematous pyelitis: findings in five patients. Radiology 2001;218:647–50.
11. Bhatt S, MacLennan G, Dogra V. Renal pseudotumors. AJR Am J Roentgenol 2007;188: 1380–7.
12. Majd M, Rushton HG. Renal cortical scintigraphy in the diagnosis of acute pyelonephritis. Semin Nucl Med 1992;22:98–111.
13. Craig WD, Wagner BJ, Travis MD. Pyelonephritis: radiologic-pathologic review. Radiographics 2008; 28:255–77 [quiz: 327–8].
14. Goldman SM, Hartman DS, Fishman EK, et al. CT of xanthogranulomatous pyelonephritis: radiologic-pathologic correlation. AJR Am J Roentgenol 1984; 142:963–9.
15. Vourganti S, Agarwal PK, Bodner DR, et al. Ultrasonographic evaluation of renal infections. Radiol Clin North Am 2006;44:763–75.
16. Takahashi N, Kawashima A, Fletcher JG, et al. Renal involvement in patients with autoimmune pancreatitis: CT and MR imaging findings. Radiology 2007; 242:791–801.
17. Sahani DV, Kalva SP, Farrell J, et al. Autoimmune pancreatitis: imaging features. Radiology 2004; 233:345–52.
18. Brennan D, Pedrosa I. Lymphoplasmacytic sclerosing pancreatitis. AJR Am J Roentgenol 2005; 185:1367–8 [author reply: 8].
19. Finkelberg DL, Sahani D, Deshpande V, et al. Autoimmune pancreatitis. N Engl J Med 2006;355: 2670–6.
20. Kawamoto S, Siegelman SS, Hruban RH, et al. Lymphoplasmacytic sclerosing pancreatitis with obstructive jaundice: CT and pathology features. AJR Am J Roentgenol 2004;183:915–21.
21. Buchbinder JH, Lipkoff CJ. Splenosis: multiple peritoneal splenic implants following abdominal injury. Surgery 1939;6:927–34.
22. Kiser JW, Fagien M, Clore FF. Splenosis mimicking a left renal mass. AJR Am J Roentgenol 1996;167: 1508–9.
23. Umemoto S, Miyoshi Y, Nakaigawa N, et al. Distinguishing splenosis from local recurrence of renal cell carcinoma using a technetium sulfur colloid scan. Int J Urol 2007;14:245–7.

24. Pumberger W, Wiesbauer P, Leitha T. Splenosis mimicking tumor recurrence in renal cell carcinoma: detection on selective spleen scintigraphy. J Pediatr Surg 2001;36:1089–91.

25. Imbriaco M, Camera L, Manciuria A, et al. A case of multiple intra-abdominal splenosis with computed tomography and magnetic resonance imaging correlative findings. World J Gastroenterol 2008;14: 1453–5.

26. Berman AJ, Zahalsky MP, Okon SA, et al. Distinguishing splenosis from renal masses using ferumoxide-enhanced magnetic resonance imaging. Urology 2003;62:748.

27. Frank PH, Nuttall J, Brander WL, et al. The cortical rim sign of renal infarction. Br J Radiol 1974;47:875–8.

28. Suzer O, Shirkhoda A, Jafri SZ, et al. CT features of renal infarction. Eur J Radiol 2002;44:59–64.

29. Yamakado K, Tanaka N, Nakagawa T, et al. Renal angiomyolipoma: relationships between tumor size, aneurysm formation, and rupture. Radiology 2002; 225:78–82.

30. Kim JK, Park SY, Shon JH, et al. Angiomyolipoma with minimal fat: differentiation from renal cell carcinoma at biphasic helical CT. Radiology 2004;230: 677–84.

31. Kim JK, Kim SH, Jang YJ, et al. Renal angiomyolipoma with minimal fat: differentiation from other neoplasms at double-echo chemical shift FLASH MR imaging. Radiology 2006;239:174–80.

32. Browne R, Meehan C, Colville J, et al. Transitional cell carcinoma of the upper urinary tract: spectrum of imaging findings. Radiographics 2005;25:1609–27.

33. Quinn MJ, Hartman DS, Friedman AC, et al. Renal oncocytoma: new observations. Radiology 1984; 153:49–53.

34. Rowsell C, Fleshner N, Marrano P, et al. Papillary renal cell carcinoma within a renal oncocytoma: case report of an incidental finding of a tumour within a tumour. J Clin Pathol 2007;60:426–8.

35. Shah RB, Bakshi N, Hafez KS, et al. Image-guided biopsy in the evaluation of renal mass lesions in contemporary urological practice: indications, adequacy, clinical impact, and limitations of the pathological diagnosis. Hum Pathol 2005;36: 1309–15.

36. Davidson AJ, Choyke PL, Hartman DS, et al. Renal medullary carcinoma associated with sickle cell trait: radiologic findings. Radiology 1995;195:83–5.

37. Blitman NM, Berkenblit RG, Rozenblit AM, et al. Renal medullary carcinoma: CT and MRI features. AJR Am J Roentgenol 2005;185:268–72.

38. Gelb AB, Simmons ML, Weidner N. Solitary fibrous tumor involving the renal capsule. Am J Surg Pathol 1996;20:1288–95.

39. Znati K, Chbani L, El Fatemi H, et al. Solitary fibrous tumor of the kidney: a case report and review of the literature. Rev Urol 2007;9:36–40.

40. Johnson TR, Pedrosa I, Goldsmith J, et al. Magnetic resonance imaging findings in solitary fibrous tumor of the kidney. J Comput Assist Tomogr 2005;29: 481–3.

41. Fukunaga M, Nikaido T. Solitary fibrous tumour of the renal peripelvis. Histopathology 1997;30:451–6.

42. Choyke PL, White EM, Zeman RK, et al. Renal metastases: clinicopathologic and radiologic correlation. Radiology 1987;162:359–63.

43. Bhatt GM, Bernardino ME, Graham SD. CT diagnosis of renal metastases. J Comput Assist Tomogr 1983;7:1032–4.

44. Bailey JE, Roubidoux MA, Dunnick NR. Secondary renal neoplasms. Abdom Imaging 1998; 23:266–74.

45. Sheth S, Ali S, Fishman E. Imaging of renal lymphoma: patterns of disease with pathologic correlation. Radiographics 2006;26:1151–68.

46. Urban BA, Fishman EK. Renal lymphoma: CT patterns with emphasis on helical CT. Radiographics 2000;20:197–212.

47. Araki T. Leukemic involvement of the kidney in children: CT features. J Comput Assist Tomogr 1982;6: 781–4.

48. Ali AA, Flombaum CD, Brochstein JA, et al. Lactic acidosis and renal enlargement at diagnosis and relapse of acute lymphoblastic leukemia. J Pediatr 1994;125:584–6.

49. Boueva A, Bouvier R. Precursor B-cell lymphoblastic leukemia as a cause of a bilateral nephromegaly. Pediatr Nephrol 2005;20:679–82.

50. Gore RM, Shkolnik A. Abdominal manifestations of pediatric leukemias: sonographic assessment. Radiology 1982;143:207–10.

51. Hilmes MA, Dillman JR, Mody RJ, et al. Pediatric renal leukemia: spectrum of CT imaging findings. Pediatr Radiol 2008;38:424–30.

52. Dimopoulos MA, Kiamouris C, Moulopoulos LA. Solitary plasmacytoma of bone and extramedullary plasmacytoma. Hematol Oncol Clin North Am 1999;13:1249–57.

53. Mongha R, Narayan S, Dutta A, et al. Plasmacytoma of the kidney. Saudi J Kidney Dis Transpl 2010;21: 931–4.

54. Zhang L, Wang T, Zheng L, et al. Primitive neuroectodermal tumor of the kidney with inferior vena cava tumor thrombus. J Natl Med Assoc 2009;101: 1291–4.

55. Lee H, Cho JY, Kim SH, et al. Imaging findings of primitive neuroectodermal tumors of the kidney. J Comput Assist Tomogr 2009;33:882–6.

Infectious and Inflammatory Diseases of the Kidney

Nancy A. Hammond, MD*, Paul Nikolaidis, MD,
Frank H. Miller, MD

KEYWORDS

- Renal tuberculosis • Xanthogranulomatous pyelonephritis
- Emphysematous pyelonephritis • Pyonephrosis
- Renal echinococcus • Renal aspergillosis

Radiographic evaluation is not typically necessary in evaluating a patient with acute pyelonephritis because the diagnosis can usually be made with clinical and laboratory data. Radiology plays a role in evaluating renal infection in high-risk patients and in evaluating for complications of pyelonephritis. This article discusses the imaging findings of some common renal infections and less common processes, including tuberculosis, xanthogranulomatous pyelonephritis (XGP), pyonephrosis, upper tract fungal infection, renal echinococcus, and renal apsergillosis. Many of these entities require urgent management, and it is imperative that the radiologist be familiar with their imaging findings.

RENAL TUBERCULOSIS

The genitourinary (GU) tract is the most common extrapulmonary site of tuberculosis. GU tuberculosis is acquired secondary to hematogenous dissemination of *Mycobacterium tuberculosis* to the kidneys after initial pulmonary inoculation. Renal tuberculosis is identified in 4% to 8% of patients with evidence of pulmonary tuberculosis.[1] From the kidneys, ureteral and bladder involvement can occur via descending infection. Although the kidneys and urinary tract are the most common site of primary GU involvement, genital organ involvement can also occur and does so secondary to hematogenous

seeding, lymphatic spread, or direct extension from the lower urinary tract. In men, the epididymis is the most common site of involvement. The seminal vesicles, vas deferens, and prostate can also be involved. In women with genital organ tuberculosis, patients most commonly present with infertility secondary to fallopian tube involvement; tubo-ovarian abscesses can also form.[2] The endometrium is involved in 50% of patients with fallopian tube involvement.[3] Adrenal gland involvement may also occur and may result in adrenal insufficiency.

Renal inoculation occurs at the time of initial exposure. Via hematogenous dissemination, tuberculous bacilli are trapped in the periglomerular capillaries resulting in the formation of small abscesses. In immunocompetent patients, these foci are suppressed and granulomas are formed by the host response. This response is confined to the renal cortex. Granulomas can remain dormant for decades, but reactivation occurs when there is a breakdown in the host's immune system. On reactivation, the granulomas enlarge, resulting in capillary rupture and progression of disease to the medulla along the loop of Henle and proximal tubules (Fig. 1). Once in the proximal collecting system, tuberculous infection can spread distally to involve the ureter and bladder and across retroperitoneal fascial planes to involve other organs.

Clinically, the diagnosis of GU tuberculosis is delayed because of the insidious onset and

Disclosures: No disclosures.
Funding support: None.
Department of Radiology, Northwestern University, Feinberg School of Medicine, 676 North Saint Clair, Suite 800, Chicago, IL 60611, USA
* Corresponding author.
E-mail address: nhammond@nmff.org

Radiol Clin N Am 50 (2012) 259–270
doi:10.1016/j.rcl.2012.02.002
0033-8389/12/$ – see front matter
© 2012 Elsevier Inc. All rights reserved.

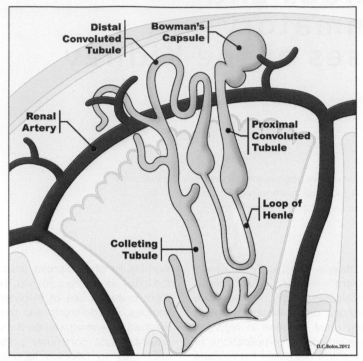

Fig. 1. Anatomy of the nephron. (*Courtesy of* DC Botos, 2012.)

nonspecific symptoms. Renal involvement can be indolent for more than 20 years. When symptoms occur, GU-related symptoms, including frequency, dysuria, microhematuria or macrohematuria, and/or back or flank pain, are usually seen. Constitutional symptoms such as weight loss, fever, and fatigue can also be present. Diagnosis of GU tuberculosis is usually established by positive urine culture results or on histologic examination of biopsy or surgical specimens.[4,5] Clinically significant renal tuberculosis is unilateral but can occur bilaterally in up to 30% of cases.[6] Imaging findings can support the diagnosis of GU tuberculosis, and, therefore, the radiologist should be aware of characteristic findings.

Imaging of GU tuberculosis depends on the stage of disease. Granuloma formation, caseous necrosis, and cavitation are stages of progressive infection and can eventually destroy the kidney.[5] The initial inoculation and granuloma formation are not radiographically evident. Early in reactivation, localized soft tissue edema and vasoconstriction secondary to acute inflammation result in focal hypoperfusion on contrast-enhanced computed tomography (CT), creating a striated nephrogram (Fig. 2). A moth-eaten calyx secondary to papillary necrosis is another finding that is seen as an early radiographic abnormality and can be best demonstrated on excretory urography but

can also be seen on contrast-enhanced CT (Fig. 3). As the parenchymal granulomas coalesce, CT demonstrates a masslike lesion (tuberculoma) with central low attenuation representing caseous necrosis (Fig. 4).[6] These cavitary lesions eventually rupture into the draining calyx, spreading the infection into the renal pelvis and further distally.

As the disease progresses, the host launches a fibrotic reaction in response to infection, causing stenosis and stricture formation of the calyceal infundibula, which leads to uneven caliectasis

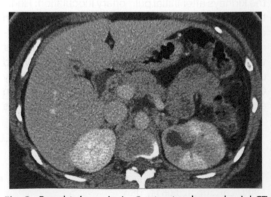

Fig. 2. Renal tuberculosis. Contrast-enhanced axial CT shows wedge-shaped areas of hypoenhancement involving the left kidney. There is focal dilatation of a calyx as can be seen in renal tuberculosis.

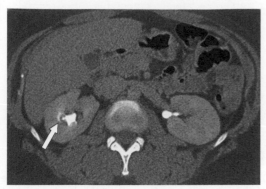

Fig. 3. Papillary necrosis. Contrast-enhanced axial CT obtained in the excretory phase shows a collection of contrast beyond the interpapillary line (*arrow*) adjacent to a midpole calyx of the right kidney.

and eventually incomplete opacification of the calyx (phantom calyx) (**Fig. 5**).[2] As the host response ensues, calcium deposition and progressive stricture formation can result in obstruction and progressive renal failure. Long-standing tuberculosis results in renal parenchymal atrophy; progressive hydronephrosis; and, eventually, autonephrectomy. CT demonstrates multiple thin-walled cysts or a multiloculated cyst along with the absence of normal enhancing renal parenchyma. The putty kidney ensues from dystrophic calcifications involving the entire kidney and is the final product of end-stage renal tuberculosis (**Fig. 6**).[7]

Ureteral involvement occurs with the passage of infected urine into the renal calyces/pelvis after rupture of the granuloma. Initially, mucosal irregularity is present, creating a "sawtooth" ureter appearance. Ureteral dilatation may be present.[6]

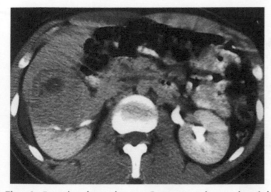

Fig. 4. Renal tuberculoma. Contrast-enhanced axial CT shows a masslike area of decreased attenuation in the right kidney. The rounded central area of low attenuation is consistent with an area of caseous necrosis.

As the disease progresses, stricturing and ureteral shortening occur. Multiple strictures can eventually form a long segment of narrowing. A "corkscrew" ureter forms because of multiple non-confluent strictures. Calcification can form along the course of the ureter. These findings can be seen with CT, excretory urography, or plain radiography, but CT can also demonstrate periureteral fibrosis and ureteral wall thickening (**Fig. 7**).[7] With tuberculous involvement of the urinary bladder, reduced bladder capacity is the most common finding.[8] Bladder wall thickening and calcification can be present.

XGP

XGP is a rare chronic destructive granulomatous disease of the kidneys that results from an atypical incomplete immune response to subacute bacterial infection. XGP occurs in a collecting system with long-standing partial obstruction. Classically, staghorn calculi are the cause of obstruction, but in 20% of cases no calculi are seen,[9] with obstruction occurring secondary to stricture or, rarely, uroepithelial tumor. The subacute infection is typically because of *Proteus mirabilis*, *Escherichia coli*, *Klebsiella*, or *Pseudomonas* species. The incomplete immune response results in deposition of lipid-laden macrophages (xanthoma cells) at the site of infection, causing irreversible destruction of the renal parenchyma. Clinically, XGP is seen in middle-aged women during their fifth to sixth decade of life. Patients with diabetes are predisposed to XGP. Symptoms include fever, flank pain, persistent bacteriuria, or history of recurrent infected nephrolithiasis.[10]

Two forms of XGP have been described. The diffuse or global form (85%) is more common than the localized or focal form (15%).[11] CT is considered the mainstay of imaging; it accurately assesses the extent of extrarenal disease, if present, and aids in surgical planning.

In the diffuse form of XGP, CT shows renal enlargement; calcifications filling the renal pelvis, often in a staghorn configuration; and replacement of the renal parenchyma by multiple oval hypodense areas representing dilated calyces and abscess cavities filled with pus and debris (**Fig. 8**).[12] The walls of these cavities may enhance after contrast administration, because of the marked vascularity of the underlying granulation tissue and compressed normal parenchyma. Cortical thinning and decrease or absence of contrast excretion can be seen in the involved kidney. Areas of fat attenuation can be present because of lipid-rich xanthomatous tissue (**Fig. 9**). In addition, less common findings may

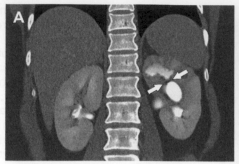
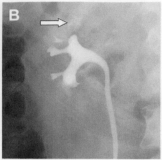

Fig. 5. Phantom calyx secondary to renal tuberculosis. (A) Contrast-enhanced axial CT shows dilatation of the upper pole calyx in the left kidney. There is narrowing of the infundibulum (arrows) at this level consistent with the CT equivalent of phantom calyx. (B) Five-minute excretory phase image from an excretory urogram in a different patient shows nonvisualization of the upper pole calyx of the right kidney. Faint calcifications (arrow) in the expected location of the calyx were present on scout images, consistent with dystrophic calcifications secondary to renal tuberculosis.

include massive pelvic dilatation, absence of stones, and renal atrophy with or without accumulation of perinephric fat.[12] It is difficult to distinguish the focal form of XGP from a renal tumor such as renal cell carcinoma, and this form of XGP is sometimes referred to as tumefactive or pseudotumoral.[11]

With diffuse disease, ultrasonography can demonstrate diffuse renal enlargement. Multiple hypoechoic masses can be present and may represent abscesses (posterior acoustic enhancement) or solid granulomatous processes (posterior acoustic shadowing).[13] Focal XGP may also mimic a masslike lesion sonographically.

Abscess formation outside the kidney secondary to the diffuse form of XGP is a common complication of the disease, but these abscesses usually appear as perinephric abscesses (Fig. 10).

The inflammatory process, however, may be widespread, sometimes extending throughout the retroperitoneum. Psoas abscesses are rare but may occur (Fig. 11).[14] In a series of 16 patients with XGP, psoas abscesses were seen in 6 patients (38%).[15] Additional complications of XGP include fistulae, with renocolic and renocutaneous fistulae described in the literature.[16]

RENAL MALAKOPLAKIA

Renal malakoplakia is a rare chronic inflammatory process usually associated with E coli infection that involves the urinary tract collecting system (most commonly the urinary bladder). Rarely, isolated renal involvement can be present. Malakoplakia is most commonly seen in middle-aged women with chronic urinary tract infections or in

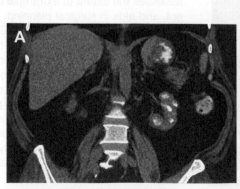
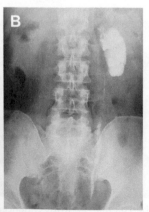

Fig. 6. End-stage renal tuberculosis. (A) Nonenhanced coronal CT shows calcifications replacing most of the atrophic left kidney. (B) Scout radiograph from an excretory urogram demonstrates replacement of the left kidney with dystrophic calcification creating a putty kidney. Note also calcification along the course of the left ureter consistent with tuberculous involvement of the ureter.

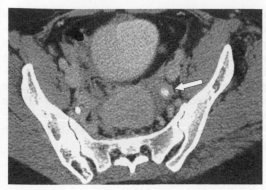

Fig. 7. Ureteritis secondary to tuberculosis. Contrast-enhanced axial CT shows marked thickening of the wall of the left ureter (*arrow*) in this patient with a known history of renal tuberculosis.

those who are immunocompromised.[10] Patients present with symptoms of urinary tract infection. The pathogenesis of malakoplakia is due to an altered host response to infection. Abnormal macrophage function prevents complete digestion of phagocytosed bacteria. These partially digested bacteria persist and form intracellular inclusion bodies or Michaelis-Gutmann bodies. The process results in the formation of tumorlike lesions in the involved portions of the GU

tract. Renal parenchymal malakoplakia is usually multifocal, resulting in a diffusely enlarged kidney and can be seen as a single lesion in less than 25% of cases. The process is unilateral, involving one kidney, but can be bilateral.[17]

Radiographically, malakoplakia can present as an enlarged kidney, a low-attenuation mass, or a diffuse infiltrative disease.[18] Sonographically, renal malakoplakia can most commonly demonstrate a diffusely enlarged kidney, poorly defined hypoechoic masses, and distortion of the renal architecture.[19] When the renal malakoplakia is multifocal, CT shows multiple hypoenhancing masses that can range in size and eventually coalesce to form larger masses. When a single lesion is present, it is difficult to distinguish renal malakoplakia from renal cell carcinoma. Although clinical features and radiographic findings are suggestive of renal malakoplakia, biopsy or surgery is required to make the diagnosis.

RENAL ASPERGILLOSIS

Renal aspergillosis is a rare entity that is seen in immunocompromised patients, including diabetic patients, human immunodeficiency virus–positive individuals, and patients on corticosteroid therapy.[20] Renal aspergillosis can be acquired via

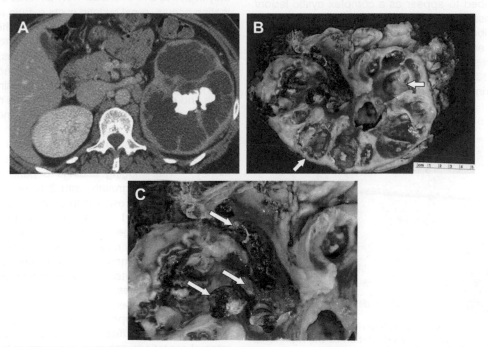

Fig. 8. XGP. (*A*) Contrast-enhanced coronal CT shows a large staghorn calculus in enlarged, poorly functioning left kidney. There is dilatation of the collecting system. (*B*) Gross specimen of XGP shows the dilated collecting system with multiple pus-filled cavities consistent with abscesses present (*arrows*). (*C*) Magnified view of the gross specimen shows the large staghorn calculus (*arrows*).

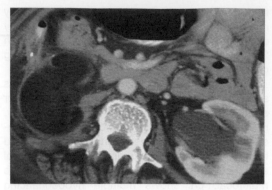

Fig. 9. XGP. Contrast-enhanced axial CT shows enlargement of the right kidney and absence of enhancement of the thinned renal cortex. Replacement of the normal renal parenchyma with fat attenuation is secondary to the presence of lipid-rich xanthomatous tissue.

3 ways, including hematogenous dissemination, from an ascending infection originating from the lower urinary tract, or secondary to an aspergillus cast in the renal pelvis.[21] Hematogenous dissemination to the kidney is the most common form of renal infection. Primary renal infection is exceedingly rare. There are relatively few reports of radiographic appearance of renal aspergillus infection in the literature. Renal aspergillosis has been described to appear as a complex cystic lesion/abscess (Fig. 12).[21] Heussel and colleagues[22] described multiple cystic lesions along with delayed enhancement of the renal parenchyma and features of accompanying local pyelonephritis (Fig. 13). Diagnosis of renal aspergillosis is made by urinalysis and aspiration of the lesion for

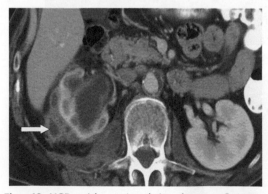

Fig. 10. XGP with perinephric abscess. Contrast-enhanced axial CT shows dilatation of the right renal collecting system with marked cortical thinning consistent with XGP. A small perinephric abscess is present along the posterolateral margin of the kidney (arrow).

microscopy and culture. Traditionally, treatment options have included antifungal therapy, nephrectomy if the disease is unilateral, and local irrigation with amphotericin B if bilateral.[23] There is a recent trend for increased use of more aggressive medical therapy, including highly active retroviral therapy and newer antifungal agents such as voriconazole in bilateral disease; concomitant percutaneous drainage has been beneficial in patients with unilateral disease.[24]

RENAL ECHINOCOCCUS

Echinococcosis is a zoonosis caused by the larvae of echinococcus tapeworms (Echinococcus granulosus). Two hosts are seen in the life cycle of E granulosus: a definitive host, usually a dog and an intermediate host, typically a sheep. The adult worms live in the proximal small bowel of the definitive host and release eggs into the host's feces. Humans can become the intermediate host through contact with the definitive host or ingestion of contaminated water or food.[25] After human contact, the liver is the first line of defense and therefore the most commonly involved organ in hydatid disease (75%); lungs are the second (15%). However, hematogenous dissemination can occur to almost any anatomic location.[26] Renal echinococcosis is extremely rare and seen only in 2% to 3% of cases.[26] When renal dissemination occurs, renal hydatid cysts remain asymptomatic for many years during which time the cysts can become quite large.[27] When symptomatic, patients usually present with flank mass, pain, and dysuria. Large cysts can rupture, leading to a strong antigenic immune response causing urticaria and even anaphylaxis.[28] When cysts rupture into the collecting system, hydatiduria and renal colic can occur.

Renal hydatid cysts are usually unilateral solitary lesions found in the upper or lower poles of the kidney.[27] The imaging findings depend on the stage of the cyst growth, with 3 types of cysts described that correspond to their imaging findings.[26,29,30] Type 1 cysts represent the initial developmental stage of the parasite and appear as unilocular cystic masses. Type 2 cysts correspond to the intermediate stage of development with multiple daughter cysts and appear as multilocular cystic masses. Type 3 cysts are completely calcified and represent quiescent disease or death of the parasite. In type 1 and type 2 cysts, the wall may be thick or calcified. The noncalcified wall and internal septations enhance after contrast administration (Fig. 14).[29]

Surgery consisting of total or partial nephrectomy is usually the treatment of choice for renal

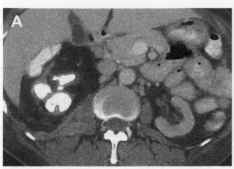
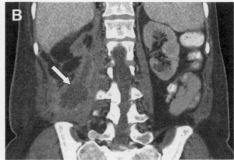

Fig. 11. XGP with psoas abscess. (*A*) Contrast-enhanced axial CT shows characteristic findings of XGP with a large staghorn calculus, thinned cortex, and absence of renal parenchymal enhancement. (*B*) Contrast-enhanced coronal CT in the same patient shows development of a rim-enhancing fluid collection along the right psoas muscle (*arrow*) consistent with a psoas abscess.

hydatid cysts. Medical therapy with antiparasitic agents has been unsuccessful.[10]

UPPER TRACT FUNGAL INFECTION

Upper tract fungal infections are uncommon in healthy individuals and are usually seen in patients with immunosuppression, diabetes mellitus, urinary tract obstruction and in those on prolonged antibiotic or steroid therapy.[1] Fungal infection is usually caused by *Candida albicans* and acquired through hematogenous dissemination

or an ascending urinary tract infection. With hematogenous dissemination, fungi are filtered by the glomerulus and become lodged in the distal tubules. The fungi proliferate and produce multiple medullary and cortical abscesses.[31] Upper tract fungal infection commonly presents as acute pyelonephritis, and patients may eventually develop multiple renal abscesses. Contrast-enhanced CT shows a striated nephrogram as seen with acute pyelonephritis. Multiple abscesses are seen on contrast-enhanced CT as multiple, small, hypodense collections.[32] Fungus

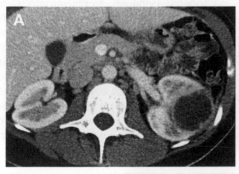
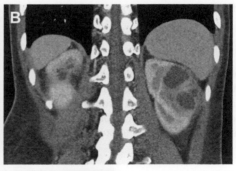
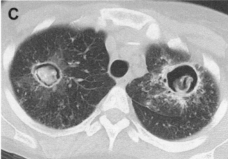

Fig. 12. Renal aspergillosis. Contrast-enhanced axial (*A*) and coronal (*B*) CT demonstrates a complex cystic mass with a thick enhancing wall and a few internal septations (best seen on the coronal image). (*C*) Contrast-enhanced axial CT shows findings consistent with pulmonary involvement of aspergillosis with mycetomas seen in both upper lobes.

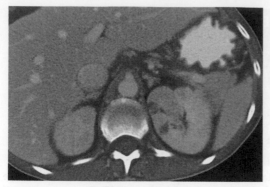

Fig. 13. Renal aspergillosis. Contrast-enhanced axial CT shows striated nephrograms involving both kidneys and small cystic foci in the left kidney representing small abscesses.

balls or mycetomas may also form and represent collections of inflammatory cells, fungus, necrotic or mucoid debris, and calculous matrix.[33] On excretory urograms or retrograde pyelograms, fungus balls appear as radiolucent filling defects in the collecting system.[34] Sonographically, fungus balls appear as echogenic masses in the renal collecting system that do not demonstrate acoustic shadowing and can mimic blood clots or pyogenic debris (**Fig. 15**).[35] On contrast-enhanced CT, a fungus ball appears as a nonspecific irregularly marginated mass of soft tissue attenuation in the collecting system.[1]

PYONEPHROSIS

Pyonephrosis is a suppurative infection that occurs in the setting of a hydronephrotic obstructed kidney and is considered a urologic emergency requiring urgent drainage. Decompression of the dilated system is necessary to prevent loss of renal function and life-threatening gram-negative bacteremia.[36] Patients present with the classic triad of fever, chills, and flank pain. Bacteriuria may not be present because of the presence of obstruction.[10] Ultrasonography demonstrates echogenic debris along the dependent portions of a dilated collecting system (**Fig. 16**).[10] If air is present in the collecting system, echogenic foci with dirty shadowing may be present.[13] Although CT is helpful in identifying hydronephrosis and underlying causes, pyonephrosis can often be indistinguishable from noninfected hydronephrosis.[31] In addition to hydronephrosis, other findings present on CT include a striated nephrogram, urothelial thickening of the renal pelvis and ureter, renal enlargement, fluid-fluid levels in the dilated collecting system, and gas in the collecting system.[1]

EMPHYSEMATOUS PYELONEPHRITIS

Emphysematous pyelonephritis is a fulminant gas-forming infection resulting in necrosis of the renal parenchyma. Patients present with symptoms of severe acute pyelonephritis, urosepsis, or shock and, almost always, diabetes (usually poorly controlled). Emphysematous pyelonephritis is seen more commonly in women than men and usually affects only one kidney. *E coli*, *Klebsiella pneumonia*, and *P mirabilis* are the most common pathogens. Because emphysematous pyelonephritis is associated with high morbidity and mortality, prompt diagnosis and treatment are necessary. Classic management includes emergent nephrectomy and the administration of broad-spectrum antibiotics. However, there has recently been a shift toward a nephron-sparing approach, including percutaneous drainage and antibiotic therapy with or without elective nephrectomy at a later stage.[37] It is important to distinguish

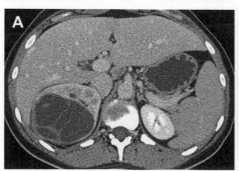
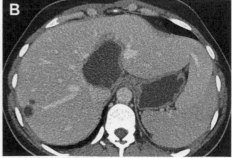

Fig. 14. Renal echinococcus. (*A*) Contrast-enhanced axial CT shows a complex cystic mass in the right kidney with thick enhancing wall and enhancing internal septations. (*B*) Contrast-enhanced axial CT in the same patient shows a dominant cystic mass with a thick enhancing wall in the left lobe of the liver. Additional areas of echinococcal infection are seen in the posterior aspect of the right hepatic lobe.

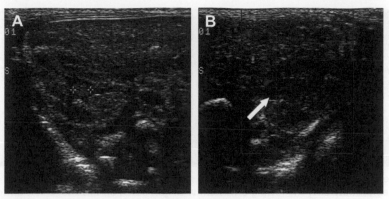

Fig. 15. Upper tract fungal infection. (*A*) Transverse sonogram of the right kidney in a newborn shows an echogenic nodule (*calipers*) in the mildly dilated collecting system consistent with a fungus ball. (*B*) Transverse sonogram of the left kidney in the same patient shows a similar-appearing echogenic nodule (*arrow*). Color Doppler confirmed the absence of flow within this nodule.

emphysematous pyelonephritis from emphysematous pyelitis because the latter has a better prognosis and can be treated with antibiotics alone.[38]

Radiographically, the presence of air in the renal parenchyma should raise suspicion of emphysematous pyelonephritis. On plain radiographs, this appears as a mottled gas collection overlying the expected location of the kidney. Ultrasonography shows an enlarged kidney with parenchymal high-amplitude echoes and posterior acoustic dirty shadowing, but may underestimate the extent of parenchymal involvement.[10] CT is considered the modality of choice in diagnosing emphysematous pyelonephritis because it accurately detects the presence of gas and assesses the extent of gas within renal parenchyma (**Fig. 17**).[1] CT also plays an important role in evaluating the effectiveness of therapy.[10]

As stated earlier, it is crucial to distinguish emphysematous pyelonephritis from emphysematous pyelitis because of prognostic and marked treatment differences. Emphysematous pyelitis demonstrates gas limited to the renal collecting system, ureter, or bladder.[1]

ACUTE PYELONEPHRITIS

Although acute pyelonephritis is not an uncommon renal infection, a brief discussion of its imaging findings, atypical presentations, and complications is warranted in this article. The diagnosis of acute pyelonephritis can be made on clinical and laboratory findings.[34] Radiologic evaluation is not necessary in uncomplicated cases but can play a role in certain scenarios: assist in diagnosis when there is a lack of response to appropriate therapy, assess patients at risk for more severe life-threatening complications, and evaluate patients for the presence of complications.

In cases of uncomplicated acute pyelonephritis, renal ultrasonography may appear normal or may demonstrate a hypoechoic region that shows

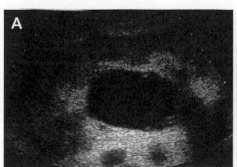
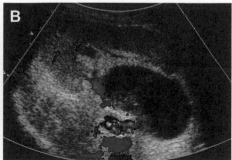

Fig. 16. Pyonephrosis. (*A*) Sagittal sonogram of the kidney shows a dilated renal pelvis with amorphous echogenic debris. (*B*) Sagittal sonogram of the kidney in the same patient shows absence of Doppler flow in the echogenic material of the dilated renal pelvis.

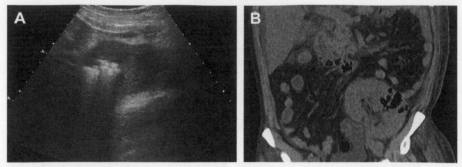

Fig. 17. Emphysematous pyelonephritis. (*A*) Transverse sonogram of a renal transplant shows multiple hypere-choic foci that demonstrate dirty shadowing consistent with gas. Based on this image, it is difficult to determine the exact location and extent of air. (*B*) Nonenhanced coronal CT confirms the presence of gas in the renal trans-plant and its involvement of the renal parenchyma.

decreased flow on power Doppler, renal enlarge-ment, and/or loss of renal sinus fat and/or cortico-medullary differentiation (Fig. 18). The classic CT finding on contrast-enhanced studies is the so-called striated nephrogram that appears as a wedge-shaped area of hypoattenuation (or hypoenhancement) extending from the papilla to the medulla (Fig. 19). Additional CT findings include focal or global renal enlargement, thick-ening of Gerota fascia, perinephric stranding, urothelial thickening of the renal pelvis and ca-lyces, calyceal effacement, and poor excretion of contrast material.[31] Hemorrhagic bacterial ne-phritis is an uncommon manifestation of py-elonephritis that demonstrates a wedge-shaped area of hyperattenuation on noncontrast CT (Fig. 20).[34] The areas of high attenuation reflect in-traparenchymal bleeding.

Acute pyelonephritis can also present as focal pyelonephritis or lobar nephronia with a masslike appearance mimicking a neoplasm such as renal cell carcinoma. Contrast-enhanced CT in these instances demonstrates an ill-defined hypoattenu-ating mass (Fig. 21). Focal pyelonephritis tends to be relatively less hypodense and have less well-defined borders than a renal abscess. Clinical history is essential in suggesting the diagnosis of focal pyelonephritis, and follow-up imaging after appropriate therapy may be necessary to exclude a renal mass.

In cases of untreated or inadequately treated pyelonephritis, tissue necrosis and liquefaction can occur and result in abscess formation.[39] Im-munocompromised patients and diabetic patients are at increased risk for abscess formation. Ultra-sonography is less sensitive than CT in evaluating for the presence of an abscess but demonstrates a hypoechoic or anechoic complex cystic mass with posterior acoustic enhancement. Internal echoes, septations, and loculations may also be evident with ultrasonography.[36] Contrast-enhanced CT demonstrates a well-defined low-attenuation mass with an irregular thick enhancing wall (Fig. 22). Gas within the collection may or may not be present; when present, it is readily identifi-able on CT. The adjacent renal parenchyma may be hypoenhanced on early phases and may retain contrast on delayed images.[1]

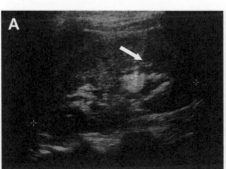
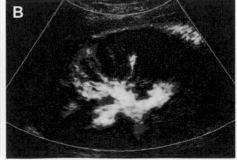

Fig. 18. Acute pyelonephritis. (*A*) Sagittal sonogram of the right kidney shows an area of decreased echogenicity involving the lower pole (*arrow*). (*B*) Sagittal power Doppler sonogram shows absence of flow to the involved portion in the lower pole of the kidney.

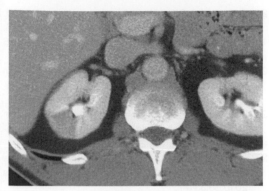

Fig. 19. Acute pyelonephritis. Contrast-enhanced axial CT shows a wedged-shape area of decreased enhancement consistent with a striated nephrogram.

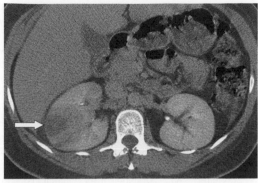

Fig. 22. Renal abscess. Contrast-enhanced axial CT shows wedge-shaped areas of decreased enhancement consistent with a striated nephrogram. A more focal rounded area of decreased attenuation (arrow) is consistent with the development of a renal abscess.

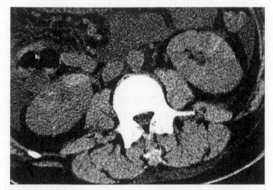

Fig. 20. Hemorrhagic pyelonephritis. Nonenhanced axial CT shows areas of increased attenuation in both kidneys in this patient with clinically diagnosed pyelonephritis.

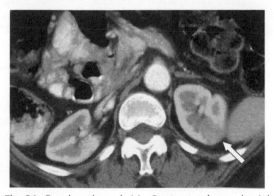

Fig. 21. Focal pyelonephritis. Contrast-enhanced axial CT shows an ill-defined masslike area of decreased enhancement involving the left kidney (arrow). The patient was clinically suspected to have pyelonephritis. Follow-up imaging after antibiotic therapy showed resolution of this finding.

SUMMARY

Although radiographic evaluation is not necessary in patients with suspected pyelonephritis, it plays a role in patients who do not respond to conventional therapy and in high-risk patients. Acute pyelonephritis is the most common renal infection but a variety of other infectious and inflammatory processes can be seen. Because many of these processes require urgent or surgical management, it is imperative that the radiologist be familiar with their imaging findings.

REFERENCES

1. Kawashima A, Sandler CM, Goldman SM, et al. CT of renal inflammatory disease. Radiographics 1997;17:851–66.
2. Engin G, Acunas B, Acunas G, et al. Imaging of extrapulmonary tuberculosis. Radiographics 2000;20: 471–88.
3. Kim SH. Genitourinary tuberculosis. In: Pollack HM, Dyer R, McClennan BL, editors. Clinical urography. 2nd edition. Philadelphia: Saunders; 2000. p. 1193–228.
4. Wang LJ, Wong YC, Chen CJ, et al. CT features of genitourinary tuberculosis. J Comput Assist Tomogr 1997;21:254–8.
5. Gibson MS, Puckett ML, Shelly ME. Renal tuberculosis. Radiographics 2004;24:254–8.
6. Matos MJ, Bacelar MT, Pinto P, et al. Genitourinary tuberculosis. Eur J Radiol 2005;55:181–7.
7. Yoon YJ, Kim JK, Cho KS. Genitourinary tuberculosis: comprehensive cross-sectional imaging. AJR Am J Roentgenol 2005;184:143–50.
8. Harisinghani MG, McLoud TC, Shepard J, et al. Tuberculosis from head to toe. Radiographics 2000;20:449–79.

9. Rabushka LS, Fishman EK, Goldman SM. Pictorial review of renal inflammatory disease. Urology 1994;44:473–80.

10. Vourganti S, Agarwal PK, Bodner DR, et al. Ultrasonographic evaluation of renal infections. Ultrasound Clin 2010;5:355–66.

11. Kim JC. US and CT findings of xanthogranulomatous pyelonephritis. Clin Imaging 2001;25:118–21.

12. Loffroy R, Guiu B, Watfa J, et al. Xanthogranulomatous pyelonephritis in adults: clinical and radiological findings in diffuse and focal forms. Clin Radiol 2007;62(9):884–90.

13. Schaeffer AJ. Urinary tract infections. In: Gillenwater JY, Grayhack JT, Howards SS, et al, editors. Adult and pediatric urology. 4th edition. Philadelphia: Lippincott Williams & Wilkins; 2002. p. 289–351.

14. Alan C, Ataus S, Tunc B. Xanthogranulamatous pyelonephritis with psoas abscess: 2 cases and review of the literature. Int Urol Nephrol 2004;36(4):489–93.

15. Goldman SM, Hartman DS, Fishman EK, et al. CT of xanthogranulomatous pyelonephritis: radiologic-pathologic correlation. AJR Am J Roentgenol 1984; 142(5):963–9.

16. Harisha RA, Nath SK, Thomas JA. Xanthogranulomatous pyelonephritis with reno-colonic and cutaneous fistulae. Br J Urol 1987;60(3):273–4.

17. Pickhardt PJ, Lonergran GJ, Davis CJ, et al. From the archives of the AFIP. Infiltrative renal lesions: radiologic-pathologic correlation. Armed Forces Institute of Pathology. Radiographics 2000;20:215–43.

18. Bhatt S, MacLennan G, Dogra V. Renal pseudotumors. AJR Am J Roentgenol 2007;188:1380–7.

19. Venkatesh SK, Mehrotra N, Gujral RB. Sonographic findings in renal parenchymal malacoplakia. J Clin Ultrasound 2000;28(7):353–7.

20. Haq J, Khan MA, Afroze N, et al. Localized primary renal aspergillosis in a diabetic patient following lithotripsy—a case report. BMC Infect Dis 2007;7:58.

21. Gupta KL. Fungal infections and the kidney. Indian J Nephrol 2001;11:147–54.

22. Heussel CP, Kauczor HU, Heussel G, et al. Multiple renal aspergillus abscesses in an AIDS patient: contrast-enhanced helical CT and MRI findings. Eur Radiol 1999;9(4):616–9.

23. Denning DW. Invasive aspergillosis. Clin Infect Dis 1998;26:781–805.

24. Oosten AW, Sprenger HG, van Leeuwen JT, et al. Bilateral renal aspergillosis in a patient with AIDS: a case report and review of reported cases. AIDS Patient Care STDS 2008;22(1):1–6.

25. Volders WK, Geert G, Stessens R. Best cases from AFIP. Hydatid cyst of the kidney: radiologic-pathologic correlation. Radiographics 2001;21:S255–60.

26. Pedrosa I, Saiz A, Arrazola L, et al. Hydatid disease: radiologic and pathologic features and complications. Radiographics 2000;20:795–817.

27. Ishimitsu DN, Saouaf R, Kallman C, et al. Best cases from the AFIP: renal hydatid disease. Radiographics 2010;30:334–7.

28. Zmerli S, Ayed M, Horchani A, et al. Hydatid cyst of the kidney: diagnosis and treatment. World J Surg 2001;25(1):68–74.

29. Polat P, Kantarci M, Alper F, et al. Hydatid disease from head to toe. Radiographics 2003;23(2): 475–94.

30. Turgut AT, Odev K, Kabaalioglu A, et al. Multitechnique evaluation of renal hydatid disease. AJR Am J Roentgenol 2009;192(2):462–7.

31. Stunnell H, Buckely O, Feeney J, et al. Imaging of acute pyelonephritis in the adult. Eur Radiol 2007; 17:1820–8.

32. Shirkohoda A. CT findings in hepatosplenic and renal candidiasis. J Comput Assist Tomogr 1987; 11:795–8.

33. Doemeny JM, Banner MP, Shapiro MJ, et al. Percutaneous extraction of renal fungus ball. AJR Am J Roentgenol 1988;150:1331–2.

34. Kawashima A, LeRoy AJ. Radiologic evaluation of patients with renal infections. Infect Dis Clin North Am 2003;17:433–56.

35. Stuck KJ, Silver TM, Jaffe MH, et al. Sonographic demonstration of renal fungus balls. Radiology 1981;142:473–4.

36. Brown RF, Zwirewich C, Torreggiani WC. Imaging of urinary tract infection in the adult. Eur Radiol 2004; 14:E169–83.

37. Ubee SS, McGlynn L, Fordham M. Emphysematous pyelonephritis. BJU Int 2010;107:1474–8.

38. Roy C, Pfleger D, Tuchmann CM, et al. Emphysematous pyelitis: findings in five patients. Radiographics 2001;218:647–50.

39. Papanicolaou N, Pfister RC. Acute renal infections. Radiol Clin North Am 1996;24:545–69.

Multimodality Imaging of Ureteric Disease

Puneet Bhargava, MD[a], Manjiri K. Dighe, MD[b],*,
Jean Hwa Lee, MD[b], Carolyn Wang, MD[b]

KEYWORDS

- Ureter • Imaging • Transitional cell carcinoma • Calculi
- Urography

The ureter is an extraperitoneal structure surrounded by fat. The ureter is divided into 3 portions: the proximal ureter (upper) extends from the ureteropelvic junction (UPJ) to where the ureter crosses the sacroiliac joint, the middle ureter courses over the bony pelvis and iliac vessels, and the distal or pelvic ureter (lower) extends from the iliac vessels to the bladder. The ureter can be imaged by a variety of modalities including CT; MR imaging; direct pyelography (DP), both antegrade pyelography (AP) and retrograde pyelography (RP); nuclear medicine diuretic scan; and voiding cystourethrography (VCUG). A wide variety of benign and malignant lesions occur in the ureter. This article provides an overview of the imaging techniques and pathology affecting the ureter.

EMBRYOLOGY AND ANATOMY

The ureter is 22 to 30 cm in length and is divided into 3 portions: the proximal ureter (upper) is the segment that extends from the UPJ to the area where the ureter crosses the sacroiliac joint, the middle ureter courses over the bony pelvis and iliac vessels, and the distal or pelvic ureter (lower) extends from the iliac vessels to the bladder. The terminal portion of the ureter may be subdivided further into the juxtavesical, intramural, and submucosal portions. The ureter's blood supply comes from the ureteral artery, which runs longitudinally along the ureter and lacks collateral flow in 80% of patients. The upper third of the ureteral artery is supplied by the aorta and renal artery, whereas branches of the iliac, lumbar, and vesicular arteries supply the middle and lower thirds of the ureter. In the abdomen, the blood supply is medial, whereas in the pelvis the blood supply is lateral, with the richest blood supply to the pelvic ureter.[1] The ureter consists of 3 distinct histologic layers. The first is an inner mucosal layer of transitional epithelium covered by lamina propria. The inner layer produces mucosal secretions to protect itself from urine. The second, or middle, layer is muscular and consists of both longitudinal and circular layers of smooth muscle, which help propel urine forward by peristalsis. The outer (adventitial) layer consists of areolar connective tissue and contains nerves, blood vessels, and lymphatic vessels. Lymphatic drainage from the ureter is through regional lymph nodes including the common iliac, external iliac, and hypogastric lymph nodes.[1] The ureter is a dynamic organ and not a simple conduit through which urine flows. It conducts urine from the renal papillae to the ureteral orifices in the bladder irrespective of the spatial orientation of the body. However, when the urinary transport system is disturbed, gravity may influence directional flow.[2] There are 3 major functions that are attributed to the renal pelvis and ureters: absorption; dynamics, which reflects the synchronous and progressive contractile

[a] Department of Radiology, VA Puget Sound Health Care System, University of Washington, Mail Box 358280, S-114/Radiology, 1660 South Columbian Way, Seattle, WA 98108-1597, USA
[b] Department of Radiology, University of Washington Medical Center, Box 357115, 1959 Northeast Pacific Street, Seattle, WA 98195-7117, USA
* Corresponding author.
E-mail address: dighe@u.washington.edu

Radiol Clin N Am 50 (2012) 271–299
doi:10.1016/j.rcl.2012.02.008
0033-8389/12/$ – see front matter Published by Elsevier Inc.

movement of the ureter away from the UPJ to the ureter-vesical orifice, produced by the intrinsic automaticity of the ureteral musculature; and tonus, which is the degree of contraction that the ureteral wall assumes for a given rate and volume of urinary output.[2]

IMAGING TECHNIQUES

Traditionally, IV urography (IVU) and RP have been used to detect and diagnose the ureteral lesions. Historically, excretory urogram (IVU) was the study of choice to evaluate all levels of the urinary tract in a single examination; however, because of rapid advances in multidetector CT technology, this has been largely replaced by CT urography as the preferred modality for evaluating the urinary tract.[3]

CT is widely available and now, with the multi-phase scanning including noncontrast, nephrographic, and pyelographic phases, CT urography allows evaluation for complications such as renal stone burden, hydronephrosis, emphysematous pyelonephritis, renal or perirenal abscesses, or other nonurologic causes of flank pain. Noncontrast CT is useful in diagnosis of ureteric calculi. Specificity and sensitivity of noncontrast CT for the detection of hydronephrosis and urolithiasis is 100%.[4] CT is already widely acknowledged to be superior to US in its ability to detect and characterize renal masses. The goal of CT urography is to obtain images of fully opacified and distended collecting systems, ureters, and bladder with the fewest scans (Fig. 1). CT urography is divided into 2 major groups: (1) hybrid CT urography–excretory urography in which CT images are combined with conventional radiographs obtained before and/or after axial image acquisition; and (2) pure CT urography, in which imaging is performed entirely with CT scanning equipment. With the advent of multislice CT scanners, pure CT

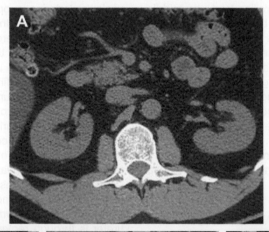

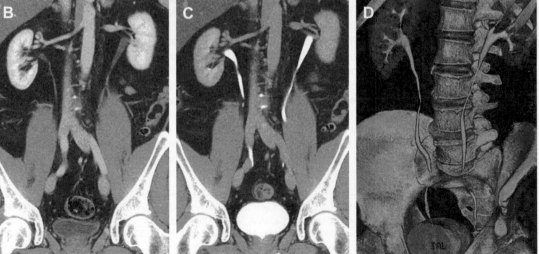

Fig. 1. Normal CT urography. Axial precontrast (A), coronal reformat from a nephrographic phase (B), and coronal reformat from a delayed phase (C) from a CT urography depicting normal bilateral ureters. (D) three-dimensional (3D) reformat showing bilateral ureters in their entirety.

urography has replaced hybrid CT urography. Two techniques are commonly performed for CT urography: the 3-phase technique and the split-bolus technique. With the 3-phase technique, 3 scans are obtained during the CT urography: an unenhanced scan, enhanced or nephrographic scan, and an excretory scan. An unenhanced CT scan is obtained to detect calculi, reveal the unenhanced appearance of masses (throughout the urinary tract), and provide a baseline attenuation value to calculate enhancement of masses and other abnormalities. Enhanced images (by using IV contrast material that contains 30–42 g of iodine) are obtained for detecting virtually all urologic abnormalities (except stones and calcifications) and are used to detect the presence of enhancement in a mass. Excretory phase images are obtained to evaluate the urothelium. Instead of obtaining 2 separate scans (nephrographic and excretory phase) after IV contrast material administration, a split-bolus technique has been described to reduce the total number of scans from 3 to 2 and, therefore, decrease radiation exposure.[5,6] With this technique, after the unenhanced CT scan, a fractionated dose of contrast material (30–50 mL, 300 mg of iodine per milliliter) is administered followed by a delay of 8 to 10 minutes before the remaining (80–100 mL) contrast material is given. A subsequent scan, obtained 100 seconds after the second dose of contrast material, contains excretory information from the first dose and nephrographic information from the second dose. Several additional maneuvers can be used when performing CT urography in an attempt to improve the renal collecting system and ureteral distention and opacification, and thereby possibly improve the sensitivity of the study in detecting urinary tract abnormalities. These maneuvers include compression bands, saline hydration, and administration of furosemide.

MR urography (Fig. 2) can be used to evaluate the urinary tract in a single imaging study as in CT urography but without radiation exposure and IV contrast administration.[7] MR urography has better contrast resolution than CT urography without exposure to ionizing radiation and does not require IV contrast administration, making it more suitable for examination of pediatric and pregnant patients.[8] Although originally thought safe, the association of gadolinium agents with nephrogenic systemic fibrosis (NSF) has limited the use of contrast-enhanced MR imaging in patients with renal impairment. Gadolinium should not be used in patients with poor renal function (glomerular filtration rate <30 mL, independent of age, race, gender, or acute kidney injury)[9] because of the risk of NSF.

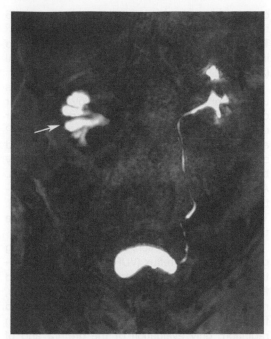

Fig. 2. MR urography. Thick-slab coronal maximum intensity projection (MIP) reformat from the excretory phase of MR urography shows normal excretion of contrast from the left kidney. The pelvicalyceal system on the right is dilated (*arrow*) and the ureter is not visualized.

Because of the capability of MR imaging to obtain multiple acquisitions, time intensity curves as a means of assessing renal function or characterizing abnormalities after IV contrast material administration may be generated. T2-weighted techniques, such as rapid acquisition with relaxation enhancement (RARE) and half-Fourier acquisition single-shot turbo spin echo (HASTE), are used to image the renal collecting systems, ureters, and bladder. However, the clinical usefulness of MR urography performed with T2-weighted imaging alone is limited in patients with nondistended urinary collecting systems. Nonpharmacologic interventions such as IV hydration and ureteral compression, and pharmacologic interventions such as IV diuretics and gadolinium chelate administration, can expand the usefulness of MR urography techniques to include the assessment of nondistended collecting systems.

US has a reported sensitivity of approximately 92% to detect a clinically relevant abnormality in patients with renal colic; however, its role in the evaluation of focal ureteral abnormalities is limited because of technical factors.[4] Color Doppler is useful to evaluate for the presence of a ureteric jet with a normal jet seen in an anteromedial direction with a peak velocity of 20 to 30 cm/s, mean duration of 15 seconds, mean frequency of 4 to 5 minutes, and interjet interval 2 to 150 seconds.[10] Three-dimensional (3D) US has been shown to improve the diagnostic ability of two-dimensional (2D) US.[11]

Direct pyelography includes RP and AP. RP is usually performed during cystoscopy or to further characterize abnormalities detected at IVU or cross-sectional imaging. Although invasive, RP allows confirmation of radiologic diagnosis and also improves diagnostic yield of urine cytology by selective lavage and localized urine collection. AP is only performed if a percutaneous nephrostomy tube is placed or RP cannot be obtained. This condition includes the inability to cannulate the ureteral orifice in a retrograde manner.

VCUG allows detection, evaluation, and grading of vesicoureteric reflux (VUR) and enables functional assessment. With modern digital and pulsed fluoroscopy and last image hold techniques, reliable documentation of the investigation and findings are possible by considerably reducing radiation; only evaluation of the urethra and of

intrarenal reflux still require additional spot films.[12–14] VCUG is still considered the gold standard for VUR and urethra evaluation.[15–18] Some centers perform a modified VCUG with intermittent imaging throughout the bladder filling for evaluation of functional disturbances and early VUR.[19,20]

Nuclear medicine diuretic scan (Fig. 3) is performed by administration of a radionuclide and mapping the progress of the radionuclide through the kidney and the ureter. The principle of diuretic renography is that the prolonged retention of a tracer seen in a nonobstructed, dilated system is caused by a reservoir effect.[21] A diuretic produces prompt washout of activity in a dilated nonobstructed system. In contrast, the capacity to augment washout is less, resulting in prolonged retention of tracer proximal to the obstruction. Diuretic renography is accepted in routine clinical practice for differentiating a dilated unobstructed urinary system from a true stenotic dilatation in the upper urinary tract and for the follow-up of patients who have hydronephrosis.[22–24] The diuretic used routinely is furosemide, which acts

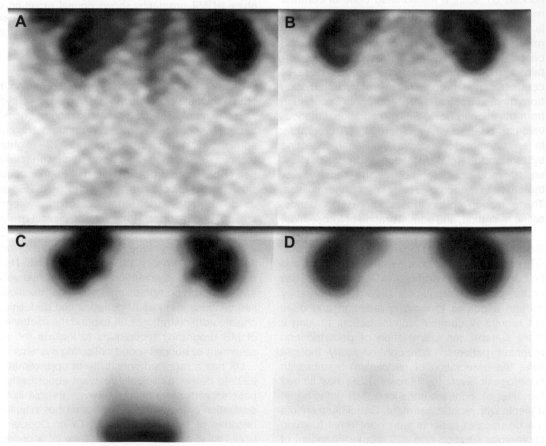

Fig. 3. Normal renal scan. Coronal images from a normal renal scan show flow (A), cortical (B), excretory phases (C), and postvoid (D) images.

at the luminal face of epithelial cells in the ascending limb of the loop of Henle, blocking active reabsorption of chloride and sodium.[25] The guidelines published by the Society of Nuclear Medicine and the European Nuclear Medicine Association recommend the use of furosemide at a dose of 1 mg/kg, up to a maximum of 20 mg in children and 40 mg in adults.[26]

CONGENITAL LESIONS
Ureteric Webs

Ureteric webs are normal developmental structures. They are postulated to form because of the reserve length of the ureter left over from the growth of the spine and the retroperitoneum after birth. It is also hypothesized that disturbances in the development of these fetal folds might be an important factor in the genesis of hydronephrosis. Histologically, these are luminal projections of lamina propria containing prominent bundles of smooth muscle. On imaging, ureteric webs are seen as linear lucencies in the proximal ureter projecting into the lumen of the ureter below the UPJ with a corkscrew appearance of the upper ureter (Fig. 4).[27,28]

UPJ Obstruction

UPJ obstruction is a benign, congenital condition defined as a functional or anatomic obstruction to urine flow from the renal pelvis into the ureter at their anatomic junction (Fig. 5).[29,30] It is the most common cause of neonatal hydronephrosis, occurring in 1 per 1500 live births. UPJ obstruction is generally sporadic; however, a familial pattern has been reported and can be inherited in an autosomal dominant pattern.[31] Boys exhibit a significantly increased frequency of UPJ obstruction compared with girls (3:1 to 4:1). It is more commonly bilateral (approximately 10%)[32] but, if unilateral, it occurs more commonly on the left[33];

however, the clinical outcome is similar in both sexes.[34] Causes of UPJ obstruction include abnormal alignment of smooth muscles at UPJ and anatomic causes like adhesions, kinking, and aberrant vessels.

During AP or RP, a vascular impression may be seen at the UPJ in these patients. Contrast-enhanced CT has proved to be 100% sensitive and 96% to 100% specific for detecting crossing arteries (Fig. 6).[35] CT angiography can usually identify the presence of a crossing vessel.

Endoscopic treatment is generally the initial surgical therapy for symptomatic UPJ obstruction because of the minimally invasive nature of the procedure and the favorable success rates. However, when crossing vessels are present, no consensus has been reached as to the appropriate treatment.[36]

Duplication and Ectopic Ureter

Ureteral duplication is one of the most common anomalies of the urinary tract and can be either complete or partial. In a complete duplication, the 2 ureters are separate in their course (Figs. 7 and 8). The insertion of the lower ends follows the Weigert-Meyer rule, which states that, in duplicated collecting systems, the upper pole ureter inserts distally and medially, whereas the lower pole ureter inserts more cranially and laterally, often in a nearly normal position.[37] In these cases, the upper pole moiety ureter commonly ends in a ureterocele, whereas reflux into the lower moiety typically occurs.[38] In women, the ectopic distal ureter may insert into the lower bladder, urethra, vestibule, vagina, or, more rarely, into the uterus or a Wolffian duct remnant such as Gartner duct or cyst. In male patients, it can empty into the lower bladder, posterior urethra, seminal vesicle, vas deferens, ejaculatory duct, or, rarely, into the rectum.[38–42] Incomplete duplications can range from bifid renal pelvis to the 2 ureters joining

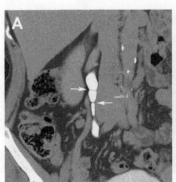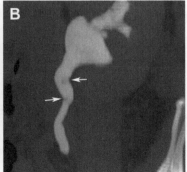

Fig. 4. Ureteric webs. Coronal excretory phase CT (A) depicts dilated right ureter with focal regions of narrowing (arrow), better seen on the thick MIP reformat (B, arrows).

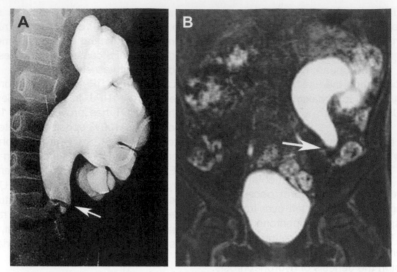

Fig. 5. UPJ obstruction. Excretory urography in a 3-year-old patient (A) and MR urography (B) show dilated left renal calyces and renal pelvis with obstruction at the UPJ (arrow).

anywhere along the course and continuing inferiorly as a single ureter.[37]

The radiologic work-up of a duplex kidney includes US and VCUG for evaluation of reflux, with US being the initial screening test of choice.[38] It usually shows the abnormal dilated ureter and can allow the ureter to be traced to its abnormally low insertion. IVU is not routinely performed because the dilated upper pole shows reduced renal function and typically does not opacify. Renal scintigraphy accurately assesses the renal function, and CT is used to localize the poorly functioning dysplastic kidney. In selected cases, MR urography may be useful because it provides an excellent overview of the malformation and can show all ectopic extravesical ureteric insertions (Fig. 9).[38,43–45]

Ureterocele

Ureterocele is a cystlike expansion of the terminal segment of the ureter projecting into the lumen of the urinary bladder. This anomaly may be associated with a single or duplicated ureter. Embryologically, these occur because of the persistence of the Chwalla membrane, which initially separates the ureteric bud from the bladder lumen.[37] The congenital defect is meatal obstruction and the ureterocele is the hyerplastic response to the obstruction.[38,46] The size of the ureterocele can vary from small (1 cm) to completely filling the bladder with prolapse through the urethra. Seventy-five percent of ureteroceles are associated with ureteral duplication.[38,47]

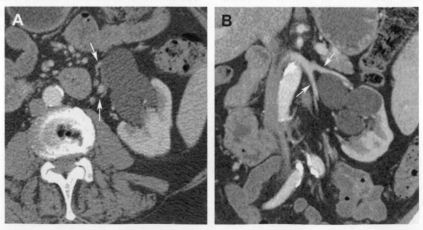

Fig. 6. UPJ obstruction caused by crossing vessels. Postcontrast CT images in a 75-year-old patient, axial (A) and coronal (B) depicting hydronephrosis to the level of the UPJ with associated cortical thinning. Crossing vessels (arrows) are identified at the transition point.

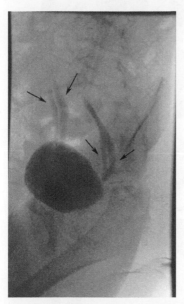

Fig. 7. Duplicated collecting system. Spot radiograph during the voiding phase of a cystourethrogram depicts duplication of both ureters (*arrows*) with bilateral grade I reflux.

Ureteroceles can be either simple or ectopic. Simple ureteroceles are presumed to be congenital in young patients and postinflammatory in adults. In simple ureteroceles, there is ballooning of the distal ureter in a normally positioned ureter immediately proximal to a distal ureteric stenosis. They usually are entirely intravesicular in location. On US, an ureterocele is seen as a cystic intravesicular mass (cyst within cyst), near the lateral margin of the trigone, contiguous with a dilated ureter and arising from a normally positioned ureteral orifice. The wall of the ureterocele is round and echogenic and the base is usually narrow (**Figs. 10** and **11**). As pressure in the bladder increases during voiding, the ureterocele may be compressed, flattened, or even everted, simulating a paraureteral diverticulum. Although IVU is rarely used for this entity, it produces a characteristic cobra-head or spring onion appearance from contrast collecting in the bladder lumen and the wall of the ureterocele forming a radiolucent halo. Dynamic MR urography can be performed for functional information as well as for complete anatomic evaluation.[37,38]

An ectopic ureterocele is located more inferiorly than a simple ureterocele, is invariably associated with a duplicated collecting system, and represents the distal portion of the ureter of the upper renal moiety.[37,48] The ectopic ureterocele represents dilatation and protrusion of the submucosal segment of the ureter at its insertion, has a broader base, is usually larger than the simple ureterocele, and its orifice is almost always in or close to the posterior urethra.[37] On US, a cystic structure is seen in or adjacent to the urinary bladder. In addition, a dysplastic upper pole of the ipsilateral kidney may also be seen on US with poor vascularity within it.[37,38]

Megaureter

Megaureter or megaloureter is a generic term that indicates dilatation of the ureter as seen on US and failure of the ureter to empty on delayed images on an IVU, retrograde urethrogram, or VCUG if the ureter is refluxed (**Fig. 12**). There may be concomitant dilatation of the upper collecting system.[37,38]

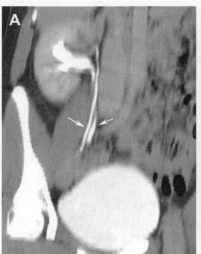
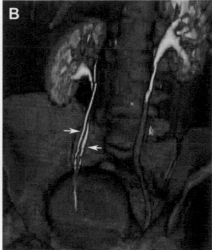

Fig. 8. Duplicated right collecting system. Coronal oblique reformat (*A*) and volume rendered (*B*) images showing complete duplication of the right ureter (*arrows*).

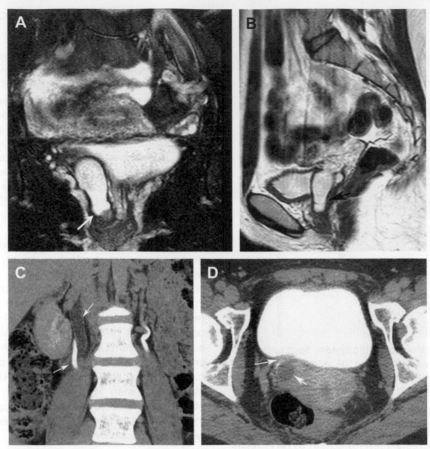

Fig. 9. Ectopic insertion of the duplicated ureter. T2-weighted MR images in a 35-year-old patient performed for pelvic discomfort to rule out prolapse; coronal (*A*) and sagittal (*B*) views show an abnormal insertion of the duplicated upper pole moiety right ureter (*large white arrow*) into the urethra. CT excretory urography performed later shows the dilated upper pole ureter and the nondilated lower pole ureter. Contrast is excreted through the nondilated lower pole ureter. (*C*) Image through the pelvis shows the normal insertion of the nondilated right lower pole ureter (*D*) and the dilated right upper pole ureter which inserts more inferiorly into the urethra (*arrows*).

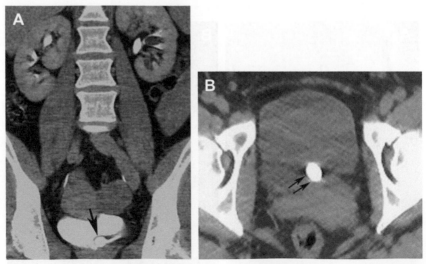

Fig. 10. Pseudoureterocele arising in the left UVJ. Coronal (*A*) postcontrast image in a 39-year-old patient shows a pseudoureterocele (*arrow*). This appearance was caused by obstruction from a calculus, as seen on the noncontrast image (*double arrow*) (*B*).

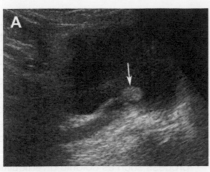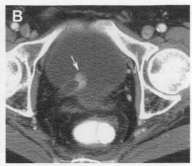

Fig. 11. Pseudoureterocele from a polyp. Transverse sonographic image (*A*) through the bladder in a 56-year-old patient shows a small echogenic mass (*arrow*) at the distal aspect of the right ureterovesicular junction (UVJ). Postcontrast axial CT image (*B*) shows an enhancing mass (*arrow*) at the distal aspect of the right UVJ. This proved to be a small polyp on resection.

The normal ureter in a child usually measures up to 5 mm in diameter. A diameter of 7 mm or more is considered a megaureter.[49,50] Primary megaureter is usually functional in origin and includes all cases of megaureter caused by an idiopathic congenital alteration at the vesicoureteral junction.[37,38,51] Causes of secondary megaureter include urethral valves, neuropathic bladder dysfunction, urethral strictures, ureteroceles, and acquired causes of obstruction.[38]

Vesicoureteral Reflux

Vesicoureteral reflux (VUR) refers to the retrograde passage of urine from the urinary bladder into the ureter or all the way to the level of the calyces. It

is a common childhood problem but is regarded as abnormal at all ages.[37] Most cases result from a primary maturation abnormality of the vesicoureteral junction or from a short distal ureteric submucosal tunnel in the bladder that alters the function of the valve mechanism. VUR can be an isolated abnormality or it can be associated with other congenital abnormalities such as posterior urethral valves or complete duplication of the urinary tract.[38,52,53] VUR predisposes to pyelonephritis because it carries bacteria from the bladder to the upper urinary tract.

VCUG remains the basic imaging technique of VUR assessment. It is indicated in all neonates with significant antenatal hydronephrosis and children after the first well-documented urinary tract

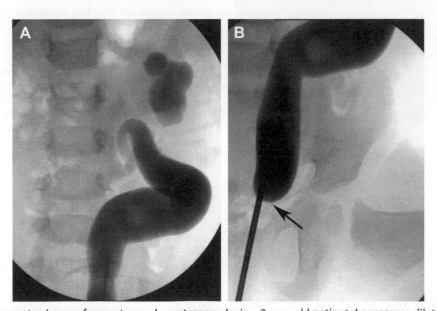

Fig. 12. Megaureter. Images from retrograde ureterography in a 2-year-old patient show severe dilatation of left ureter and hydronephrosis (*A*). No obstructing lesion is present; however, persistent narrowing (*arrow*) was seen in the distal portion of the ureter (*B*).

infection.[37] VCUG documents presence and grade of VUR, and defines the urethral anatomy in male patients (**Fig. 13**). Grading of reflux is based on the International Reflux Committee Study (**Fig. 14**).[54] Reflux can also be graded, although less precisely, with nuclear cystography and the conventional grades used are mild, moderate, and severe.

INFECTIOUS DISEASES
Ureteritis Cystica

Ureteritis cystica is a rare condition first described by Morgagni in 1761, with the first radiographic description by Jacoby and Joelson in 1929. It is caused by degeneration of the basal layer of the urothelium, which results in proliferation of surface epithelial cells that form fluid-filled cysts. An association with bacterial urinary tract infection, nephrolithiasis, and, less commonly, cyclophosphamide-induced hemorrhagic cystitis and schistosomiasis has been shown.[55,56] On IVU or retrograde imaging, ureteritis cystica is seen as multiple, small (2–3 mm), radiolucent filling defects in the ureter with a slight predilection for the proximal third of the ureter (**Fig. 15**). There are limited reports on the CT, US, and MR appearance of ureteritis cystica. The process may regress or disappear with treatment of underlying inflammatory condition.[55]

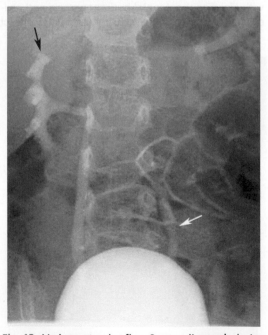

Fig. 13. Vesicoureteral reflux. Spot radiograph during the voiding phase of a VCUG depicts grade III reflux in the right ureter (*black arrow*) and grade I reflux in the left ureter (*arrow*).

Ureteritis

Primary ureteritis is rare without systemic or regional disease in the urinary tract, retroperitoneum, or pelvis and is usually secondary to pyelonephritis or cystitis. The symptoms are also typically derived from the contiguous spread of a primary infection in the kidney or bladder. Treatment of the primary infection also treats the ureter. The ureteral inflammation can occasionally be secondary to another adjacent inflammatory process such as colonic diverticulitis, from inflammatory elements excreted into the urine, or hematogenous embolism from a distant site.[57] Complications from ureteritis also typically evolve from contiguous spread from other urinary tract infections such as renal or perirenal abscesses and septic shock. Ureteritis is best evaluated radiographically by CT. The imaging characteristics include ureteral wall thickening, adjacent fat stranding, associated hydronephrosis, and possible presence of an obstructing lesion such as a stone or mass (**Figs. 16** and **17**). US has a limited role in the assessment of ureteral abnormalities because portions of the ureter are often obscured by overlying bowel gas. However, US can assess the degree and sometimes the level of obstruction.[57] Mitterberg and colleagues[58] assessed the sonographic measurement of renal pelvis wall thickness as a diagnostic criterion for acute pyelonephritis in adults and suggested that 2 mm was an appropriate cutoff. However, it cannot differentiate acute from chronic inflammation of the urothelium. The presence of dirty shadowing on US should raise suspicion for the presence of gas. MR imaging, specifically MR urography, has a limited support role in evaluating the ureters, particularly in the setting of complicated urinary tract infections, because it is costly, not widely available, requires a longer imaging time, and requires more patient cooperation to avoid significant artifact. However, the findings are similar to those of CT of smooth wall thickening and adjacent fat stranding. MR urography can also assess the degree and level of obstruction or any complications such as renal/perirenal abscesses.[59]

Tuberculosis

The incidence of tuberculosis is increasing because of the emergence of human immunodeficiency virus (HIV). It usually reaches the urinary tract by hematogenous spread to the kidneys from a pulmonary source, although pulmonary findings are seen in only 30% of patients.[57] Patients usually present with lower urinary tract symptoms including hematuria and sterile pyuria. The infection usually first involves the kidneys

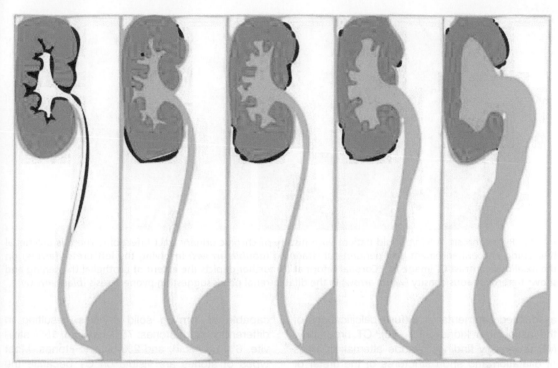

Fig. 14. Vesicoureteral reflux grading system showing the 5 grades of reflux in the ureter (grades 1–5).

and secondarily the ureter and bladder. When the infection affects the ureteral wall, initial changes are ulceration and wall edema, with thickening resulting in dilatation of the ureter and upper collecting system.[60] Even with adequate treatment, it commonly progresses to fibrous stricture. The noncontrast phase of the CT urography may also show calcification of the ureter with or without

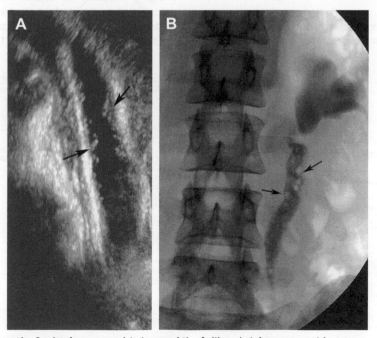

Fig. 15. Ureteritis cystic. Sagittal sonographic image (*A*) of dilated right ureter with numerous smooth-walled, rounded, lucent filling defects projecting into the lumen (*arrows*). AP radiograph of a retrograde ureter shows numerous lucencies (*arrows*) in the left ureter (*B*) consistent with ureteritis cystica.

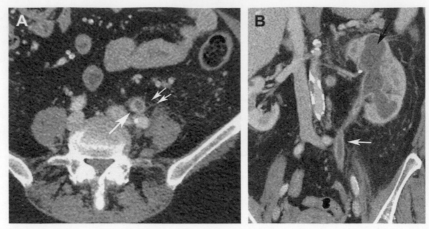

Fig. 16. Pyonephrosis. A 51-year-old patient with history of chronic urinary tract infections. There is urothelial thickening and enhancement and periureteral stranding (*double arrows*) involving the left ureter (*arrow*) on the axial postcontrast CT image (*A*). Coronal reformat (*B*) further depicts the extent of urothelial thickening and shows heterogeneous density (*white arrow*) in the dilated renal pelvis suggesting pyonephrosis (*black arrow*).

associated segmental or diffuse calcifications of the associated kidney (Fig. 18). CT urography/ MR urography findings include alternating areas of dilatation and short strictures of the ureter or long straight stricture (pipe-stem ureter) or isolated stricture (Fig. 19).[57] MR urography is less sensitive at identifying calcifications of the ureter but can identify the multiple strictures that are characteristic for tuberculosis.[59]

CALCULI

Ureterolithiasis originates in the kidney when the urine becomes supersaturated with a salt that is capable of forming solid crystals, resulting in different types of stones: 75% calcium, 15% struvite, 6% uric acid, and 2% cystine stones. Most types of stones are visible on CT because the density of even radiolucent stones like uric acid is greater than that of soft tissue or blood clot[61]; however, stones formed in patients on protease inhibitors as a side effect of the medicine may not be visible on CT.[62]

Noncontrast CT has supplanted IVU as the imaging modality of choice to detect ureteral calculi and associated renal obstruction because of its lack of need for IV contrast, high sensitivity for renal calculi (approaching 100%), and ability

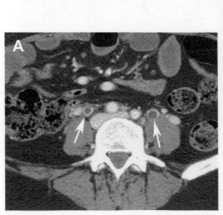
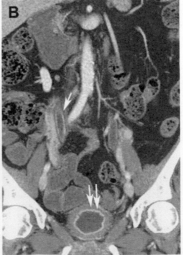

Fig. 17. Ureteral mucositis. A 46-year-old patient with a history of breast cancer on chemotherapy. Axial (*A*) and coronal reformat (*B*) from postcontrast CT shows urothelial enhancement involving both ureters (*arrows*). Note mucosal enhancement in the bladder (*double arrow*), caused by mucositis from patient's chemotherapy.

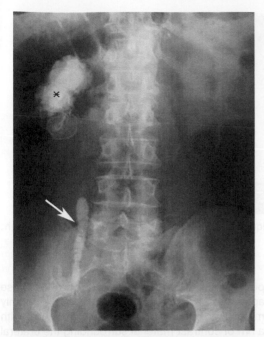

Fig. 18. Renal tuberculosis. Abdominal radiograph in a 45-year-old patient with known tuberculosis shows calcification of the right ureter (*arrow*). Dystrophic calcification of the right kidney (so-called putty kidney) is also present (*asterisk*).

to detect nonurologic causes of flank pain (Fig. 20).[4,63,64] Stones greater than 5 mm may require surgical retrieval because they may not pass spontaneously. Secondary signs of ureterolithiasis such as ureteral dilatation, dilatation of the

intrarenal collecting system, and renal enlargement are well depicted on CT, US, and MR imaging. On MR urography, the ureteral stone can be seen as a round or ovoid signal void filling defect that causes a variable degree of dilatation of the urinary tract. Small calculi can be obscured by the hyperintense urine on maximum intensity projection images for both excretory and T2-weighted sequences, therefore the source images must be assessed for subtle filling defects.[59] Perinephric fat stranding can also be seen on both MR urography and CT urography as a secondary finding. Findings on US include a constant echogenic focus within the ureter that may show twinkling artifact on Doppler imaging, with a variable degree of proximal collecting system dilatation.[65] Additional Doppler imaging of the bladder at the ureterovesicular junction (UVJ) may assess for a unilateral absence of the ureteral jet, which would suggest an obstructing ureteral stone. However, the presence of a jet does not necessarily exclude ureterolithiasis; Sheafor and colleagues[4] noted that 30% of their patients with documented ureteral calculi had normal ureteral jets. Sheafor and colleagues[4] prospectively compared nonenhanced helical CT with US for the depiction of urolithiasis and found that CT had a 96% sensitivity and US 61% sensitivity for detecting ureteral calculi directly, and that the sensitivity improved (100% for CT and 92% for US) if they only considered detection of associated relevant abnormalities (such as unilateral hydronephrosis and absence of an ureteral jet).

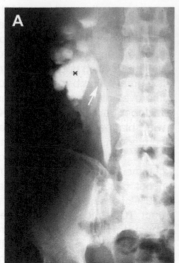

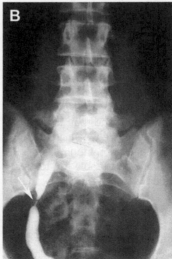

Fig. 19. Renal tuberculosis. IV pyelogram (*A*) and retrograde ureterogram (*B*) performed in a 57-year-old patient with known tuberculosis depicts multiple strictures in the right ureter (*arrows*). Papillary necrosis and uneven calyceal dilatation is also seen in the right kidney (*asterisk*), findings characteristic of renal tuberculosis.

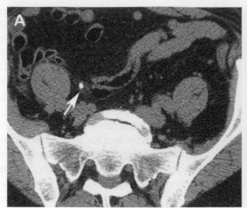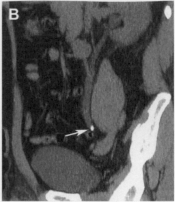

Fig. 20. Ureteral calculus. Axial (*A*) noncontrast CT and oblique reformat (*B*) shows a calculus (*arrow*) in the right midureter with dilatation of the proximal ureter.

NEOPLASTIC CAUSES
Fibroepithelial Polyps

Fibroepithelial polyps are the most common benign tumors of the ureter; however, they are rare tumors that occur in younger adults (20–40 years old) more commonly than in children and older patients. There is slight male predominance. The cause for the polyps is unknown, although some have suggested congenital factors in children and chronic inflammation in adults. The typical size of the polyps is 1 to 5 cm, but they may occasionally exceed 10 cm. Histologically, fibroepithelial polyps are of mesodermal origin and have a loose fibrovascular stromal core, covered with benign transitional epithelium. Although fibroepithelial polyps are benign, progressive growth and coexistent transitional cell carcinoma have been reported. Despite the benign nature, most fibroepithelial polyps reported in the literature were discovered at the time of nephroureterectomy for a presumed ureteral malignancy.[66–68] Conventional excretory urograms show a fibroepithelial polyp as an elongated, smooth ureteral filling defect surrounded by contrast material. A ureteral polyp can be mobile and may change in configuration and position between images.[69] Hematuria and flank pain are common presenting symptoms that may be attributable to torsion, intermittent intussusception of the polyp, or intermittent obstruction. Dysuria and urinary tract infection may rarely occur in patients with fibroepithelial polyps.[68] On IVU and RP, fibroepithelial polyps are typically shown as slender, elongated, smooth ureteral filling defects with mobility. A corkscrew appearance of the polyp within the ureter has also been described.[68] There have been limited reports of fibroepithelial polyps on CT; however, described CT appearances of polyps are similar to those of IVU and RP. These appearances include an elongated, smoothly marginated intraluminal tubular structure with a rim of contrast material surrounding the ureteral lesion, with an attachment of the lesion to the wall of the ureter (**Fig. 21**).[67] US has a limited role in detection of fibroepithelial polyps; however, they may appear as mobile soft tissue masses with elongated and smooth margins extending into the renal pelvis, if located in the proximal ureter, or into the urinary bladder if located in the distal ureter.[66] Treatment of choice for fibroepithelial polyp is complete excision.

Transitional Cell Carcinoma

Transitional cell carcinoma (TCC) is the most common malignant tumor of the ureter. Although it is rare among genitourinary carcinomas, the incidence has increased because of improved survival rates of patients with bladder cancer who subsequently develop upper urinary tract TCC, and there is a greater number of detected cases because of improved diagnostic techniques.

Upper tract TCC occur in 2% to 4% of patients with bladder cancer.[70] Ureteral TCC is more common in men than women and typically occurs in the sixth and seventh decades of life. It is commonly multifocal and multicentric. Simultaneous bilateral ureteral TCCs are reported in 2% to 9% of cases; 11% to 13% of patients with upper tract TCC subsequently develop metachronous upper tract TCC. Furthermore, up to 50% of patients initially presenting with upper tract TCC eventually develop metachronous bladder TCC within 2 years of surgery.[71] The risk factors for TCC include smoking; exposure to certain chemical carcinogens such as aniline, benzidine, and aromatic amines; cyclosporine therapy; heavy

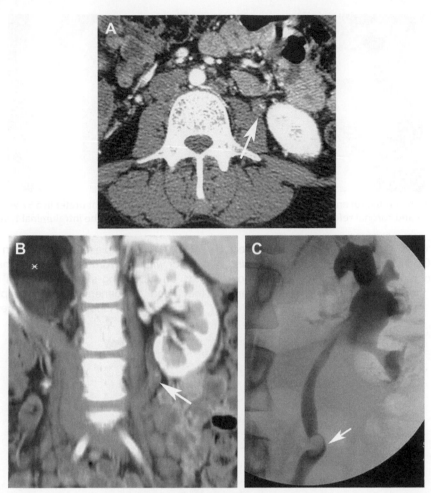

Fig. 21. Fibroepithelial polyp. A soft tissue mass with calcification (*arrow*) was seen in the left ureter in a 57-year-old patient with hematuria on axial postcontrast image (*A*) and coronal reformat (*B*). A retrograde urogram image (*C*) shows a filling defect in the left ureter, which was shown to be a fibroepithelial polyp. An incidental myelolipoma was seen on CT in the right adrenal gland (*asterisk*).

caffeine consumption; analgesic abuse; and long-term use of phenacetin. Stasis of urine and structural abnormalities such as horseshoe kidney also increase the risk of developing TCC. Certain familial diseases such as Balkan endemic nephropathy are associated with high risk of TCC.[71]

TCCs are classified as papillary, infiltrating, papillary and infiltrating, and carcinoma in situ. Eighty-five percent of ureteral TCCs are low-stage, superficial, papillary lesions with a broad base and frondlike morphologic features. These TCCs are usually small at diagnosis and typically are slow-growing tumors. The other 15% are either pedunculated (**Fig. 22**), masslike with intraluminal and extraluminal components (**Fig. 23**), or diffusely infiltrating tumors (**Fig. 24**) with more aggressive behavior and are more advanced at the time of diagnosis. Infiltrating tumors are characterized by thickening and induration of ureteric or renal pelvic wall (**Fig. 25**). If the renal pelvis is involved, there is often invasion into the renal parenchyma.[71,72] Ureteral TCCs spread by direct invasion and via lymphatics secondary to the thin wall and rich lymphatic drainage of the ureter. Retroperitoneal lymph nodes are commonly involved. Invasion of the renal vein and inferior vena cava is rare.[70]

The most common presenting symptom for TCC is hematuria. Initial diagnosis of TCC is usually made from urine cytology. However, unlike bladder TCCs, which are diagnosed using cystoscopy, ureteral TCCs are detected primarily using radiological procedures including IVU, direct pyelography (either RP or AP), CT urography, and MR urography. Traditionally, IVU was the most

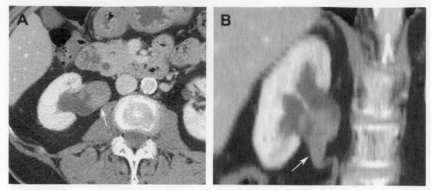

Fig. 22. TCC of the ureter. An enhancing mass (*arrow*) is seen within the upper right ureter in a 57-year-old patient on the axial (*A*) and coronal reformat (*B*) images. This finding is consistent with the intraluminal type of TCC.

commonly used radiologic modality to detect ureteral TCCs in the setting of hematuria. With the advent of multislice CT, CT urography is now considered the standard for evaluating ureteral TCCs.

Single or multiple filling defects in the ureter, with or without hydronephrosis, are the main findings on IVU. Long-standing ureteral obstruction may lead to generalized hydronephrosis and poor excretion. Findings that suggest TCC on

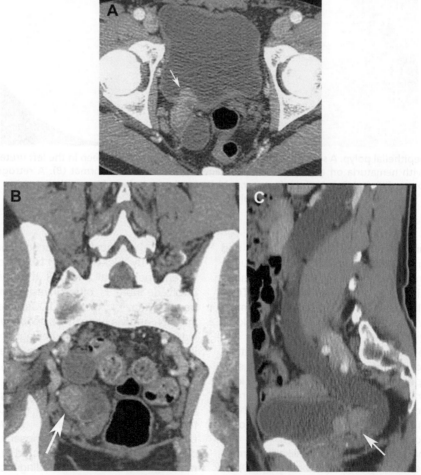

Fig. 23. TCC of the ureter. Axial (*A*), coronal (*B*), and sagittal oblique reformat (*C*) images from postcontrast CT in a 66-year-old patient show enhancing mass (*arrow*) in the distal right ureter.

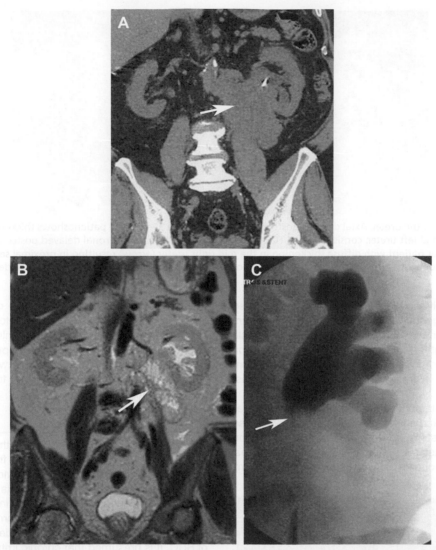

Fig. 24. TCC of the ureter. Coronal reformat from noncontrast CT (*A*) and coronal T2-weighted (*B*) images from noncontrast MR in a 71-year-old patient shows a large mass (*arrow*) in the mid right ureter with extension outside the ureter. Retrograde examination (*C*) shows irregularity and narrowing (*arrow*) in this region. Biopsy showed this mass to be a TCC.

direct pyelography are similar to IVU. A filling defect with or without hydronephrosis and ureteral stricture with an apple-core appearance have been described. At RP, localized ureteric dilatation distal to the filling defect may give rise to the goblet sign, which occurs because of slow tumor growth with resultant lumen expansion.[70,71]

CT urography allows primary tumor detection and tumor staging with a single examination. Multiple studies have confirmed that CT urography has higher detection rates for upper and lower urinary tract malignancies compared with IVU.[70,73] Small TCCs typically appear as a small filling defect/mass or ureteral wall thickening

(circumferential or eccentric) on CT urography. Thinner slices and improved resolution allow the detection of small lesions on CT urography. Hydronephrosis and hydroureter to the point of obstruction can also be seen. A thickened ureteral wall with periureteric fat stranding suggests extramural spread.

MR urography is less commonly used in the primary detection of ureteral TCC and is still an evolving technique. MR urography suffers from significant limitations of poorer spatial resolution than CT urography and various artifacts including motion artifacts from breathing and peristalsis. Therefore, MR urography currently is used as an

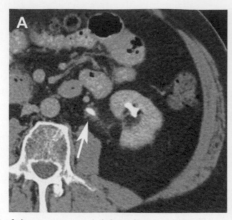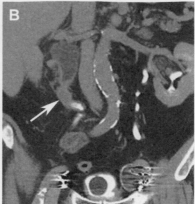

Fig. 25. TCC of the ureter. Axial delayed postcontrast image (*A*) in a 51-year-old patient shows thickening (*arrow*) in the proximal left ureter, consistent with TCC on retrograde brush biopsy. Coronal delayed postcontrast image (*B*) in another patient with diffuse thickening in the mid right ureter (*arrow*) resulting in proximal severe hydronephrosis. Contrast seen in the distal ureter was thought to be secondary to reflux from the bladder.

alternative if a patient is allergic to iodine-based contrast agents. Ureteric TCC typically appears an irregular mass that is isointense to muscle on T1-weighted images, slightly hyperintense on T2-weighted images, with tumor enhancement after administration of gadolinium contrast material.[71]

Tumor staging at diagnosis predicts overall prognosis and survival. The most commonly used staging system in ureteric TCC is the tumor, node, metastasis system (**Fig. 26**). The traditional treatment choice is total nephroureterectomy

with excision of ipsilateral ureteric orifice and a contiguous cuff of bladder tissue. However, the development of endoscopic and minimally invasive surgical techniques allows renal preservation in selected patients, including those with solitary kidney, bilateral tumor, low-grade tumor, and significant surgical risk.[71]

Squamous Cell Carcinoma

Squamous cell carcinoma (SCC) of the ureter is rare. The reported incidence ranges from 6% to 15% among malignant ureteral tumors.[74] Men and women are equally affected. It is frequently associated with nephrolithiasis, including staghorn stones and hydronephrosis. Long-term phenacetin abuse may also contribute to development of SCC. It is presumed that chronic irritation of urothelium may result in squamous metaplasia that later may develop into SCC. Early metastatic spread is common and the prognosis is poor, with few patients surviving longer than 5 years. SCC may appear as a solid mass with hydronephrosis and calcifications on radiologic examinations (**Fig. 27**). Hence, the diagnosis of SCC is usually not established before the histopathologic examination of the surgical specimen.[74]

Adenocarcinoma

Adenocarcinoma of ureter is also rare. There are 3 histologic subtypes: tubulovillous, mucinous, and papillary nonintestinal.[75,76] Tubulovillous and mucinous types are more common than the papillary nonintestinal type. Tubulovillous and mucinous types often occur with intestinal metaplasia, therefore it is suspected that they may have resulted from chronic irritation. Treatment

Fig. 26. Staging of TCC of the ureter.

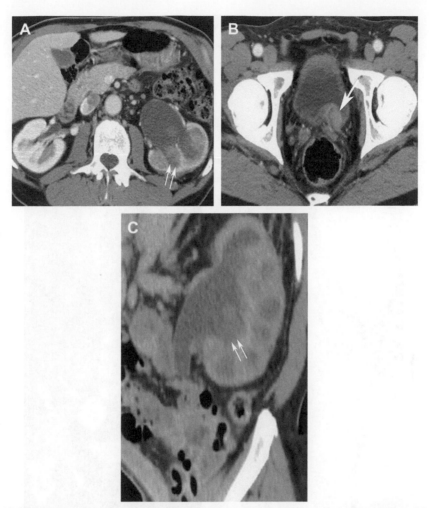

Fig. 27. SCC of the ureter. Axial postcontrast CT (*A, B*) in a patient with hematuria shows dilated left collecting system with an enhancing lesion in the left renal pelvis (*double arrow*). Coronal (*C*) postcontrast CT in the same patient also shows the lesion in the left collecting system (*arrow*). This lesion was shown to be SCC on nephroureterectomy.

depends on the histologic subtypes. The papillary nonintestinal type is treated with surgery only, whereas the tubulovillous and mucinous types are treated with surgery and adjuvant chemoradiation therapy. Tubulovillous adenocarcinomas are the most aggressive, followed by mucinous and papillary nonintestinal adenocarcinomas. Papillary nonintestinal tumors are associated with a nearly 100% survival rate.[75] No specific radiologic findings are reported and imaging findings are similar to those of TCC (**Fig. 28**).

Lymphoma

Lymphomatous involvement of the ureter is rare, with a reported incidence of 0.86% (±7%)[77] and 1% (±16%)[78] of cases in patients with lymphomas examined postmortem. Involvement of the ureter is usually caused by non-Hodgkin lymphoma and is usually seen with renal involvement or retroperitoneal adenopathy. Although rare, symptoms may include lumbar or hip pain, dysuria, oliguria, anuresis, and, more rarely, hematuria and pollakiuria. Imaging findings in ureteral lymphoma include multiple masses and diffuse infiltration of the ureter (**Figs. 29 and 30**). Contiguous retroperitoneal disease is seen in these cases. The upper third of the ureter is typically displaced laterally by lymph nodes, whereas the lower third is displaced medially.[79]

Metastasis

Ureteral metastasis can be the result of direct tumor extension, lymphatic spread, or hematogenous spread. Direct extension usually results

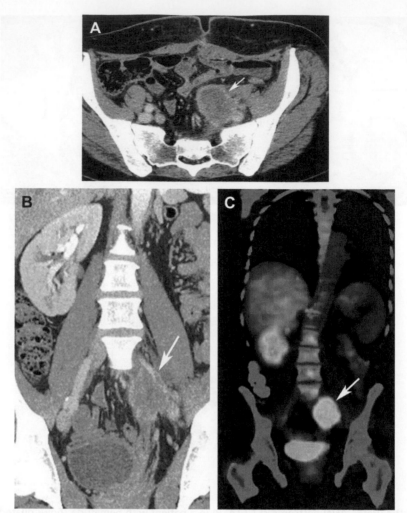

Fig. 28. Adenocarcinoma of the ureter. Postcontrast CT images (*A*, axial; *B*, coronal reformat) in a 67-year-old patient with a history of left nephrectomy for severe infection show heterogeneously enhancing mass centered in the expected location of the left ureteral remnant (*arrow*). Coronal positron emission tomography (PET) CT (*C*) shows diffusely increased fluorodeoxyglucose (FDG) uptake. Biopsy confirmed adenocarcinoma of ureter.

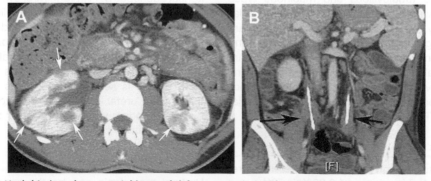

Fig. 29. Non-Hodgkin lymphoma. Axial image (*A*) from a staging CT in a 57-year-old patient shows multiple focal lesions in both kidneys (*arrow*). Coronal image (*B*) shows dilated ureters and bilateral ureteric thickening (*black arrow*).

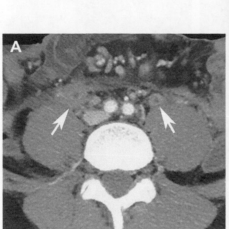
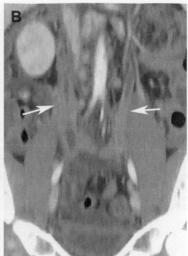

Fig. 30. Lymphoma. Axial postcontrast CT image (*A*) and coronal reformat image (*B*) shows periureteral thickening bilaterally (*arrows*).

from primary pelvic tumors (such as carcinomas of the urinary bladder, prostate, and cervix) or from bulky retroperitoneal lymphadenopathy. Ureteral metastasis most commonly arises from the carcinomas of breast, stomach, pancreas, colon, bladder, prostate, and cervix.[80,81] Extrinsic compression resulting in obstruction is the main finding on radiologic examination. On direct pyelography, ureteral metastasis may appear as filliform or corkscrewlike narrowing of the ureteral lumen with extraluminal obstruction. On CT, lesions may appear as ill-defined ureteral wall thickening with associated ureteral obstruction (Figs. 31–33). Discrete streaky density may be present surrounding the obstructed ureter. Ureteral metastasis may be either unifocal or

multifocal, and is bilateral in 25% to 30% of cases. Metastatic spread with desmoplastic reaction may occur in metastatic scirrhous adenocarcinoma of the prostate, stomach, and colon.[82]

TRAUMA

Ureteral trauma is rare, accounting for less than 1% of all urologic traumas.[83] The ureter is well protected by the structures in the retroperitoneum, such as the psoas muscles, vertebrae, and bony pelvis.[84,85] The ureter can be injured by external trauma or iatrogenically. External trauma could be caused by blunt avulsion or transection by a stab wound or a gunshot wound. Blunt trauma represents 4.1% of all ureteral traumas, is related

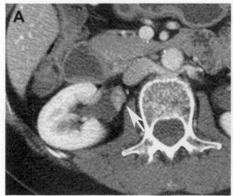
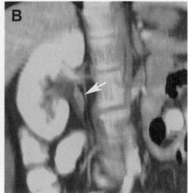

Fig. 31. Ureteral metastasis. A 34-year-old patient with history of uveal melanoma, after enucleation, presented with new-onset hematuria. A new enhancing lesion in the right renal pelvis (*arrow*) was seen on axial postcontrast image (*A*) and coronal oblique reformat (*B*). Nephrectomy revealed metastatic melanoma involving the proximal ureter and right renal pelvis.

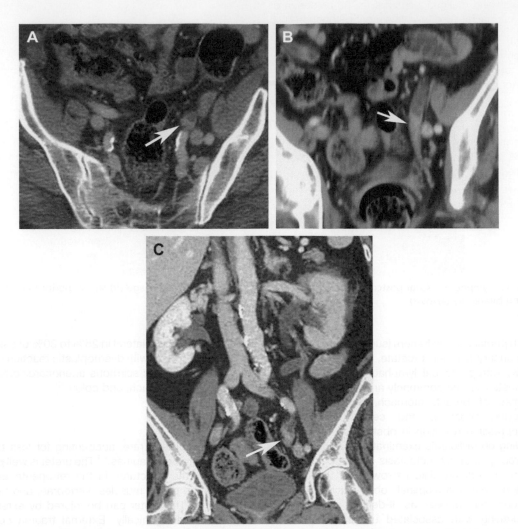

Fig. 32. Ureteral metastasis. A 43-year-old patient with known breast carcinoma. Axial postcontrast CT (*A*), coronal oblique reformat (*B*), and coronal reformat (*C*) from staging CT show a soft tissue mass in the left ureter (*arrow*) representing a breast carcinoma metastasis.

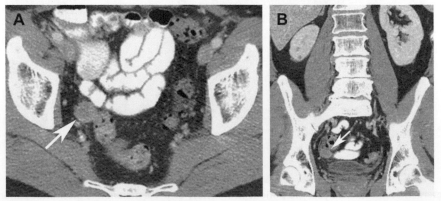

Fig. 33. Ureteral metastasis. Axial (*A*) and coronal (*B*) postcontrast CT images in a 36-year-old patient with history of thyroid carcinoma show a soft tissue mass occluding the right ureter (*arrow*). Biopsy was consistent with a metastatic thyroid cancer.

to rapid deceleration, and usually affects the UPJ.[41] Stab wounds represent about 5.2% of such ureteral traumas. Gunshot wounds account for the greatest number of external traumatic ureteral injuries (90.7%).[86,87] Iatrogenic injury can occur secondary to suture ligation, sharp incision or transection, avulsion, devascularization and heat from microwave, electrocautery or vibratory energy, or cryoablative therapy. Approximately 52% to 82% of iatrogenic injuries occur during gynecologic surgery.[88,89] Low anterior resection (LAR) and abdominal perineal resection (APR) of the colon account for 9% of all ureteral injuries.[89] Vascular surgery, including aortoiliac and aortofemoral bypass, can result in intraoperative ureteral injury to the middle and distal third of the ureter; however, injuries during these procedures are less commonly seen. Ureteroscopy results in ureteral avulsion in 0.3% and perforation in 2% to 6% of cases. A missed ureteral injury can result in significant morbidity and mortality.

Presentation of ureteral trauma can be variable, with hematuria being an unreliable indicator that may be absent in many patients.[85,90] The American Association for the Surgery of Trauma Organ Injury Severity grades of ureteral injuries are as follows: grade 1, ureteral contusion; grade 2, less than 50% partial transection; grade 3, more than 50% partial transection; grade 4, complete transection; and grade 5, complete transection and extensive devascularization.[91] In the acute setting, imaging may not be routinely performed, particularly in patients with penetrating trauma, because these patients are often rapidly transferred to the operating room for exploration.[85] One-shot intraoperative or preoperative IVU may be performed in these patients to assess for extravasation of contrast. However, because of the poor diagnostic performance and delay in performing the examination in an unstable patient, this is not commonly performed.[85,90,92] In stable patients, CT urography is the modality of choice to evaluate for ureteral injury, showing extravasation of contrast from the ureter or partial or complete ureteral obstruction.[93] Urinary ascites or urinoma may also be seen in these patients.

In stable patients with blunt trauma, CT urography is a reliable tool for evaluation. UPJ injury should be suspected with predominantly medial perirenal contrast extravasation in the absence of renal parenchymal injury (Fig. 34).[94] If the UPJ is lacerated, contrast material will be present in the distal ureter; however, with transection, the distal ureter will not be opacified. The distinction between laceration and transection is important for management because lacerations are managed with a ureteral stent, whereas transections require surgical repair. Retrograde pyelography may be necessary in distinguishing partial laceration from complete transection.[90]

MISCELLANEOUS DISEASES
Retroperitoneal Fibrosis

Retroperitoneal fibrosis is a rare disease characterized by chronic inflammation and marked fibrosis of the retroperitoneal tissue that often entraps the ureters or other abdominal organs.[95] Two forms of retroperitoneal fibrosis are seen: the idiopathic form and the secondary form. The idiopathic form of the disease accounts for more than two-thirds of cases, with the rest being secondary to other factors that include neoplasms, infections, trauma, radiotherapy, surgery, and use of certain drugs.[96] Idiopathic retroperitoneal fibrosis is seen more commonly in men, with a 2:1 to 3:1 ratio compared with women, and the mean age at presentation is 50 to 60 years, but reports of the condition in children and older adults are common.[97]

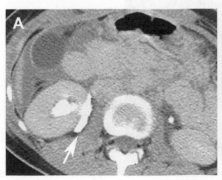
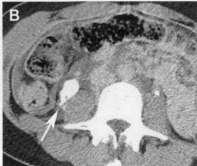

Fig. 34. Traumatic rupture of the right ureter. Axial images (*A*, *B*) from delayed postcontrast CT in a 36-year-old patient with a history of trauma and hematuria show extravasation of contrast around the right kidney and ureter (*arrow*). This extravasation was secondary to a traumatic rupture of the right ureter at the level of the UPJ.

Imaging studies are essential in the diagnosis and management of retroperitoneal fibrosis, and can help to differentiate between idiopathic and secondary disease. CT or MR imaging is the modality of choice for the diagnosis and follow-up of the disease. However, US can also be used when the patient is azotemic because of ureteral obstruction. The finding of a soft tissue mass surrounding the abdominal aorta and the iliac arteries, and with the possible encasement of neighboring structures, usually suggests a diagnosis of retroperitoneal fibrosis. On unenhanced CT, idiopathic retroperitoneal fibrosis usually appears as a homogeneous plaque, isodense with muscle, surrounding the lower abdominal aorta and the iliac arteries, and often enveloping the ureters and the inferior vena cava (**Fig. 35**).[98,99] On MR imaging, idiopathic retroperitoneal fibrosis is hypointense on T1-weighted images; on T2-weighted images it should appear hyperintense in the early or active stages of disease because of tissue edema and hypercellularity and low signal in the later stages.[98,99] The presence of an inhomogeneous signal on T2-weighted images suggests malignant retroperitoneal fibrosis.[100]

Endometriosis

Ureteral endometriosis is unusual and occurs in about 1% of patients with endometriosis, with a higher prevalence in women between the ages of 30 and 35 years.[101,102] Frequency, dysuria, urgency, cyclic hematuria, and renal colic are the common symptoms of urinary tract endometriosis. Other uncommon presentations of ureteral endometriosis include unilateral or bilateral ureteral obstruction, hypertension, anuria in a solitary kidney, and cyclical ureteral obstruction.[103–105]

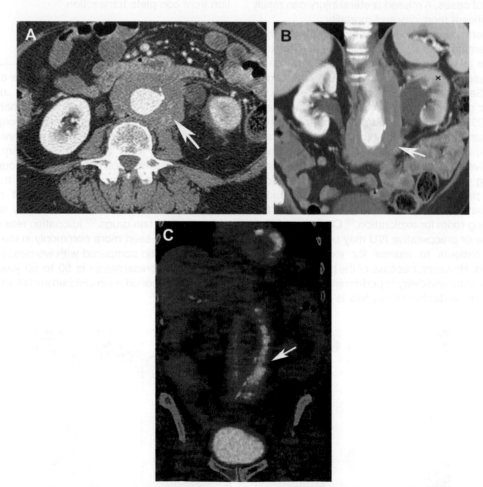

Fig. 35. Retroperitoneal fibrosis. Axial (*A*) and coronal (*B*) postcontrast CT images in a 68-year-old patient, obtained during the nephrographic phase, show soft tissue attenuation encasing the abdominal aorta (*arrow*). There is also delayed enhancement of the left kidney (*asterisk*) with bilateral hydronephrosis. Fused coronal PET CT image (*C*) shows circumferential periaortic FDG uptake (*arrow*) suggesting active inflammation in the retroperitoneal fibrosis.

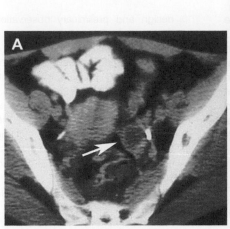

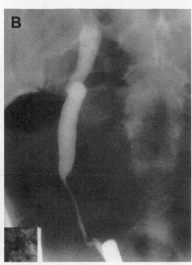

Fig. 36. Endometriosis of the ureter. Axial (A) postcontrast CT image in a 43-year-old patient with a history of endometriosis and hematuria shows thickening around the left ureter (*arrow*). Retrograde image (B) shows a stricture involving the distal third of the ureter. Cytology was negative for malignancy and the stricture was thought to be secondary to endometriosis.

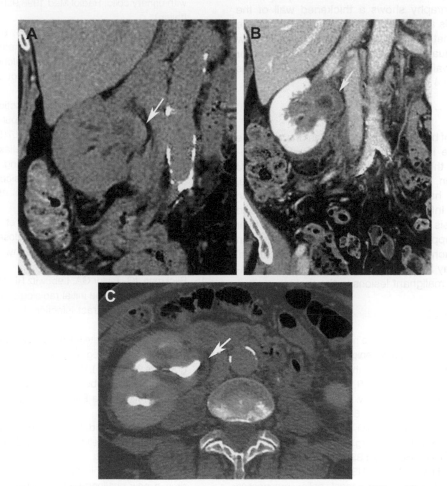

Fig. 37. Spontaneous urothelial hemorrhage. Coronal reformat from a noncontrast CT in a 56-year-old patient with hematuria (A) shows high density around the right ureter (*arrow*). Postcontrast nephrographic phase coronal (B) and delayed phase axial (C) images show diffuse circumferential thickening and enhancement of the mucosa of the ureter (*arrow*), which resolved on follow-up imaging and was consistent with urothelial hemorrhage.

CT findings of ureteral endometriosis can be nonspecific and can be mistaken for a TCC (**Fig. 36**). Because the ureter is usually involved by transmural spread from the peritoneum, a larger soft tissue density component maybe seen outside the ureter. Multiple sites of involvement are commonly seen.[106] MR imaging would show a characteristic appearance with high signal on T1-weighted images and shading on T2-weighted images.[107]

Urothelial Hemorrhage

Intramural renal pelvic and ureteral hemorrhage is seen most commonly in patients treated with anti-coagulant therapy.[108] The incidence of hemorrhage in these patients is 4% to 24%, with urinary tract hemorrhage seen in 40% of these patients.[108] Spontaneous renal pelvic or ureteral hemorrhage can also occur in renal neoplasms.[109] Ultrasonography shows a thickened wall of the renal pelvis and/or ureter. CT is the most valuable imaging method and unenhanced CT scans show high-attenuation thickening of the pelvic and/or ureteral wall, with resolution of these findings within 3 to 4 weeks (**Fig. 37**).[108]

SUMMARY

A variety of benign and malignant lesions affect the ureter, the imaging appearance of which is reviewed in this article. Congenital lesions like UPJ obstruction, ureteric webs, duplicated ureters, and VUR have a characteristic appearance on imaging. Infectious lesions like ureteritis and tuberculosis can also be diagnosed by their imaging appearance and clinical history. Benign lesions such as endometriosis and fibroepithelial polyps may in some cases be difficult to differentiate from malignant lesions in the ureter.

REFERENCES

1. Gray H. Anatomy of the human body. 20th edition. Philadelphia: Lea & Febiger; 2000.
2. Narath P. Physiology of the renal pelvis and ureter. In: Wein AJ, Kavoussi LR, Novick AC, et al, editors. Campbell-Walsh urology. 3rd edition. Philadelphia: WB Saunders; 1954. p. 61–108.
3. Demertzis J, Menias CO. State of the art: imaging of renal infections. Emerg Radiol 2007;14(1):13–22.
4. Sheafor DH, Hertzberg BS, Freed KS, et al. Nonenhanced helical CT and US in the emergency evaluation of patients with renal colic: prospective comparison. Radiology 2000;217(3):792–7.
5. Chai RY, Jhaveri K, Saini S, et al. Comprehensive evaluation of patients with haematuria on multislice computed tomography scanner: protocol design and preliminary observations. Australas Radiol 2001;45(4):536–8.
6. Chow LC, Kwan SW, Olcott EW, et al. Split-bolus MDCT urography with synchronous nephrographic and excretory phase enhancement. AJR Am J Roentgenol 2007;189(2):314–22.
7. Leyendecker JR, Gianini JW. Magnetic resonance urography. Abdom Imaging 2009;34(4):527–40.
8. O'Regan KN, O'Connor OJ, McLoughlin P, et al. The role of imaging in the investigation of painless hematuria in adults. Semin Ultrasound CT MR 2009;30(4):258–70.
9. ACR manual on contrast media - Version 7, 2011. ACR; [cited December 31, 2011]. Available at: http://www.acr.org/SecondaryMainMenuCategories/quality_safety/contrast_manual.aspx. Accessed November, 2011.
10. Catalano O, De Sena G, Nunziata A. The color Doppler US evaluation of the ureteral jet in patients with urinary colic. Radiol Med 1998;95(6):614–7 [in Italian].
11. Elwagdy S, Ghoneim S, Moussa S, et al. Three-dimensional ultrasound (3D US) methods in the evaluation of calcular and non-calcular ureteric obstructive uropathy. World J Urol 2008;26(3): 263–74.
12. Hernandez RJ, Goodsitt MM. Reduction of radiation dose in pediatric patients using pulsed fluoroscopy. AJR Am J Roentgenol 1996;167(5):1247–53.
13. Kleinman PK, Diamond DA, Karellas A, et al. Tailored low-dose fluoroscopic voiding cystourethrography for the reevaluation of vesicoureteral reflux in girls. AJR Am J Roentgenol 1994;162(5): 1151–4 [discussion: 5–6].
14. Ward VL, Strauss KJ, Barnewolt CE, et al. Pediatric radiation exposure and effective dose reduction during voiding cystourethrography. Radiology 2008;249(3):1002–9.
15. Blickman JG, Taylor GA, Lebowitz RL. Voiding cystourethrography: the initial radiologic study in children with urinary tract infection. Radiology 1985; 156(3):659–62.
16. Fernbach SK, Feinstein KA, Schmidt MB. Pediatric voiding cystourethrography: a pictorial guide. Radiographics 2000;20(1):155–68 [discussion: 68–71].
17. Hellström M, Jacobsson B. Diagnosis of vesicoureteric reflux. Acta Paediatr Suppl 1999;88(431): 3–12.
18. Lebowitz RL. The detection and characterization of vesicoureteral reflux in the child. J Urol 1992; 148(5 Pt 2):1640–2.
19. Fotter R. Neurogenic bladder in infants and children–a new challenge for the radiologist. Abdom Imaging 1996;21(6):534–40.
20. Fotter R, Kopp W, Klein E, et al. Unstable bladder in children: functional evaluation by modified voiding cystourethrography. Radiology 1986;161(3):811–3.

21. Thrall JH, Koff SA, Keyes JW. Diuretic radionuclide renography and scintigraphy in the differential diagnosis of hydroureteronephrosis. Semin Nucl Med 1981;11(2):89–104.

22. O'Reilly PH. Standardization of diuresis renography techniques. Nucl Med Commun 1998;19(1):1–2.

23. O'Reilly PH, Lawson RS, Shields RA, et al. Idiopathic hydronephrosis–the diuresis renogram: a new non-invasive method of assessing equivocal pelviureteral junction obstruction. J Urol 1979; 121(2):153–5.

24. English PJ, Testa HJ, Lawson RS, et al. Modified method of diuresis renography for the assessment of equivocal pelviureteric junction obstruction. Br J Urol 1987;59(1):10–4.

25. Imai M. Effect of bumetanide and furosemide on the thick ascending limb of Henle's loop of rabbits and rats perfused in vitro. Eur J Pharmacol 1977; 41(4):409–16.

26. Gordon I, Colarinha P, Fettich J, et al. Guidelines for standard and diuretic renography in children. Eur J Nucl Med 2001;28(3):BP21–30.

27. Kirks DR, Currarino G, Weinberg AG. Transverse folds in the proximal ureter: a normal variant in infants. AJR Am J Roentgenol 1978;130(3):463–4.

28. Dorph S, Horn T, Steven K. Transverse folds of the adult obstructed ureter. Case report. Scand J Urol Nephrol Suppl 1994;157:153–8.

29. Park JM, Bloom DA. The pathophysiology of UPJ obstruction. Current concepts. Urol Clin North Am 1998;25(2):161–9.

30. Gupta M, Moore RG, Nadler RB, et al. Symptomatic ureteropelvic junction (UPJ) obstruction. J Endourol 1999;13(6):413–6.

31. Atwell J. Familial pelviureteric junction hydronephrosis and its association with a duplex pelvicaliceal system and vesicoureteric reflux. A family study. Br J Urol 1985;57(4):365–9.

32. Havutcu A, Nikolopoulos G, Adinkra P, et al. The association between fetal pyelectasis on second trimester ultrasound scan and aneuploidy among 25,586 low risk unselected women. Prenat Diagn 2002;22(13):1201–6.

33. Ouzounian J, Castro M, Fresquez M, et al. Prognostic significance of antenatally detected fetal pyelectasis. Ultrasound Obstet Gynecol 1996; 7(6):424–8.

34. Guys J, Borella F, Monfort G. Ureteropelvic junction obstructions: prenatal diagnosis and neonatal surgery in 47 cases. J Pediatr Surg 1988;23(2):156–8.

35. Braun P, Guilabert JP, Kazmi F. Multidetector computed tomography arteriography in the preoperative assessment of patients with ureteropelvic junction obstruction. Eur J Radiol 2007;61(1):170–5.

36. Khaira HS, Platt JF, Cohan RH, et al. Helical computed tomography for identification of crossing vessels in ureteropelvic junction obstruction-comparison with operative findings. Urology 2003;62(1):35–9.

37. Riccabona M. The ureter and vesicoureteral reflux. In: Slovis TL, editor. Caffey's pediatric diagnostic imaging. 11th edition. Philadelphia: Mosby; 2008. p. 2315–55.

38. Berrocal T, Lopez-Pereira P, Arjonilla A, et al. Anomalies of the distal ureter, bladder, and urethra in children: embryologic, radiologic, and pathologic features. Radiographics 2002;22(5):1139–64.

39. Van Houtte JJ. Ureteral ectopia into a Wolffian duct remnant (Gartner's ducts or cysts) presenting as a urethral diverticulum in two girls. AJR Am J Roentgenol 1970;110:540–5.

40. Fernbach SK, Feinstein KA, Spencer K, et al. Ureteral duplication and its complications. Radiographics 1997;17(1):109–27.

41. Gharagozloo AM, Lebowitz RL. Detection of a poorly functioning malpositioned kidney with single ectopic ureter in girls with urinary dribbling: imaging evaluation in five patients. AJR Am J Roentgenol 1995;164(4):957–61.

42. Ahmed S, Barker A. Single-system ectopic ureters: a review of 12 cases. J Pediatr Surg 1992;27(4): 491–6.

43. Korogi Y, Takahashi M, Fujimura N, et al. Computed tomography demonstration of renal dysplasia with a vaginal ectopic ureter. J Comput Tomogr 1986; 10(3):273–5.

44. Avni FE, Nicaise N, Hall M, et al. The role of MR imaging for the assessment of complicated duplex kidneys in children: preliminary report. Pediatr Radiol 2001;31(4):215–23.

45. Staatz G, Rohrmann D, Nolte-Ernsting CC, et al. Magnetic resonance urography in children: evaluation of suspected ureteral ectopia in duplex systems. J Urol 2001;166(6):2346–50.

46. Friedland GW, Cunningham J. The elusive ectopic ureteroceles. AJR Am J Roentgenol 1972;116: 792–811.

47. Brock WA, Kaplan WG. Ectopic ureteroceles in children. J Urol 1878;119:800–4.

48. Berdon WE, Baker DH, Becker JA. Ectopic ureterocele. Radiol Clin North Am 1968;6:205–14.

49. Hellstrom M, Hjalmas K, Jacobsson B, et al. Ureteral diameter in low-risk vesicoureteral reflux in infancy and childhood. Acta Radiol Diagn (Stockh) 1986;27(1):77–83.

50. Kass EJ. Megaureter. In: Kelalis PP, King LR, Belman AB, editors. Clinical pediatric urology. 3rd edition. Philadelphia: Saunders; 1992. p. 781–821.

51. Belman BA. A perspective on vesicoureteral reflux. Urol Clin North Am 1995;22:139–50.

52. Gross GW, Lebowitz RL. Infection does not cause reflux. AJR Am J Roentgenol 1981;137(5):929–32.

53. Smellie JM, Normand IC. Bacteriuria, reflux, and renal scarring. Arch Dis Child 1975;50(8):581–5.

54. Lebowitz RL, Olbing H, Parkkulainen KV, et al. International system of radiographic grading of vesicoureteric reflux. International Reflux Study in Children. Pediatr Radiol 1985;15(2):105–9.

55. Amos AM, Figlesthaler WM, Cookson MS. Bilateral ureteritis cystica with unilateral ureteropelvic junction obstruction. Tech Urol 1999;5(2):108–12.

56. Petersen UE, Kvist E, Friis M, et al. Ureteritis cystica. Scand J Urol Nephrol 1991;25(1):1–4.

57. Wasserman NF. Inflammatory disease of the ureter. Radiol Clin North Am 1996;34(6):1131–56.

58. Mitterberger M, Pinggera GM, Feuchtner G, et al. Sonographic measurement of renal pelvis wall thickness as diagnostic criterion for acute pyelonephritis in adults. Ultraschall Med 2007;28(6): 593–7.

59. Blandino A, Gaeta M, Minutoli F, et al. MR urography of the ureter. AJR Am J Roentgenol 2002; 179(5):1307–14.

60. Muttarak M, ChiangMai WN, Lojanapiwat B. Tuberculosis of the genitourinary tract: imaging features with pathological correlation. Singapore Med J 2005;46(10):568–74 [quiz: 75].

61. Bechtold RB, Chen MY, Dyer RB, et al. CT of the ureteral wall. AJR Am J Roentgenol 1998;170(5): 1283–9.

62. Dalrymple NC, Casford B, Raiken DP, et al. Pearls and pitfalls in the diagnosis of ureterolithiasis with unenhanced helical CT. Radiographics 2000; 20(2):439–47 [quiz: 527–8, 32].

63. Smith RC, Verga M, McCarthy S, et al. Diagnosis of acute flank pain: value of unenhanced helical CT. AJR Am J Roentgenol 1996;166(1):97–101.

64. Chen MY, Zagoria RJ. Can noncontrast helical computed tomography replace intravenous urography for evaluation of patients with acute urinary tract colic? J Emerg Med 1999;17(2):299–303.

65. Park SJ, Yi BH, Lee HK, et al. Evaluation of patients with suspected ureteral calculi using sonography as an initial diagnostic tool: how can we improve diagnostic accuracy? J Ultrasound Med 2008; 27(10):1441–50.

66. Wang ZJ, Meng MV, Yeh BM, et al. Ureteral fibroepithelial polyp. J Ultrasound Med 2008;27(11): 1647–9.

67. Harvin HJ. Ureteral fibroepithelial polyp on MDCT urography. AJR Am J Roentgenol 2006;187(4): W434–5.

68. Bellin MF, Springer O, Mourey-Gerosa I, et al. CT diagnosis of ureteral fibroepithelial polyps. Eur Radiol 2002;12(1):125–8.

69. Plante P, Smayra T, Bouchard L, et al. Ureteral tumors. In: Joffre F, Otal P, Soulie M, editors. Radiological imaging of the ureter. Berlin: Springer-Verlag; 2003. p. 127–53.

70. Vikram R, Sandler CM, Ng CS. Imaging and staging of transitional cell carcinoma: part 2, upper urinary tract. AJR Am J Roentgenol 2009;192(6): 1488–93.

71. Browne RF, Meehan CP, Colville J, et al. Transitional cell carcinoma of the upper urinary tract: spectrum of imaging findings. Radiographics 2005;25(6): 1609–27.

72. Wong-You-Cheong JJ, Wagner BJ, Davis CJ Jr. Transitional cell carcinoma of the urinary tract: radiologic-pathologic correlation. Radiographics 1998;18(1):123–42 [quiz: 48].

73. Caoili EM, Cohan RH, Inampudi P, et al. MDCT urography of upper tract urothelial neoplasms. AJR Am J Roentgenol 2005;184(6):1873–81.

74. Holmäng S, Lele SM, Johansson SL. Squamous cell carcinoma of the renal pelvis and ureter: incidence, symptoms, treatment and outcome. J Urol 2007;178(1):51–6.

75. Busby JE, Brown GA, Tamboli P, et al. Upper urinary tract tumors with nontransitional histology: a single-center experience. Urology 2006;67(3):518–23.

76. Spires SE, Banks ER, Cibull ML, et al. Adenocarcinoma of renal pelvis. Arch Pathol Lab Med 1993; 117(11):1156–60.

77. McMillin KI, Gross BH. CT demonstration of peripelvic and periureteral non-Hodgkin lymphoma. AJR Am J Roentgenol 1985;144(5):945–6.

78. Curry NS, Chung CJ, Potts W, et al. Isolated lymphoma of genitourinary tract and adrenals. Urology 1993;41(5):494–8.

79. Connor SE, Umaria N, Guest PJ. Case report: extranodal peripelvic and periureteric lymphoma–demonstration with computed tomography. Clin Radiol 2001;56(5):422–4.

80. Gakis G, Merseburger AS, Sotlar K, et al. Metastasis of malignant melanoma in the ureter: possible algorithms for a therapeutic approach. Int J Urol 2009;16(4):407–9.

81. Winalski CS, Lipman JC, Tumeh SS. Ureteral neoplasms. Radiographics 1990;10(2):271–83.

82. Marincek B, Scheidegger JR, Studer UE, et al. Metastatic disease of the ureter: patterns of tumoral spread and radiologic findings. Abdom Imaging 1993;18(1):88–94.

83. Presti JC, Carroll PR, McAninch JW. Ureteral and renal pelvic injuries from external trauma: diagnosis and management. J Trauma 1989;29(3): 370–4.

84. Lynch TH, Martínez-Piñeiro L, Plas E, et al. EAU guidelines on urological trauma. Eur Urol 2005; 47(1):1–15.

85. Best CD, Petrone P, Buscarini M, et al. Traumatic ureteral injuries: a single institution experience validating the American Association for the Surgery of Trauma-Organ Injury Scale grading scale. J Urol 2005;173(4):1202–5.

86. Elliott SP, McAninch JW. Ureteral injuries from external violence: the 25-year experience at San

Francisco General Hospital. J Urol 2003;170(4 Pt 1): 1213–6.

87. Perez-Brayfield MR, Keane TE, Krishnan A, et al. Gunshot wounds to the ureter: a 40-year experience at Grady Memorial Hospital. J Urol 2001; 166(1):119–21.

88. Lee RA, Symmonds RE, Williams TJ. Current status of genitourinary fistula. Obstet Gynecol 1988;72(3 Pt 1): 313–9.

89. St Lezin MA, Stoller ML. Surgical ureteral injuries. Urology 1991;38(6):497–506.

90. Brandes S, Coburn M, Armenakas N, et al. Diagnosis and management of ureteric injury: an evidence-based analysis. BJU Int 2004;94(3): 277–89.

91. Moore EE, Cogbill TH, Jurkovich GJ, et al. Organ injury scaling. III: chest wall, abdominal vascular, ureter, bladder, and urethra. J Trauma 1992;33(3): 337–9.

92. Stevenson J, Battistella FD. The 'one-shot' intravenous pyelogram: is it indicated in unstable trauma patients before celiotomy? J Trauma 1994;36(6): 828–33 [discussion: 33–4].

93. Ramchandani P, Buckler PM. Imaging of genitourinary trauma. AJR Am J Roentgenol 2009;192(6): 1514–23.

94. Kawashima A, Sandler CM, Corriere JN, et al. Ureteropelvic junction injuries secondary to blunt abdominal trauma. Radiology 1997;205(2): 487–92.

95. Gilkeson GS, Allen NB. Retroperitoneal fibrosis. A true connective tissue disease. Rheum Dis Clin North Am 1996;22(1):23–38.

96. Koep L, Zuidema GD. The clinical significance of retroperitoneal fibrosis. Surgery 1977;81(3):250–7.

97. Miller OF, Smith LJ, Ferrara EX, et al. Presentation of idiopathic retroperitoneal fibrosis in the pediatric population. J Pediatr Surg 2003;38(11):1685–8.

98. Kottra JJ, Dunnick NR. Retroperitoneal fibrosis. Radiol Clin North Am 1996;34(6):1259–75.

99. Vivas I, Nicolás AI, Velázquez P, et al. Retroperitoneal fibrosis: typical and atypical manifestations. Br J Radiol 2000;73(866):214–22.

100. Arrivé L, Hricak H, Tavares NJ, et al. Malignant versus nonmalignant retroperitoneal fibrosis: differentiation with MR imaging. Radiology 1989;172(1): 139–43.

101. Nezhat C, Nezhat F, Nezhat CH, et al. Urinary tract endometriosis treated by laparoscopy. Fertil Steril 1996;66(6):920–4.

102. Stanley KE, Utz DC, Dockerty MB. Clinically significant endometriosis of the urinary tract. Surg Gynecol Obstet 1965;120:491–8.

103. Kyriakidis A, Pappas I. Ureteral endometriosis in a female patient presenting with single-kidney anuria. Eur Urol 1995;28(2):175–6.

104. Lam AM, French M, Charnock FM. Bilateral ureteric obstruction due to recurrent endometriosis associated with hormone replacement therapy. Aust N Z J Obstet Gynaecol 1992;32(1):83–4.

105. Esen T, Akinci M, Ander H, et al. Bilateral ureteric obstruction secondary to endometriosis. Br J Urol 1990;66(1):98–9.

106. Wang LJ, Wong YC, Chuang CK, et al. Diagnostic accuracy of transitional cell carcinoma on multidetector computerized tomography urography in patients with gross hematuria. J Urol 2009;181(2): 524–31 [discussion: 31].

107. Bazot M, Darai E, Hourani R, et al. Deep pelvic endometriosis: MR imaging for diagnosis and prediction of extension of disease. Radiology 2004;232(2):379–89.

108. Phinney A, Hanson J, Talner LB. Diagnosis of renal pelvis subepithelial hemorrhage using unenhanced helical CT. AJR Am J Roentgenol 2000;174(4): 1023–4.

109. Fishman MC, Pollack HM, Arger PH, et al. Radiographic manifestations of spontaneous renal sinus hemorrhage. AJR Am J Roentgenol 1984;142(6): 1161–4.

Imaging Features of Common and Uncommon Bladder Neoplasms

Samdeep Mouli, MD, MS[a],*, David D. Casalino, MD[a],
Paul Nikolaidis, MD[b]

KEYWORDS

- Bladder neoplasms • Computed tomography
- Magnetic resonance imaging • Transitional cell carcinoma
- Squamous cell carcinoma

The urinary bladder is located within the extraperitoneal space, surrounded by pelvic fat. Four layers compose the bladder wall: mucosa (urothelium); a vascular submucosa (lamina propria); muscularis propria (inner and outer longitudinal smooth muscle, with an intervening circular layer); and adventitia. The peritoneum serves as a serosal covering, bolstering the bladder dome.[1–3] The bladder trigone contains an extra layer of detrusor muscle, lending it a slightly thicker appearance than the adjacent bladder wall.[2]

The urothelium is lined by layers of transitional cells, which can transform into a variety of benign and malignant tumors. Most tumors (90% to 95%) are epithelial in origin.[4] Benign entities include papillomas and adenomas. Malignant tumors are more common and include entities, such as urothelial cell carcinoma, squamous cell carcinoma, and adenocarcinoma, and rarer entities, including small cell or neuroendocrine carcinoma and carcinoid tumors.[3,5–7] Furthermore, epithelial tumors may exhibit mixed cell types, such as concomitant urothelial and squamous cell carcinoma or urothelial carcinoma and adenocarcinoma.[8]

Nonepithelial tumors, or mesenchymal tumors, include benign entities, such as leiomyoma and neurofibroma, and malignant entities, including leiomyosarcoma and lymphoma.[9]

Although there is considerable overlap in the clinical and radiologic presentation of these neoplasms, biopsy provides definitive diagnosis. However, many of these entities have specific radiologic features that may dictate clinical management.

IMAGING TECHNIQUES

Evaluation of the bladder begins with direct visualization of the mucosa using cystoscopy. However, clinical staging with cystoscopy cannot reliably determine the depth of invasion or histologic diagnosis, both critical prognostic factors. Clinical staging is inaccurate in 25% to 50% of patients with muscle invasive malignancies.[10,11] Therefore, imaging strategies using computed tomography (CT) or magnetic resonance (MR) imaging are used to complement cystoscopic examinations.

CT has become the imaging modality of choice for the evaluation of hematuria, supplanting previous strategies, including excretory urography.[12] CT urography (CTU) protocols permit the evaluation of the lower urinary tract as well as evaluate for direct perirenal, periureteral, and extravesical tumor extension, in addition to lymphadenopathy and distant metastasis.[13] The use of multidetector helical CT permits fast volumetric acquisition of

Disclosures: No disclosures.
Funding support: None.
[a] Department of Radiology, Northwestern University, 676 North Saint Clair, Suite 800, Chicago, IL 60611, USA
[b] Department of Radiology, Northwestern University, Feinberg School of Medicine, 676 North Saint Clair, Suite 800, Chicago, IL 60611, USA
* Corresponding author.
E-mail address: s-mouli@northwestern.edu

Radiol Clin N Am 50 (2012) 301–316
doi:10.1016/j.rcl.2012.02.001
0033-8389/12/$ – see front matter © 2012 Elsevier Inc. All rights reserved.

high-resolution images in addition to multiplanar reconstruction capabilities.

CTU has a reported sensitivity and specificity of 79% and 94% respectively for bladder malignancies.[14] However, CTU is primarily useful in the evaluation of advanced stage disease. Specifically, CTU cannot determine the depth of invasion[15] or microscopic perivesical invasion.[1] Overall accuracy for local bladder cancer staging is approximately 60%, with a tendency to overstage.[3]

MR imaging has several advantages for evaluating bladder neoplasms because of its superior soft tissue resolution and direct multiplanar imaging capabilities.[16] Additionally, contrast between perivesical fat, bladder wall soft tissue, and urine permits excellent soft tissue detail, allowing improved local staging over CTU. Reported accuracy for overall staging ranges from 60% to 85%, with local staging accuracy ranging from 73% to 96%.[17]

MR imaging is performed using a pelvic phased array coil to permit high resolution for local staging.[1] Standard sequences include T2-weighted imaging (T2WI) and precontrast and postcontrast T1-weighted imaging (T1WI). T1WI images allow the depiction of the tumor, perivesical invasion, and lymph node or bone marrow involvement.[1,18] On T1WI, the bladder tumor typically has a low to intermediate signal intensity similar to that of the bladder wall.[16] With the use of gadolinium contrast, tumors involving the urothelium and submucosa demonstrate prominent enhancement compared with the uninvolved bladder wall.[19,20] T2WI allows the assessment of bladder wall invasion, or invasion into surrounding structures, such as the prostate or seminal vesicles, and uterus or cervix.[1] On T2WI, the tumors tend to be more conspicuous because they contrast with surrounding structures (because the signal intensity of tumors is typically intermediate between that of the darker bladder wall muscle and the brighter high-signal-intensity urine).[16]

Diffusion-weighted imaging is a newer MR imaging technique that evaluates thermally

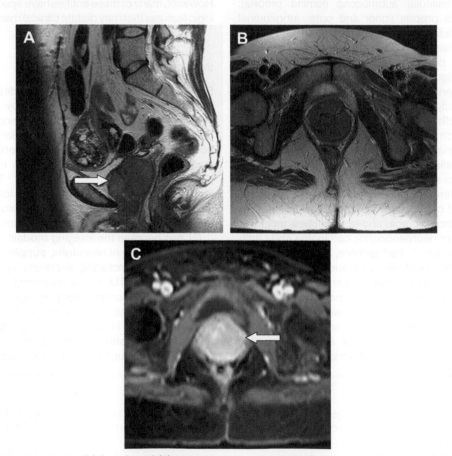

Fig. 1. Leiomyoma. Sagittal (A) and axial (B) T2WI demonstrate a smooth intramural mass (A–arrow) along the posterior superior bladder wall. The mass demonstrates homogenous low signal intensity. (C) Axial contrast-enhanced T1WI shows uniform avid enhancement (arrow).

induced Brownian motion in cellular tissues.[21] With the increased cellularity of tissues (which is seen in malignancy), there is a proportional increase in water molecule diffusion restriction. An apparent diffusion coefficient map can be calculated reflecting the diffusion properties of the tissue; this may then be used as an imaging biomarker for tissue characterization, cancer detection, and to assess response to treatment.[22] This technique is still under investigation, but several investigators have validated its utility.[23–25]

BENIGN BLADDER NEOPLASMS
Leiomyoma

Leiomyomas of the bladder are rare (0.43% of bladder neoplasms); however, they are the most-common benign bladder tumors. Patients present with a wide age range, spanning from 20 to 80 years,[26] and equal incidence between men and women. Most lesions are small and asymptomatic. Larger lesions typically present with symptoms caused by mass effect or urinary obstruction, such as hesitancy, frequency, and hematuria.[27] Although these tumors originate from the

submucosa, growth may be intravesical (63%), extravesical (30%), or intramural (7%).[28]

Tumors are usually found incidentally on CT and appear as homogenous, solid masses that cause smooth compression of the bladder or extend intraluminally.[1] Cystic components indicate degeneration or necrosis. MR imaging is superior to CT for characterization, better demonstrating their submucosal origin and muscular preservation.[9] T1WI demonstrates intermediate signal intensity, whereas T2WI shows low signal intensity. In the presence of cystic degeneration, high signal intensity may be seen on T2WI.[29] Enhancement is variable following contrast administration (Fig. 1).[9] Although these are benign tumors without malignant potential, histologic evaluation is necessary to exclude leiomyosarcoma. The treatment of choice is, therefore, local excision; preoperative imaging may demonstrate benign features that may obviate radical surgery.[9]

Paraganglioma

Extra-adrenal pheochromocytomas, or paragangliomas, compose 0.1% of all bladder tumors and 1% of all pheochromocytomas. The mean

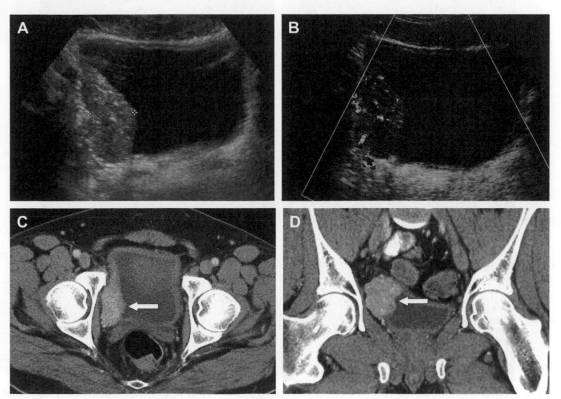

Fig. 2. Bladder paraganglioma. Transverse sonogram of the bladder (A) demonstrates a right lateral intramural mass projecting into the bladder lumen, demarcated by the calipers. Transverse color Doppler sonogram (B) shows the mass to be markedly hypervascular. Axial (C) and coronal (D) contrast-enhanced CT demonstrates the mass to be homogenously enhancing (arrow).

age of diagnosis is 41 years, with a wide age range, and higher female prevalence.[9] These lesions originate from the chromaffin cells in the sympathetic chain found in the detrusor muscle layer at the bladder trigone.[9] Most lesions are metabolically active, with a characteristic catecholamine release during micturition, or micturition attack, seen in 50% of patients. Patients present with hematuria, headache, sweating, anxiety, palpitation, syncope, and hypertension. Most lesions are sporadic; however, they can also be associated with familial syndromes, including neurofibromatosis, von Hippel-Lindau syndrome, Sturge-Weber syndrome, tuberous sclerosis, and multiple endocrine neoplasia.[30]

Radiologically, these lesions appear as homogenous, solid, intramural or submucosal masses, demonstrating marked enhancement following contrast administration (Fig. 2). Heterogeneity is seen with cystic necrosis or hemorrhage. Additionally, peripheral ring calcification is highly suggestive of these lesions.[31] These lesions also demonstrate characteristic MR imaging features:

T1WI shows low signal intensity, whereas T2WI and submucosal location. They enhance avidly following gadolinium administration. Iodine-131-metaiodobenzylguandine (MIBG) scanning is highly specific for their diagnosis (96%); however, MR imaging remains more sensitive than either MIBG or CT.[32] Treatment involves local excision under adrenergic blockade. Long-term follow-up is necessary because histology in not predictive of malignancy, which can be seen in up to 18% of cases.[31,33]

Neurofibroma

The bladder is the most-common site of genitourinary neurofibroma, a rare entity. These lesions may be sporadic or may be seen with neurofibromatosis type I.[9] These lesions originate from neural plexus tissue found at the trigone[34] and can present in localized, diffuse, or plexiform forms. The plexiform variant involves thickened neural nodules, which cause bladder wall thickening. An intraluminal bladder mass may be

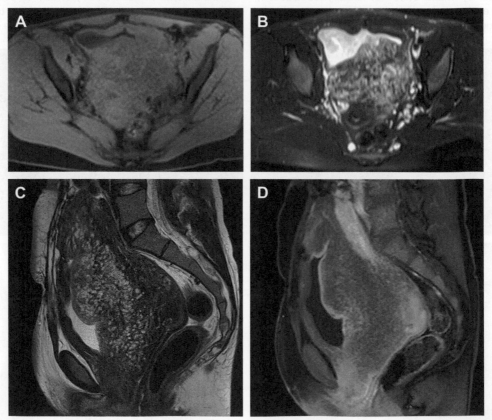

Fig. 3. Plexiform neurofibroma. Axial noncontrast T1WI (A) shows a large ill-defined predominantly isointense mass that is inseparable from the bladder. Axial T2WI with fat saturation (B) demonstrates marked heterogeneity of the mass with areas of increased signal intensity. Sagittal T2WI (C) shows a large pelvic mass and numerous characteristic target signs. Sagittal contrast-enhanced T1WI (D) shows the mass to be relatively hypointense and hypoenhancing. On subsequent axial postcontrast images, increased enhancement was seen (not shown).

seen, which may result in ureteral obstruction and hydronephrosis. There may be involvement of contiguous surrounding structures, such as the prostate in men, vagina or uterus in women, or the rectum.[34] Patients may present with urinary tract infections and irritative voiding symptoms.

On CT, a low-attenuation, heterogeneously enhancing, nodular bladder wall mass is often seen, with extension into the pelvic side wall.[35] MR demonstrates low T1 signal and a characteristic target sign on T2WI,[36] seen with the plexiform variant (**Fig. 3**). The lesions enhance following contrast administration.

MALIGNANT BLADDER NEOPLASMS

Most bladder tumors are malignant, representing the fourth most-common type of cancer in men (6%–8%), with a 4:1 male-to-female predominance. The peak incidence is in the sixth to seventh decades; however, the incidence in younger patients is rising.[37–40] Most tumors, approximately 90%, are uroepithelial in origin, with urothelial tumors (previously known as transitional cell carcinoma) composing 90%. The remaining cell types include squamous cell carcinoma (6%–8%) and adenocarcinoma (1%–2%).[3,4,41] Rare entities include small cell or neuroendocrine carcinoma (<1%).[42] Nonepithelial malignancies compose less than 10% of bladder neoplasms and include non-Hodgkin lymphoma and leiomyosarcoma, among others.

Prognosis depends on the pathologic stage, which is determined by the TNM staging system by the American Joint Committee on Cancer (**Table 1**). Increased depth of invasion is associated with poorer prognosis.[2,43–46] With tumors confined to the lamina propria, 5-year survival ranges from 55% to 80%. Five-year survival decreases to 40% with muscular invasion, 20% with perivesical extension, and 5% with metastatic disease.[47]

The cause of most of these lesions stems from prolonged urothelial contact with carcinogens.[9] Thus, there is a propensity for bladder malignancies, especially urothelial carcinoma, to be multicentric with synchronous and metachronous involvement of the urinary tract.[9] Cigarette smoking is the most well-established risk factor for bladder cancer, causing 50% to 66% of cancers in men and 35% of cancers in women.[48,49] Other chemical carcinogens, found through occupational exposures, include aniline, benzidine, aromatic amines, and azo dyes, which account for 20% of the cases.[4] Finally, bladder tumors can be hereditary in 8% of cases.[1] These lesions are typically managed surgically, with the extent of resection determined by the pathologic stage.

Table 1 TNM classification from AJCC	
TX	Primary tumor cannot be assessed
T0	No tumor
Tis	Carcinoma in situ
Ta	Papillary tumor confined to the epithelium
T1	Tumor invades superficial connective tissue (lamina propria)
T2a	Tumor invades superficial muscle layer (inner half)
T2b	Tumor invades deep muscle layer (outer half)
T3a	Tumor invades perivesical fat (microscopic)
T3b	Tumor invades perivesical fat (macroscopic)
T4a	Tumor invades surrounding organs
T4b	Tumor invades pelvic or abdominal wall
N1	Metastasis in single pelvic lymph node ≤2 cm
N2	Metastasis in single pelvic lymph node >2 cm and ≤5 cm or multiple nodes ≤5 cm
N3	Metastasis in single node >5 cm
N4	Lymph node metastases above the bifurcation of the common iliac arteries
M1	Distant metastases

Used with the permission of the American Joint Committee on Cancer (AJCC), Chicago, Illinois. The original source for this material is the AJCC Cancer Staging Manual, Seventh Edition (2010) published by Springer-Verlag New York, www.springer.com.

Urothelial Carcinoma

Urothelial carcinoma accounts for most bladder neoplasms, malignant or otherwise. Most patients present with painless microscopic hematuria. Other symptoms may result from irritation and reduced bladder capacity, including urinary frequency, urgency, and dysuria. Advanced lesions may present with urinary obstruction, pelvic pain, or a palpable mass.[4,50]

On CT, T1 lesions are seen as either asymmetric bladder wall thickening or a pedunculated or polypoid mass. T2 neoplasms generally appear as sessile lesions; however, CT imaging cannot distinguish muscle invasion, as seen with T2b lesions. CT can differentiate T3a and T3b lesions by demonstrating perivesical soft tissue infiltration in the latter stage. T4 lesions demonstrate invasion of adjacent organs and structures. Overdistension of the bladder limits the accuracy of staging, which ranges from 40% to 60% for CT.[51] Nodular calcification may be seen along the surface of tumors on noncontrast CT (Fig. 4).[52] Early enhancement is seen with contrast administration.[53]

MR imaging provides superior soft tissue resolution compared with CT, permitting improved localization and characterization of neoplasms. The use of phase array coils allows for a high signal-to-noise ratio and smaller field-of-view high-resolution imaging.[54] The inherent high contrast on MR imaging examinations permits the differentiation of the different bladder wall layers. On T1WI, the bladder wall and tumor should demonstrate intermediate signal intensity, whereas the urine is dark. With T2WI, tumors demonstrate intermediate to high signal intensity, whereas the adjacent bladder wall is low in signal (Fig. 5). T2WI is, thus, ideal for determining the depth of invasion, both into the muscle and perivesical fat (T3b) and into surrounding organs (T4).[55] A search for additional lesions should be undertaken on imaging given their propensity to be multicentric with synchronous and metachronous involvement of the urinary tract and for complications, such as hydronephrosis and hydroureter (Fig. 6).

Tumors may also arise in bladder diverticula, which may develop secondary to chronic bladder outlet obstruction or increased intravesical pressure. In this setting, urinary stasis within the diverticula occurs, leading to a 10% risk of development of a malignancy. Although these patients have a propensity to develop squamous cell carcinomas, most of these lesions are urothelial carcinomas. Prognosis is generally poor because of the difficulty in diagnosis and early invasion caused by the lack of a muscular layer of the diverticulum.[9] These lesions are often not evident on cystoscopy because the neck of the diverticulum, if narrow, may not be seen and there may be difficulty in passing the cystoscope into the diverticulum. Cross-sectional imaging may be necessary for diagnosis (Figs. 7 and 8).

Squamous Cell Carcinoma

Squamous cell carcinoma accounts for 6% to 8% of bladder cancers.[1,56] The pathogenesis of this lesion stems from chronic bladder irritation. It can be seen in the setting of recurrent urinary tract infections, bladder calculi, or chronic indwelling catheterization.[57] These tumors are especially prevalent in patients with spinal cord injuries, who are at increased risk.[4] Furthermore, in regions

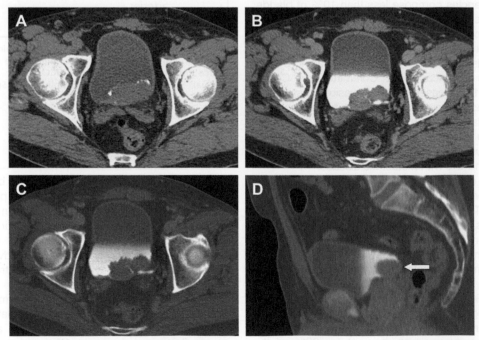

Fig. 4. Transitional cell carcinoma. Axial noncontrast CT (*A*) shows an irregular left posterior bladder wall mass with multiple superficial calcifications. Corresponding axial contrast-enhanced CT (*B*) obtained during the excretory phase demonstrates enhancement of this mass. Axial (*C*) and sagittal (*D*) contrast-enhanced CT during the excretory phase from the same patient, using bone window algorithms, demonstrates the mass as an irregular filling defect within the bladder (*arrow*).

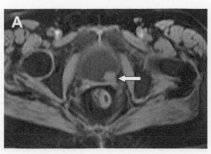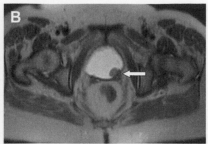

Fig. 5. Transitional cell carcinoma. Axial precontrast T1WI (*A*) demonstrates an isointense, small polypoid mass arising from right posterior bladder wall (*arrow*). Corresponding axial T2WI (*B*) shows the mass to be of intermediate signal intensity (*arrow*). On T2WI, these tumors tend to be quite conspicuous because they contrast with the surrounding darker bladder wall muscle and the high-signal-intensity urine.

where schistosomiasis is endemic, squamous cell carcinomas compose 50% of bladder cancers.[58]

Tumors are typically high grade and locally aggressive, presenting with muscular invasion in 80% of patients at diagnosis.[59] Tumors preferentially arise from the trigone and lateral walls and can be seen in bladder diverticula.[60] On CT, imaging characteristics for these lesions are nonspecific: tumors present as either focal or diffuse bladder wall thickening or a single enhancing mass (**Fig. 9**).[61,62] Unlike urothelial carcinoma, squamous cell carcinoma typically demonstrates sessile, not papillary, growth. Lesions within diverticula appear as soft tissue masses with occasional overlying calcification.[60]

On MR imaging, squamous cell carcinomas typically demonstrate intermediate signal intensity on T1WI and T2WI and avid enhancement following contrast administration (**Fig. 10**).

Adenocarcinoma

Adenocarcinoma accounts for less than 2% of bladder cancers. Tumors are categorized as primary, urachal, or secondary (metastatic) malignancies.[63] The mean age at presentation of primary adenocarcinoma is 60 years, with urachal lesions seen 10 years earlier. Most patients present with hematuria (90%), whereas irritative voiding symptoms can be seen in up to half of patients. Lesions are associated with bladder

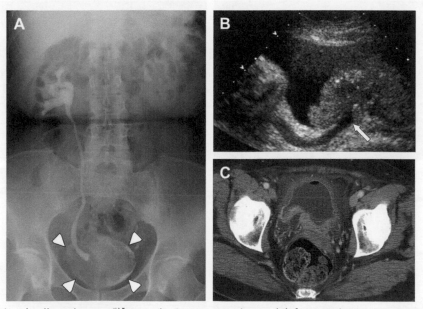

Fig. 6. Transitional cell carcinoma. Fifteen-minute excretory image (*A*) from an intravenous urogram demonstrates a large irregular filling defect within the bladder (*arrowheads*) along with dilatation of the right collecting system. Longitudinal sonogram (*B*) on the same patient demonstrates an irregular mural mass involving the posterior bladder wall with resultant distal hydroureter (*arrow*). Axial contrast-enhanced CT (*C*) shows an irregular right posterior bladder wall mass involving the right ureterovesicular junction with resulting obstruction. Note the dilatation of the adjacent distal right ureter.

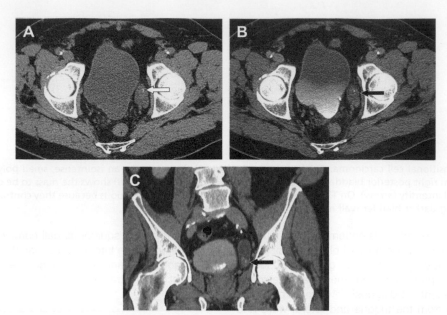

Fig. 7. Transitional cell carcinoma in a bladder diverticulum. Axial noncontrast CT (*A*) shows a left lateral bladder wall diverticulum with a subtle area of increased density and faint punctate calcification (*arrow*). Corresponding axial (*B*) and coronal (*C*) contrast-enhanced CT images obtained during the excretory phase show a small enhancing mass within the diverticulum (*arrows*).

exstrophy and a persistent urachus.[9] Primary adenocarcinoma may be subdivided into mucinous and signet ring cell types. Signet ring cancers can present with diffuse infiltration, producing linitis plastica of the bladder.[64] Urachal lesions may present with urinary mucus (25%) or umbilical discharge. Secondary, or metastatic, lesions are typically from direct invasion by

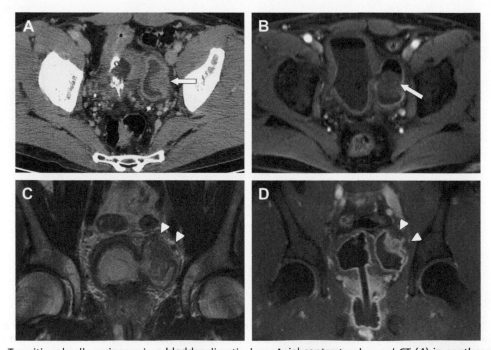

Fig. 8. Transitional cell carcinoma in a bladder diverticulum. Axial contrast-enhanced CT (*A*) in another patient shows a large left-sided bladder diverticulum with an enhancing mass (*arrow*). Corresponding axial noncontrast T1WI (*B*) shows the isointense mass within the diverticulum (*arrow*). Coronal T2WI (*C*) and contrast-enhanced T1WI (*D*) nicely depict invasion of the perivesical fat (*arrowheads*).

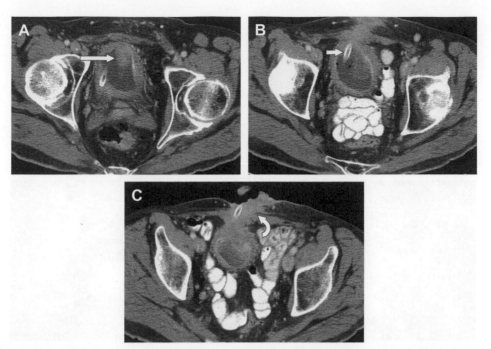

Fig. 9. Squamous cell carcinoma. Sequential axial contrast-enhanced CT images (*A–C*) in a patient with paraplegia with a chronic indwelling suprapubic bladder catheter (*short arrow*) show diffuse bladder wall thickening and a large enhancing bladder mass extending from the anterior aspect of the bladder (*long arrow*) to the subcutaneous tissues and skin surface (*curved arrow*).

adjacent pelvic neoplasms, particularly tumors of the prostate, colon, and rectum.[65,66]

Urachal adenocarcinomas are typically seen midline at the bladder dome (**Fig. 11**). Most (90%) are seen adjacent to the bladder, with the remainder seen along the course of the urachus.[9] CT will also often demonstrate peripheral calcification, seen in 72% of lesions. Characteristically, a midline, infraumbilical soft tissue mass with calcifications is seen.[66] A prominent extravesical component is usually seen, with lesions often exceeding 5 cm.[67] On CT, 84% of tumors will show mixed solid and cystic components because of the underlying mucin production (**Fig. 12**).[9]

On sagittal T2-weighted MR images, focal areas of high signal intensity, secondary to mucin, are a distinctive feature of adenocarcinomas.[68] The solid components are typically isointense on T1WI and enhance with contrast. Prognosis is generally poor because these lesions tend to be high grade and diffusely infiltrative at presentation, especially urachal subtypes.[4]

Small Cell Tumors

Composing less than 0.5% of bladder neoplasms, small cell tumors are a rare entity. They are derived from dedifferentiated neuroendocrine cells and are

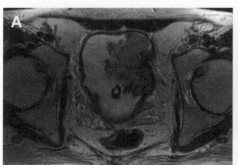
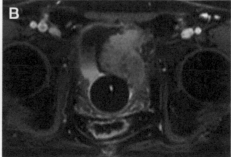

Fig. 10. Squamous cell carcinoma. Axial T2WI (*A*) in another patient with a chronic indwelling Foley catheter shows a large heterogeneous lobulated mass arising from the left lateral wall of the bladder. Corresponding post-contrast T1WI (*B*) shows avid enhancement of the large bladder mass.

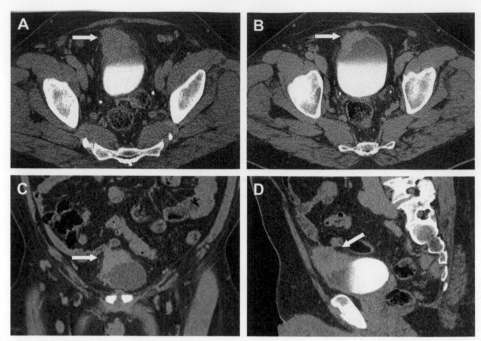

Fig. 11. Urachal adenocarcinoma. Sequential axial contrast-enhanced CT images (*A, B*) show an enhancing mass arising from the superior aspect of the bladder (*arrow*). The classic midline location of this tumor, continuity with the bladder dome, and extravesical extension (*arrows*) are all best appreciated on the coronal (*C*) and sagittal (*D*) contrast-enhanced CT reformations.

highly aggressive lesions, typically presenting with invasive disease at the time of diagnosis.[4,69,70] Early lymph node metastasis is seen in 66%, and distant metastases to liver, lung, and bone occur.[4] Hematuria is present in 85% of patients and 65% are smokers.[55,56] These tumors show a male predominance, with a male-to-female ratio of 4:1.

Imaging reveals large nodular or polypoid invasive bladder masses (**Figs. 13** and **14**). Central necrosis and cystic changes are characteristic findings,[71] along with patchy enhancement.[72] Aggressive local invasion and diffuse peritoneal

metastases are often seen.[70] Despite radical surgical excision, prognosis is generally poor, with a 5-year survival of 16%.[70,73]

Leiomyosarcoma

Leiomyosarcoma is the most-common malignant mesenchymal tumor of the bladder, representing less than 1% of bladder malignancies. Increased prevalence is seen in patients with a history of pelvic irradiation or prior cyclophosphamide chemotherapy. These lesions have a male-to-female ratio of 2:1, and most patients present

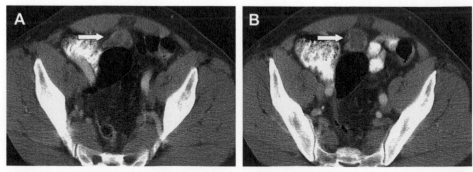

Fig. 12. Urachal adenocarcinoma. Sequential axial contrast-enhanced CT images (*A, B*) show a heterogeneous midline mass immediately superior to the bladder with an area of central low attenuation (*arrows*), representing an area of cystic change with a high mucin content.

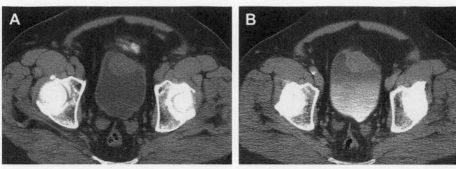

Fig. 13. Small cell tumor of the bladder. Axial noncontrast CT (*A*) shows an irregular anterior bladder wall mass without calcifications. Corresponding axial contrast-enhanced CT (*B*) during the excretory phase demonstrates slightly heterogeneous enhancement of this mass.

between the ages of 60 and 80 years.[26] Tumors are often high grade and aggressive, with local recurrence and metastatic disease seen in 16% and 53% of patients respectively.[9] Gross hematuria is the most-common presenting symptom, but patients may also exhibit urinary obstruction or a pelvic mass on examination. Lesions are typically located at the bladder dome but can occur at other sites. Tumors are often large and polypoid and extend into the bladder lumen and extravesical space.[26]

It may be difficult to distinguish leiomyosarcoma from its benign counterpart, leiomyoma. On CT, leiomyosarcoma may demonstrate more ill-defined margins; following iodinated contrast administration, central areas of necrosis or nonenhancement may be present (**Fig. 15**). On MR imaging, both lesions exhibit low T2 signal intensity.[19] However, leiomyosarcoma will more often demonstrate necrosis and poorly defined margins, heterogeneous signal intensity, and embedded areas of high T2 signal. Following contrast

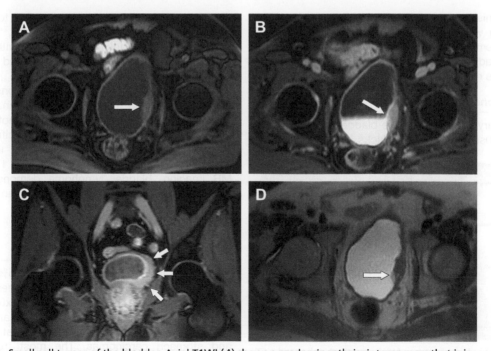

Fig. 14. Small cell tumor of the bladder. Axial T1WI (*A*) shows a predominantly isointense mass that is inseparable from the left lateral bladder wall (*arrow*). Axial contrast-enhanced T1WI (*B*) demonstrates avid enhancement of the mass (*arrow*). Coronal contrast-enhanced T1WI (*C*) shows diffuse irregularity and thickening of left lateral wall and subtle invasion of the perivesical fat (*short arrows*). The mass is slightly hyperintense to bladder muscle (*arrow*) on T2WI (*D*).

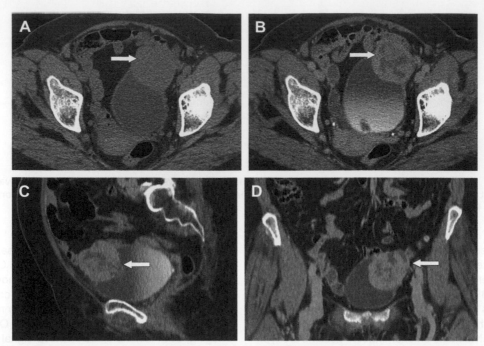

Fig. 15. Leiomyosarcoma. Axial noncontrast CT (*A*) and corresponding axial contrast-enhanced CT (*B*) show a large, heterogeneously enhancing mass (*arrows*) involving the anterior aspect of the bladder dome. The mass extends into the bladder lumen and into the extravesical space. Sagittal (*C*) and coronal (*D*) contrast-enhanced CT reformations nicely depict the anatomic location of the mass (*arrows*) and its relationship to adjacent bowel. Several hypodense, nonenhancing areas of internal degeneration are seen within the mass.

administration, patchy enhancement may be seen along with central areas of necrosis or nonenhancement. Treatment involves surgical excision with adjuvant chemotherapy. The 5-year survival rate is reported to be 62%.[27]

Lymphoma

Primary lymphoma of the bladder is a rare entity because the bladder lacks lymphoid tissue.

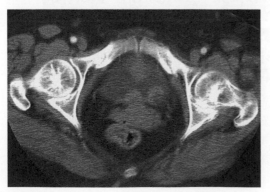

Fig. 16. Lymphoma. Axial contrast-enhanced CT shows multiple enhancing nodular lesions in the bladder in a woman with history of breast cancer and lung cancer. Lymphoma was diagnosed by biopsy performed at time of cystoscopy.

Secondary involvement is seen in 10% to 25% of patients with leukemia and lymphoma.[74] Most lesions are non-Hodgkin lymphoma,[75] with low-grade B-cell mucosa-associated lymphoid tissue and diffuse, large B-cell being the most-common histologic subtypes.[74] Lesions are most common in middle-aged women, who present with hematuria and irritative symptoms.[9] On CT, imaging findings are nonspecific but may include well-defined masses that involve the dome or lateral walls (**Figs. 16** and **17**). On MR imaging, bladder lymphoma demonstrates intermediate T1 and T2 signal intensity and mild enhancement with contrast.[76]

Metastases to the Bladder

Metastases to the bladder account for 15% of all malignant bladder tumors (**Fig. 18**).[77] These are most often seen in the setting of local extension from colonic, prostatic, or cervical malignancies.[1] Other sources include melanoma, breast, lung, and stomach carcinomas. The most frequent sites of involvement are the bladder neck and trigone.[77] Multifocal, predominantly submucosal vascular lesions may point to a metastatic origin.[78]

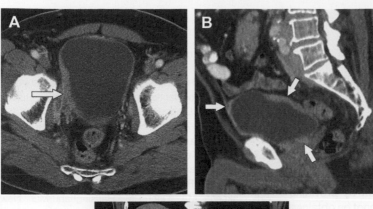

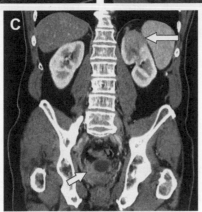

Fig. 17. Lymphoma. Axial contrast-enhanced CT image (*A*) demonstrates irregular thickening along the posterolateral bladder wall on the right (*arrow*). Sagittal contrast-enhanced CT reformatted image (*B*) from the same patient shows additional areas of nodularity and asymmetry involving the inferior, anterior, and superior bladder wall (*short arrows*). Lymphoma was diagnosed following cystoscopic biopsy. Coronal contrast-enhanced CT reformation in the same patient (*C*) only partially shows the bladder abnormalities (*short arrow*) but demonstrates an infiltrating lesion in the upper pole of the left kidney (*long arrow*), also representing lymphoma.

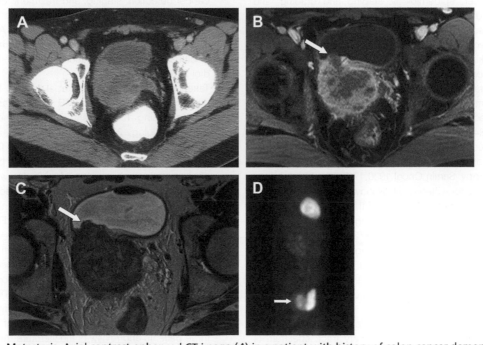

Fig. 18. Metastasis. Axial contrast-enhanced CT image (*A*) in a patient with history of colon cancer demonstrates a large exophytic heterogeneous mass along the posterolateral bladder wall on the right. The mass shows invasion into the bladder wall (*arrow*) on T2WI (*B*). Axial contrast-enhanced T1WI (*C*) better demonstrates invasion through the bladder wall into the bladder lumen (*arrow*). Note the marked heterogeneity of the mass with large areas of necrosis. Sagittal image from a positron emission tomography scan in the same patient (*D*) shows a large area of abnormal hypermetabolic activity posterior to the bladder (*arrow*). This mass was separate from the adjacent rectum, and endoscopic biopsy proved adenocarcinoma metastasis.

SUMMARY

Although urothelial carcinoma represents the most-common bladder neoplasm, other epithelial and mesenchymal tumors can be seen. Clinical presentation can be similar for many lesions, and cystoscopic examination with biopsy is often needed for diagnosis. However, improved imaging capabilities of multidetector CT and MR imaging allow these imaging modalities to be useful adjuncts to cystoscopic evaluation by providing critical staging information that cannot be obtained from clinical evaluation alone. As such, imaging plays an important role in directing clinical management of these patients.

REFERENCES

1. Dighe MK, Bhargava P, Wright J. Urinary bladder masses: techniques, imaging spectrum, and staging. J Comput Assist Tomogr 2011;35(4):411–24.
2. Lawler LP. MR imaging of the bladder. Radiol Clin North Am 2003;41(1):161–77.
3. Zhang J, Gerst S, Lefkowitz RA, et al. Imaging of bladder cancer. Radiol Clin North Am 2007;45(1): 183–205.
4. Kirkali Z, Chan T, Manoharan M, et al. Bladder cancer: epidemiology, staging and grading, and diagnosis. Urology 2005;66(6 Suppl 1):4–34.
5. Wilson TG, Pritchett TR, Lieskovsky G, et al. Primary adenocarcinoma of bladder. Urology 1991;38(3):223–6.
6. Kakizoe T, Matsumoto K, Andoh M, et al. Adenocarcinoma of urachus. Report of 7 cases and review of literature. Urology 1983;21(4):360–6.
7. Kantor AF, Hartge P, Hoover RN, et al. Urinary tract infection and risk of bladder cancer. Am J Epidemiol 1984;119(4):510–5.
8. Reuter VE. Pathology of bladder cancer: assessment of prognostic variables and response to therapy. Semin Oncol 1990;17(5):524–32.
9. Wong-You-Cheong JJ, Woodward PJ, Manning MA, et al. From the Archives of the AFIP: neoplasms of the urinary bladder: radiologic-pathologic correlation. Radiographics 2006;26(2):553–80.
10. Cowan NC, Crew JP. Imaging bladder cancer. Curr Opin Urol 2010;20(5):409–13.
11. Totaro A, Pinto F, Brescia A, et al. Imaging in bladder cancer: present role and future perspectives. Urol Int 2010;85(4):373–80.
12. Browne RF, Meehan CP, Colville J, et al. Transitional cell carcinoma of the upper urinary tract: spectrum of imaging findings. Radiographics 2005;25(6):1609–27.
13. Kawashima A, Vrtiska TJ, LeRoy AJ, et al. CT urography. Radiographics 2004;24(Suppl 1):S35–54 [discussion: S5–8].
14. Sadow CA, Silverman SG, O'Leary MP, et al. Bladder cancer detection with CT urography in an academic medical center. Radiology 2008;249(1): 195–202.
15. Setty BN, Holalkere NS, Sahani DV, et al. State-of-the-art cross-sectional imaging in bladder cancer. Curr Probl Diagn Radiol 2007;36(2):83–96.
16. Moses KA, Zhang J, Hricak H, et al. Bladder cancer imaging: an update. Curr Opin Urol 2011;21(5):393–7.
17. Tekes A, Kamel I, Imam K, et al. Dynamic MRI of bladder cancer: evaluation of staging accuracy. AJR Am J Roentgenol 2005;184(1):121–7.
18. Saksena MA, Dahl DM, Harisinghani MG. New imaging modalities in bladder cancer. World J Urol 2006;24(5):473–80.
19. Mallampati GK, Siegelman ES. MR imaging of the bladder. Magn Reson Imaging Clin N Am 2004; 12(3):545–55, vii.
20. Barentsz JO, Jager GJ, van Vierzen PB, et al. Staging urinary bladder cancer after transurethral biopsy: value of fast dynamic contrast-enhanced MR imaging. Radiology 1996;201(1):185–93.
21. Gass A, Niendorf T, Hirsch JG. Acute and chronic changes of the apparent diffusion coefficient in neurological disorders–biophysical mechanisms and possible underlying histopathology. J Neurol Sci 2001;186(Suppl 1):S15–23.
22. Malayeri AA, El Khouli RH, Zaheer A, et al. Principles and applications of diffusion-weighted imaging in cancer detection, staging, and treatment follow-up. Radiographics 2011;31(6):1773–91.
23. El-Assmy A, Abou-El-Ghar ME, Mosbah A, et al. Ibrahiem el H. Bladder tumour staging: comparison of diffusion- and T2-weighted MR imaging. Eur Radiol 2009;19(7):1575–81.
24. Takeuchi M, Sasaki S, Ito M, et al. Urinary bladder cancer: diffusion-weighted MR imaging–accuracy for diagnosing T stage and estimating histologic grade. Radiology 2009;251(1):112–21.
25. Thoeny HC, Triantafyllou M, Birkhaeuser FD, et al. Combined ultrasmall superparamagnetic particles of iron oxide-enhanced and diffusion-weighted magnetic resonance imaging reliably detect pelvic lymph node metastases in normal-sized nodes of bladder and prostate cancer patients. Eur Urol 2009;55(4):761–9.
26. Martin SA, Sears DL, Sebo TJ, et al. Smooth muscle neoplasms of the urinary bladder: a clinicopathologic comparison of leiomyoma and leiomyosarcoma. Am J Surg Pathol 2002;26(3):292–300.
27. Cornella JL, Larson TR, Lee RA, et al. Leiomyoma of the female urethra and bladder: report of twenty-three patients and review of the literature. Am J Obstet Gynecol 1997;176(6):1278–85.
28. Knoll LD, Segura JW, Scheithauer BW. Leiomyoma of the bladder. J Urol 1986;136(4):906–8.
29. Sundaram CP, Rawal A, Saltzman B. Characteristics of bladder leiomyoma as noted on magnetic resonance imaging. Urology 1998;52(6):1142–3.

30. Crecelius SA, Bellah R. Pheochromocytoma of the bladder in an adolescent: sonographic and MR imaging findings. AJR Am J Roentgenol 1995; 165(1):101–3.

31. Asbury WL Jr, Hatcher PA, Gould HR, et al. Bladder pheochromocytoma with ring calcification. Abdom Imaging 1996;21(3):275–7.

32. Jalil ND, Pattou FN, Combemale F, et al. Effectiveness and limits of preoperative imaging studies for the localisation of pheochromocytomas and paragangliomas: a review of 282 cases. French Association of Surgery (AFC), and The French Association of Endocrine Surgeons (AFCE). Eur J Surg 1998; 164(1):23–8.

33. Doran F, Varinli S, Bayazit Y, et al. Pheochromocytoma of the urinary bladder. APMIS 2002;110(10): 733–6.

34. Levy AD, Patel N, Dow N, et al. From the archives of the AFIP: abdominal neoplasms in patients with neurofibromatosis type 1: radiologic-pathologic correlation. Radiographics 2005;25(2):455–80.

35. Shonnard KM, Jelinek JS, Benedikt RA, et al. CT and MR of neurofibromatosis of the bladder. J Comput Assist Tomogr 1992;16(3):433–8.

36. Wilkinson LM, Manson D, Smith CR. Best cases from the AFIP: plexiform neurofibroma of the bladder. Radiographics 2004;24(Suppl 1):S237–42.

37. MacVicar D, Husband JE. Radiology in the staging of bladder cancer. Br J Hosp Med 1994;51(9):454–8.

38. Husband JE. Staging bladder cancer. Clin Radiol 1992;46(3):153–9.

39. Husband JE, Olliff JF, Williams MP, et al. Bladder cancer: staging with CT and MR imaging. Radiology 1989;173(2):435–40.

40. Jewett MA, Pereira G, Nijmeh P, et al. Increasing incidence, but stable mortality, of bladder cancer in Ontario. Analysis of a population sample. Urology 1991;37(Suppl 5):4–7.

41. Bradford TJ, Montie JE, Hafez KS. The role of imaging in the surveillance of urologic malignancies. Urol Clin North Am 2006;33(3):377–96.

42. Heney NM, Nocks BN, Daly JJ, et al. Ta and T1 bladder cancer: location, recurrence and progression. Br J Urol 1982;54(2):152–7.

43. Buy JN, Moss AA, Guinet C, et al. MR staging of bladder carcinoma: correlation with pathologic findings. Radiology 1988;169(3):695–700.

44. Fisher MR, Hricak H, Tanagho EA. Urinary bladder MR imaging. Part II. Neoplasm. Radiology 1985; 157(2):471–7.

45. Rholl KS, Lee JK, Heiken JP, et al. Primary bladder carcinoma: evaluation with MR imaging. Radiology 1987;163(1):117–21.

46. Tachibana M, Baba S, Deguchi N, et al. Efficacy of gadolinium-diethylenetriamine pentaacetic acid-enhanced magnetic resonance imaging for differentiation between superficial and muscle-invasive tumor of the bladder: a comparative study with computerized tomography and transurethral ultrasonography. J Urol 1991;145(6):1169–73.

47. Reuter VE. Bladder. Risk and prognostic factors–a pathologist's perspective. Urol Clin North Am 1999;26(3):481–92.

48. Zeegers MP, Tan FE, Dorant E, et al. The impact of characteristics of cigarette smoking on urinary tract cancer risk: a meta-analysis of epidemiologic studies. Cancer 2000;89(3):630–9.

49. Steiner H, Bergmeister M, Verdorfer I, et al. Early results of bladder-cancer screening in a high-risk population of heavy smokers. BJU Int 2008;102(3): 291–6.

50. Pashos CL, Botteman MF, Laskin BL, et al. Bladder cancer: epidemiology, diagnosis, and management. Cancer Pract 2002;10(6):311–22.

51. Ng CS. Radiologic diagnosis and staging of renal and bladder cancer. Semin Roentgenol 2006;41(2): 121–38.

52. Moon WK, Kim SH, Cho JM, et al. Calcified bladder tumors. CT features. Acta Radiol 1992;33(5):440–3.

53. MacVicar AD. Bladder cancer staging. BJU Int 2000;86(Suppl 1):111–22.

54. Maeda H, Kinukawa T, Hattori R, et al. Detection of muscle layer invasion with submillimeter pixel MR images: staging of bladder carcinoma. Magn Reson Imaging 1995;13(1):9–19.

55. Barentsz JO, Witjes JA, Ruijs JH. What is new in bladder cancer imaging. Urol Clin North Am 1997; 24(3):583–602.

56. Wong-You-Cheong JJ, Woodward PJ, Manning MA, et al. From the archives of the AFIP: inflammatory and nonneoplastic bladder masses: radiologic-pathologic correlation. Radiographics 2006;26(6): 1847–68.

57. Stein JP, Skinner EC, Boyd SD, et al. Squamous cell carcinoma of the bladder associated with cyclophosphamide therapy for Wegener's granulomatosis: a report of 2 cases. J Urol 1993;149(3):588–9.

58. Shokeir AA. Squamous cell carcinoma of the bladder: pathology, diagnosis and treatment. BJU Int 2004;93(2):216–20.

59. Serretta V, Pomara G, Piazza F, et al. Pure squamous cell carcinoma of the bladder in Western countries. Report on 19 consecutive cases. Eur Urol 2000; 37(1):85–9.

60. Dondalski M, White EM, Ghahremani GG, et al. Carcinoma arising in urinary bladder diverticula: imaging findings in six patients. AJR Am J Roentgenol 1993;161(4):817–20.

61. Narumi Y, Sato T, Hori S, et al. Squamous cell carcinoma of the uroepithelium: CT evaluation. Radiology 1989;173(3):853–6.

62. Wong JT, Wasserman NF, Padurean AM. Bladder squamous cell carcinoma. Radiographics 2004; 24(3):855–60.

63. Barentsz JO, Ruijs SH, Strijk SP. The role of MR imaging in carcinoma of the urinary bladder. AJR Am J Roentgenol 1993;160(5):937–47.

64. Blute ML, Engen DE, Travis WD, et al. Primary signet ring cell adenocarcinoma of the bladder. J Urol 1989;141(1):17–21.

65. Grignon DJ, Ro JY, Ayala AG, et al. Primary adenocarcinoma of the urinary bladder. A clinicopathologic analysis of 72 cases. Cancer 1991;67(8): 2165–72.

66. Sheldon CA, Clayman RV, Gonzalez R, et al. Malignant urachal lesions. J Urol 1984;131(1):1–8.

67. Thali-Schwab CM, Woodward PJ, Wagner BJ. Computed tomographic appearance of urachal adenocarcinomas: review of 25 cases. Eur Radiol 2005;15(1):79–84.

68. Rafal RB, Markisz JA. Urachal carcinoma: the role of magnetic resonance imaging. Urol Radiol 1991; 12(4):184–7.

69. Sved P, Gomez P, Manoharan M, et al. Small cell carcinoma of the bladder. BJU Int 2004; 94(1):12–7.

70. Cheng L, Pan CX, Yang XJ, et al. Small cell carcinoma of the urinary bladder: a clinicopathologic analysis of 64 patients. Cancer 2004;101(5):957–62.

71. Kim JC, Kim KH, Jung S. Small cell carcinoma of the urinary bladder: CT and MR imaging findings. Korean J Radiol 2003;4(2):130–5.

72. Kim JC. CT features of bladder small cell carcinoma. Clin Imaging 2004;28(3):201–5.

73. Dahm P, Gschwend JE. Malignant non-urothelial neoplasms of the urinary bladder: a review. Eur Urol 2003;44(6):672–81.

74. Bates AW, Norton AJ, Baithun SI. Malignant lymphoma of the urinary bladder: a clinicopathological study of 11 cases. J Clin Pathol 2000;53(6):458–61.

75. Sufrin G, Keogh B, Moore RH, et al. Secondary involvement of the bladder in malignant lymphoma. J Urol 1977;118(2):251–3.

76. Yeoman LJ, Mason MD, Olliff JF. Non-Hodgkin's lymphoma of the bladder–CT and MRI appearances. Clin Radiol 1991;44(6):389–92.

77. Morichetti D, Mazzucchelli R, Lopez-Beltran A, et al. Secondary neoplasms of the urinary system and male genital organs. BJU Int 2009;104(6):770–6.

78. Bates AW, Baithun SI. Secondary neoplasms of the bladder are histological mimics of nontransitional cell primary tumours: clinicopathological and histological features of 282 cases. Histopathology 2000; 36(1):32–40.

Ultrasound Evaluation of Scrotal Pathology

Brandon Mirochnik, MD[a], Puneet Bhargava, MD[b],*,
Manjiri K. Dighe, MD[c], Nalini Kanth, MD[a]

KEYWORDS

- Ultrasound • Testis • Scrotum imaging • Scrotal imaging
- Torsion • Orchitis

A palpable scrotal mass, acute scrotal pain, and an enlarged scrotum are common scenarios in clinical practice. Evaluation of these patients includes an ultrasound (US) examination with gray-scale and color Doppler.[1] US is essential in determining if there is an intratesticular or extratesticular mass and the characteristics of the mass (solid vs cystic). This information helps narrow the differential to benign or malignant etiologies.[2] Extratesticular lesions are more common and are usually benign, especially if the lesion is cystic.[2,3] Approximately 3% of extratesticular solid lesions are malignant.[3] Intratesticular solid lesions are typically considered malignant; however, accurately diagnosing the rare benign intratesticular lesion is vital to avoid an unnecessary orchiectomy.[2,3] This article reviews the common extratesticular and intratesticular lesions presenting as a palpable mass and other scrotal pathologies seen commonly in practice. Specific US features that help classify the lesions as benign or malignant are emphasized.

ANATOMY

The scrotum consists of 2 sacs divided by a median raphe and contains the testis, epididymis, spermatic cord, and fascial covering.[2] The testis is enclosed by the tunica albuginea, a fibrous capsule, beneath the tunica vaginalis. Its posterior aspect invests inside of the testis and forms an incomplete septum called the mediastinum testis, which serves as a passageway for ducts, nerves, and blood vessels.[1,3,4] The tunica albuginea has contractile properties and functions in the transport of spermatozoa from the seminiferous tubules to the epididymis via the mediastinum testis.[1,4] The tunica albuginea is surrounded by the tunica vaginalis, a 2-layered covering consisting of an inner visceral layer and an outer parietal layer, which lines the inner scrotal wall.[1,3,4] Each testis is divided into lobules by fibrous septa; each lobule contains seminiferous tubules, the site of spermatogenesis and the principal functioning unit of the testes.[1] The seminiferous tubules converge to form ducts, the tubuli recti, which open into the rete testis.[1,4] The rete testes are converging spaces, which form efferent ductules that exit through the mediastinum testis and form the head of the epididymis.[1,4,5] The epididymis consists of a head, body, and tail. The efferent ductules converge into a single larger duct, which becomes the vas deferens as it enters the spermatic cord.[1,2,4] The vas deferens joins the seminal vesicle duct and forms the ejaculatory duct.[2]

Testicular arteries are branches from the abdominal aorta, which provide the primary vascular supply to the testes. After coursing through the spermatic cord, they continue along the posterior surface of the testes and form capsular arteries after penetrating the tunica albuginea. Capsular arteries branch into centrifugal branches that carry blood toward the mediastinum. A transmediastinal arterial branch of the testicular artery is identified

[a] Department of Radiology, Nassau University Medical Center, East Meadow, NY 11554, USA
[b] Department of Radiology, VA Puget Sound Health Care System, University of Washington, Mail Box 358280, S-114/Radiology, 1660 South Columbian Way, Seattle, WA 98108-1597, USA
[c] Department of Radiology, University of Washington Medical Center, Box 356510, 1959 Northeast Pacific Street, Seattle, WA 98195-7117, USA
* Corresponding author.
E-mail address: bhargp@uw.edu

Radiol Clin N Am 50 (2012) 317–332
doi:10.1016/j.rcl.2012.02.005
0033-8389/12/$ – see front matter Published by Elsevier Inc.

radiologic.theclinics.com

in approximately half the normal testes. The epididymis and the vas deferens receive blood supply from the deferential artery, which is a branch of the superior vesical artery, and the cremasteric artery, which is a branch of the inferior epigastric artery. The scrotal wall receives its blood supply from the branches of the pudendal artery. Venous drainage of the testes is via the papiniform plexus of draining veins, which further continues as the testicular vein in the deep inguinal canal. The right testicular vein empties into the inferior vena cava and the left testicular vein empties into the left renal vein.[1]

IMAGING TECHNIQUE

Radiologic evaluation of scrotal pathology is primarily accomplished by US examination using a high-frequency (5–10 MHz) linear transducer.[1,2,4] Patients are usually examined in the supine position and the testes are imaged in the sagittal and transverse planes. A midline transverse image, including a portion of each testis, is essential in the comparison of echotexture and vascular flow. Scanning a patient in the upright position or during a Valsalva maneuver may help in the detection of a varicocele.[1,2] The sensitivity of US in the detection of scrotal masses nears 100% and is 98% to 100% for the classification of a mass as extratesticular or intratesticular.[2,4] On US, the testes are normally homogenous with a granular echotexture.[2,3] The mediastinum testis is seen as a linear area of increased echogenicity in the posterior part of the testis.[4] The epididymis is best evaluated in the sagittal plane and is isoechoic to hyperechoic in relation to the testis.[2,4] The majority of testicular tumors are hypoechoic. Some, however, may be more heterogeneous with internal calcifications, cystic change, and increased vascularity. When the results of the US study are ambiguous, as in large scrotal masses, where it is difficult to assess the origin of the scrotal mass and assess its relationship to the testis, further evaluation with MR imaging should be performed.[4]

SCROTAL WALL PATHOLOGY

Scrotal wall swelling appears as layers of alternating hypoechogenicity and hyperechogenicity within a thickened scrotal wall. Noninflammatory causes of scrotal edema include liver and heart failure, lymphatic and venous obstruction, and idiopathic lymphedema.[1]

Inflammatory causes of scrotal wall edema include cellulitis and Fournier gangrene. Obese patients, diabetics, and immunocompromised patients are predisposed to scrotal wall cellulitis.

On US, there is increased scrotal wall thickening that demonstrates increased flow on color Doppler interrogation (Fig. 1). An abscess should be suspected when fluid collections with low-level internal echoes and irregular walls are present.[1]

Fournier gangrene is a polymicrobial necrotizing fasciitis caused by *Klebsiella*, *Proteus*, *Streptococcus*, *Staphylococcus*, *Peptostreptococcus*, *Escherichia coli*, and *Clostridium perfringens*. It is a urologic emergency that should be recognized early due to its high mortality rate of up to 75%. Diagnosis of this condition is primarily clinical (crepitus on palpation) although US may be useful if the clinical findings are nonspecific. Identification of subcutaneous gas in the scrotum is the key finding. On US, gas is seen as echogenic foci demonstrating posterior acoustic dirty shadowing. Scrotal wall thickening is usually present (Fig. 2). Subcutaneous gas from an infection needs to be distinguished from bowel gas in an inguinal scrotal hernia. Often, conventional radiography or CT is required to determine the exact location and cause of the scrotal gas.[1]

BENIGN INTRATESTICULAR CYSTIC LESIONS
Tunica Albuginea Cysts

Tunica albuginea cysts present as firm, palpable masses and are approximately 2 mm to 5 mm in diameter. The mean age at presentation is 40 years.[3,6] The cysts may be unilocular or multilocular and are usually found at the upper anterior or lateral part of the testis. Although uncommon, knowledge of their specific US characteristics is important to distinguish this entity from a possible malignant process.[6] Tunica albuginea cysts are

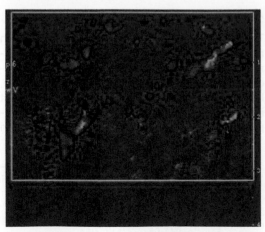

Fig. 1. Cellulitis. A 20-year-old man with scrotal swelling. Longitudinal color Doppler US image shows increased scrotal wall thickening and increased flow consistent with cellulitis.

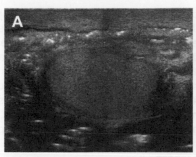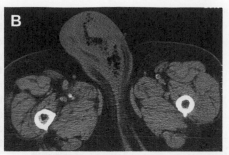

Fig. 2. Fournier gangrene. A 45-year-old man with scrotal swelling and crepitus on physical examination. Transverse US image (A) shows echogenic foci in the subcutaneous tissue consistent with gas along with scrotal wall thickening. The left testis was normal. Contrast-enhanced axial CT image (B) through the scrotum confirms scrotal wall thickening and subcutaneous gas, consistent with Fournier gangrene. Small reactive hydroceles are also seen.

extratesticular. The pathogenesis of tunica albuginea cysts has not been completely elucidated, but they are thought to arise from mesothelial embryonic remnants or from dilated efferent ducts after an initial traumatic or infectious insult.[1,3,6] On US, the tunica albuginea may be appreciated as a thin echogenic line encompassing the testis.[1] Cysts in the tunica albuginea are well-circumscribed cystic lesions with an anechoic center and smooth contours and are increased through transmission (Fig. 3).[4,6] Milk of calcium may be present in tunica albuginea cysts and may appear as a precipitate of echogenic material casting an acoustic shadow.[7] Tunica albuginea cysts can be distinguished from intratesticular simple cysts, because the latter are usually not palpable.[3] Tunica albuginea cysts, however, sometimes are large, have complex characteristics, and appear to be intratesticular, making

their separation from simple cysts or tunica vaginalis cysts difficult.[3,6]

Epidermoid Cyst

Epidermoid cysts, also known as keratocysts, are rare benign tumors of germ cell origin that compose less than 1% of all intratesticular tumors.[1,8,9] Patients are usually 20 to 40 years of age and present with an incidentally discovered firm, smooth, nontender nodule. Epidermoid cysts more commonly involve the right testis.[8,10] It is hypothesized that epidermoid cysts arise from either the development of the ectodermal cell line of a teratoma with the elimination of the endodermal layer or from squamous metaplasia of the epithelium lining the seminiferous tubules or the rete testis.[4,8] US characteristics of an epidermoid cyst vary with its maturation, amount of keratin, and compactness.[1] There are 4 US characteristics that define epidermoid cysts and either 1 or up to all 4 of the features may be present within a single lesion.[1,10] The classic appearance is of alternating hyperechoic and hypoechoic layers forming an onion ring pattern (Fig. 4). Grossly this corresponds to the multiple layers of keratin.[1,4,10] Other patterns include a halo with a central area of increased echogenicity forming a target appearance, an echogenic rim surrounding a solid mass, and a well-defined mass with rim calcification.[1,10] Although epidermoid cysts are considered benign lesions, teratomas and other tumors with malignant potential can have a similar radiologic appearance, making the treatment of epidermoid cysts controversial. If malignancy cannot be ruled out, orchiectomy is usually performed. Testis-sparing enucleation, however, can be done if there is strong evidence for an epidermoid cyst based on the absence of tumor markers and classic US appearance.[4,8]

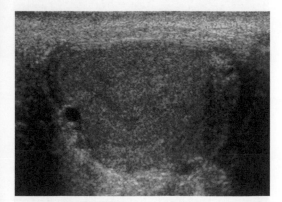

Fig. 3. Tunica albuginea cyst. A 33-year-old man with a palpable nodule in the left hemiscrotum. Transverse US image shows a small cystic lesion along the medial aspect of the left testis consistent with a tunica albuginea cyst. No vascularity was seen on the color Doppler US image (not shown). (Courtesy of Dr Paul Nikolaidis, Northwestern University, Chicago, IL.)

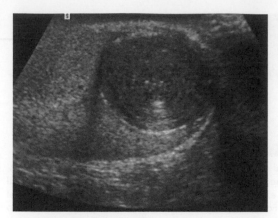

Fig. 4. Epidermoid cyst. A 43-year-old with a palpable mass in left testis. Longitudinal US image through the testis shows a hypoechoic mass with peripheral ring calcifications and the onion-ring appearance typical of an epidermoid. Color Doppler US (not shown) did not demonstrate vascularity.

Tubular Ectasia of the Rete Testis

Tubular ectasia of the rete testis are sperm-containing, intratesticular lesions, frequently associated with a spermatocele or epididymal cysts, and usually bilateral.[1,11–13] On US, the rete testes are hypoechoic and have a striated configuration along the mediastinum testis.[1] Tubular ectasia of the rete testis is a benign condition, caused by partial or complete obstruction of the epididymis or efferent ductules, resulting in dilation of the rete testis.[1,5,11,12] Patients are usually over 55 years of age and commonly present with painless scrotal swelling.[1,11,12] On US, tubular ectasia of the rete testis is characterized by anechoic, elongated, tubular or spherical cystic spaces adjacent to the mediastinum testis (**Fig. 5**).[1,3,5,11–13] The

presence of epididymal cysts in conjunction with the US findings supports the diagnosis of tubular ectasia of the rete testis.[1,11] Doppler US fails to demonstrate vascular flow in tubular ectasia of the rete testis, which distinguishes it from the rare entity of intratesticular varicocele.[5,11] The lack of a sonographically demonstrable solid mass, older age group at presentation, and location adjacent to mediastinum testis help distinguish tubular ectasia of the rete testis from a neoplastic process.[1,5]

BENIGN EXTRATESTICULAR LESIONS
Spermatocele

A spermatocele is a fluid-filled, extratesticular cyst usually measuring 1 cm to 2 cm, containing spermatozoa, lymphocytes, and cellular debris. It result from dilation and obstruction of the efferent ductules in the head of the epididymis.[1,2] Spermatoceles may be seen in a male adult of any age, are almost always found at the head of the epididymis, are usually unilocular, and occur with increased frequency after a vasectomy.[1,2,14] On US, spermatoceles are well-defined, hypoechoic structures with posterior acoustic enhancement (**Fig. 6**).[1] Internal low-level echoes are present in many instances. Occasionally, a spermatocele may crystallize and appear hyperechoic.[14] Spermatoceles and epididymal cysts are not distinguishable on US; however, the latter may be seen anywhere in the epididymis, and the distinction between the two is of little clinical significance.[1]

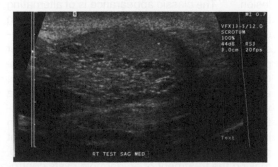

Fig. 5. Tubular ectasia of the rete testis. A 40-year-old man with a palpable mass in the right testis. Longitudinal US image images show multiple channels of cystic spaces in the right testis along the mediastinum testis, an appearance classic for tubular ectasia of the rete testis. This mass was avascular on color Doppler US images (not shown).

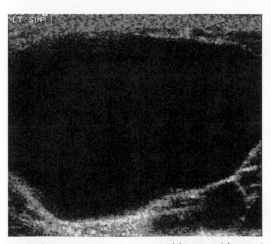

Fig. 6. Spermatocele. A 47-year-old man with a palpable mass in the region of the left testis. The patient had a vasectomy 5 years ago. Longitudinal US image shows a large extratesticular cyst in the region of the epididymal head containing internal echoes consistent with a spermatocele.

Sperm Granulomas

Granulomatous reaction to extravasated sperms, most commonly seen in patients postvasectomy, leads to sperm granuloma or epididymitis nodosa formation. It is a type of chronic epididymitis, and other causes include inflammation and trauma. On US, sperm granuloma is a well-demarcated hypoechoic intraepididymal lesion, which may be inhomogeneous with cystic change (Fig. 7).[1]

Varicocele

A varicocele refers to the abnormal dilation of the intrascrotal veins composing the pampiniform plexus and is the most common palpable mass of the spermatic cord.[2,14] Varicoceles can either be idiopathic or secondary.[2] An idiopathic varicocele results from incompetent valves in the intrascrotal veins, is usually seen in boys and men 15 to 25 years of age, and becomes more pronounced during a Valsalva maneuver and upright posture.[1] Idiopathic varcioceles are usually seen on the left side; unlike the right testicular vein, which drains into the inferior vena cava, the left testicular vein travels a longer course before reaching the left renal vein and inserts at a right angle, resulting in a higher pressure system. Secondary varicoceles can be caused by hydronephrosis, cirrhosis, or an abdominal mass, usually renal cell carcinoma, which causes an increase in the pressure in the spermatic veins.[1,2] When attempting to diagnose a varicocele, patients should be evaluated with US in supine and upright positions with the examination also performed using the Valsalva maneuver.[1] On US, varicoceles are identified as multiple hypoechoic/anechoic serpiginous and tubular structures larger than 2 mm in diameter and are best seen superior

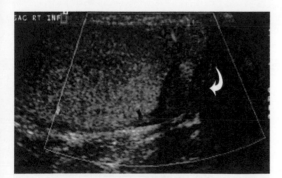

Fig. 7. Sperm granuloma. A 45-year-old man with history of previous vastectomy. Longitudinal color Doppler US image shows an avascular isoechoic to mildly hyperechoic mass inferior to the right testis (*curved arrow*). This lesion was surgically removed and pathology confirmed a sperm granuloma.

and posterior to the testis.[1,2] Color Doppler shows flow reversal during the Valsalva maneuver and helps in the diagnosis (Fig. 8).[2] Treatment of a varicocele helps improve fertility by improving sperm quality (number, morphology, and motility). If a varicocele is noncompressible or if there is an isolated right varicocele, patients should be evaluated for a retroperitoneal mass, tumor extension into the renal veins, and renal vein thrombosis.[1]

Hydrocele

A hydrocele is a large collection of serous fluid in the potential space between the visceral and parietal layers of the tunica vaginalis and is the most common cause of painless scrotal swelling. Hydroceles are seen secondary to an underlying pathologic process, are a congenital anomaly, or are idiopathic. Secondary causes include trauma, infection, torsion, or tumor.[1,2] Congenital hydroceles arise from a patent processus vaginalis, which acts as a portal of entry for peritoneal fluid into the scrotum, and usually resolve by 18 months of age. Idiopathic hydroceles can be due to overproduction or decreased absorption of serous fluid.[2] In adults presenting with a hydrocele, a secondary pathologic process should be elucidated.[1] On US, a hydrocele is seen as a collection of anechoic fluid surrounding the anterolateral part of the testis, with good through transmission; internal echoes sometimes are seen, related to protein or cholesterol within the hydrocele (Fig. 9).[1,2]

Hematocele

A hematocele is a collection of blood within the tunica vaginalis. They are usually due to either trauma, torsion, surgery, or tumor and may be acute or chronic.[1,2] Patients may present with a hard mass and discomfort. A hematocele can exert mass effect on the testis, distorting its contour. The majority of hematoceles respond to conservative treatment and show resolution; however, there is a possibility of a chronic hematocele that may become fibrotic and calcified.[2] US shows a complex, heterogeneous fluid collection with septations or a lace-like appearance (Fig. 10). Echogenic debris and calcifications may be seen in chronic cases.[1,2]

TESTICULAR CALCIFICATION
Microlithiasis

Testicular microlithiasis is usually discovered incidentally on US. These represent intratubular calcifications and are seen on US as multiple echogenic foci without acoustic shadowing (Fig. 11). More than 5 echogenic foci in a single US image is the main criterion for diagnosing this condition. Although

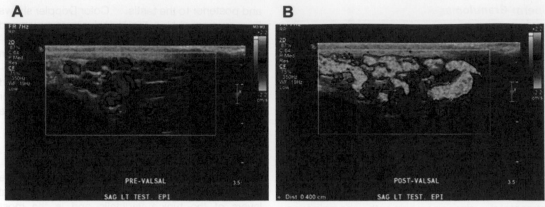

A PRE-VALSAL
SAG LT TEST. EPI

B POST-VALSAL
SAG LT TEST. EPI

Fig. 8. Varicocele. (*A*) A 55-year-old man with a palpable mass and heaviness in the left hemiscrotum. Color Doppler US images prevalsalva and (*B*) postvalsalva show multiple tubular structures in the left hemiscrotum with flow reversal during Valsalva maneuver. On gray-scale US (not shown) these measure greater than 2 mm in diameter.

controversial, there is no definite evidence in the literature to suggest that testicular microlithiasis is definitely premalignant and a precursor to testicular neoplasia. In the past, US follow-up has been recommended after the diagnosis of microlithiasis due to the possible association with testicular malignancy. More recent literature, however, suggests that this may not be necessary.[15] Testicular microlithiasis has also been associated with cryptorchism, infertility, pseudohermaphroditism, Klinefelter syndrome, and pulmonary alveolar microlithiasis.[1]

Scrotolith

Scrotoliths, or scrotal pearls, are calcifications in the scrotum, with no clinical significance and a typical US appearance.[1] Their pathogenesis may be secondary to the calcification of loose bodies formed after torsion of the appendix testes or epididymis. Repetitive trauma has also been postulated as a cause, with increased incidence seen in mountain bikers.[1,16] US demonstrates extratesticular, echogenic nodules that are usually mobile and demonstrate acoustic shadowing (**Fig. 12**).[1] They can reach sizes of up to 1 cm and may be associated with a hydrocele, which facilitates their identification on US and assessment of mobility.[16]

INGUINAL SWELLING
Inguinal Hernia

Inguinal hernias are either indirect or direct; the former is lateral to the inferior epigastric artery,

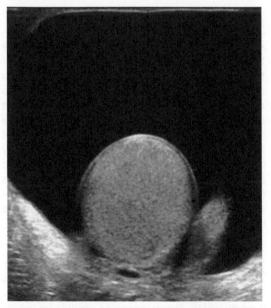

Fig. 9. Hydrocele. A 52-year-old man with painless scrotal swelling. Transverse US image of the right testis shows large amount of anechoic fluid surrounding the right testis consistent with a hydrocele. The ipsilateral testis and epididymis are normal in appearance.

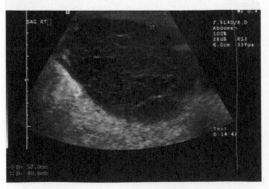

Fig. 10. Hematocele. A 45-year-old man who sat on his testicle. Longitudinal US image of the right testicle demonstrates a complex fluid collection with multiple internal septations consistent with a hematocele.

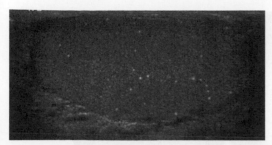

Fig. 11. Testicular microlithiasis. A 25-year-old man with testicular pain. Longitudinal US image shows multiple tiny 1-mm to 2-mm sized echogenic foci without discrete shadowing consistent with microlithiasis (diagnostic criteria >5 echogenic foci in a single US image).

whereas the latter is located medial to it. An inguinal hernia is usually a clinical diagnosis; however, occasionally, it may present as a hard, irreducible mass that cannot be differentiated from a scrotal mass and may require imaging to differentiate. Indirect inguinal hernias pass through the internal inguinal ring and inguinal canal and enter the scrotum. They are more common in children and are associated with a patent processus vaginalis. Direct hernias are more common in adults and protrude through an area of weakness in the anterior abdominal wall. The US characteristics of an inguinal hernia depend on the herniated visceral structure.[1,2] Hernias involving omentum are hyperechoic, corresponding to omental fat (Fig. 13). Hernias containing bowel are fluid-filled or air-filled and have multiple bright echoes; the presence of air or gas results in shadowing. Occasionally the valvulae conniventes or haustra is seen and peristalsis may be visualized.[2] A strangulated hernia is seen as an akinetic, dilated loop of bowel within the hernial sac.[1] Often evaluation with a curvilinear

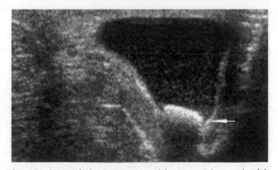

Fig. 12. Scrotolith. A 30-year-old man with a palpable hard mass in the left scrotum. Longitudinal US image show an extratesticular hyperechoic mobile mass with posterior acoustic shadowing in the left scrotum, consistent with a scrotolith (arrow). A small chronic hydrocele with low-level internal echoes is also seen.

US probe is needed to evaluate the contents of a large inguinal hernia due to limited penetration of the linear US probe.

Acute Scrotal Pain: Epididymo-orchitis and Torsion

Epididymo-orchitis and epididymitis are common causes of acute scrotal pain in adolescent boys and in adults. In adolescents and young adults, many cases are secondary to sexually transmitted organisms, such as Chlamydia trachomatis and Neisseria gonorrhoeae. In prepubertal boys and in men over 35 years of age, the disease is most frequently caused by Escherichia coli and Proteus mirabilis. Rare causes, such as sarcoidosis, brucellosis, tuberculosis, cryptococcus, and mumps, may also cause epididymitis and orchitis. Drugs, such as amiodarone hydrochloride, may also cause epididymitis (chemical epididymitis). Complications of acute epididymitis include chronic pain, infarction, abscess, gangrene, infertility, atrophy, and pyocele.[17]

Gray-scale US findings of acute epididymitis include an enlarged hypoechoic or hyperechoic (presumably secondary to hemorrhage) epididymis.[18] An associated hydrocele or pyocele with scrotal wall thickening is often present. Orchitis develops in 20% to 40% of cases due to direct spread of infection. Diffuse testicular involvement is confirmed by the presence of testicular enlargement and an inhomogeneous testicular echotexture, which may be diffuse or multifocal.[19] Marked increased flow is usually seen on color Doppler US evaluation (Fig. 14). Differential diagnosis includes scrotal trauma, which may also present with epididymal enlargement and hyperemia.[20]

Testicular torsion can occur at any age; however, it is most frequently encountered in adolescent boys. In testicular torsion, venous obstruction occurs first, followed by obstruction of arterial flow and ultimately by testicular ischemia. The testicular salvage rate depends on the degree of torsion and the duration of ischemia. A nearly 100% salvage rate exists within the first 6 hours after the onset of symptoms, a 70% rate within 6 to 12 hours, and a 20% rate within 12 to 24 hours.[21]

Torsion is extravaginal or intravaginal. Extravaginal testicular torsion occurs exclusively in newborns. Torsion occurs outside the tunica vaginalis when the testes and gubernacula are not fixed and are free to rotate.[22] The affected neonate presents with swelling, discoloration of the scrotum on the affected side and a firm painless mass in the scrotum.[23,24] The testis is typically infarcted and necrotic at birth. US findings include an enlarged heterogeneous testis, ipsilateral hydrocele, skin

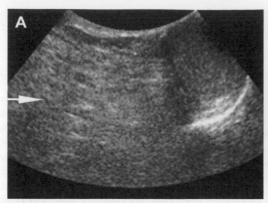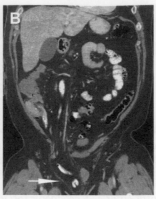

Fig. 13. Inguinoscrotal hernia. A 56-year-old man with an enlarged right hemiscrotum. Longitudinal US image (A) shows a hyperechoic heterogenous mass (arrow) extending from the inguinal region into the scrotum extending up to the testis, which is displaced to the left side. This was thought to represent a hernia and CT was performed for better definition of the extent of the hernia. Coronal contrast-enhanced CT image (B) shows a large right inguinal hernia (arrow) extending into the right scrotum and containing fat and bowel.

thickening, and no color Doppler flow signal in the testis or spermatic cord.[25]

In children, power Doppler US is more sensitive than color Doppler US for detection of intratesticular blood flow. Scintigraphy remains a reasonable alternative for evaluation of acute scrotal pain and should be used when color Doppler US sensitivity for low-velocity, low-volume testicular blood flow is inadequate and if the diagnosis of torsion remains in question.

Intravaginal torsion is caused by a long and narrow mesentery or a bell-clapper deformity, bilateral in most cases, in which the tunica vaginalis completely encircles the epididymis, distal spermatic cord, and testis rather than attaching to the posterolateral aspect of the testis. The deformity leaves the testis free to swing and rotate within the tunica vaginalis much like a clapper inside a bell.[26]

Patients with acute torsion (children or adults) typically present after a sudden onset of pain followed by nausea, vomiting, and a low-grade fever. US is the first step in evaluation. The main US findings include an enlarged heterogeneous testis, ipsilateral hydrocele, skin thickening, and lack of color Doppler flow signal in the affected testis (Fig. 15). Lack of demonstrable intratesticular flow on color Doppler US is 86% sensitive, 100% specific, and 97% accurate in the diagnosis of torsion and ischemia in painful scrotum.[27] The high degree of accuracy is due to the superiority of power Doppler US depiction of intratesticular vessels compared with that of color Doppler US.[28]

Torsion of Testicular Appendages

Testicular appendages are remnants of the embryonic ducts. Four appendages have been described: the appendix testes, the appendix epididymis, the vas aberrans, and the paradidymis. The appendix testis and the appendix epididymis are usually seen on scrotal US. The appendix testis is seen in the groove between the testis and the epididymis along the upper pole. The appendix epididymis is attached to the head of the epididymis. Torsion of the appendix testes and the appendix epididymis presents with acute scrotal pain. On physical examination, a small firm nodule is usually palpable in the superior aspect of the testes and may exhibit the classic blue dot sign. Nearly all torsed appendages involve the appendix testes and typically occur

Fig. 14. Epididymo-orchitis. A 36-year-old man with scrotal pain and fever. Longitudinal color Doppler US image shows an enlarged heterogeneous testis and epididymis with increased flow and scrotal wall thickening, findings consistent with acute epididymo-orchitis.

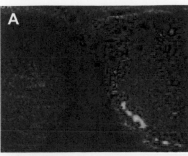
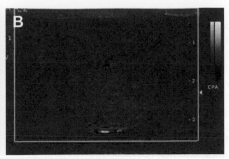

Fig. 15. Acute testicular torsion. A 38-year-old man who presented to the emergency room with acute testicular pain. Transverse color Doppler US image (A) shows an enlarged right testicle with subtle increased echogenicity compared with the left side and no internal vascular flow. Power Doppler US image (B) shows no appreciable flow within the right testis. Trace flow was noted at the periphery of this testis.

between the ages of 7 and 14 years. On US, a round hyperechoic mass with a central hypoechoic area adjacent to the testis or epididymis is identified. A reactive hydrocele and scrotal wall thickening are usually present (Fig. 16). Doppler interrogation is of limited value because internal flow is not normally present in the normal appendage. Increased peripheral flow may be present in cases of torsion. The role of US is to exclude acute testicular torsion and acute epididymo-orchitis. Management of torsion of the appendix is conservative (pain management) with the pain resolving within a few days.[1]

THE UNDESCENDED TESTIS

Cryptorchidism is defined as complete or partial failure of the intra-abdominal testes to descend into the scrotal sac. The undescended testis may be positioned anywhere along the normal path of descent. The most common location is in the inguinal canal (72%), followed by prescrotal (20%) and abdominal (8%) locations. The ectopic testis may also lie in the perineum, femoral canal, superficial inguinal pouch, or contralateral hemiscrotum. The most common ectopic location is in the superficial inguinal pouch, a subcutaneous pocket in front of, and lateral to, the external ring.[1] The undescended testis most commonly appears as a hypoechoic oval structure (Fig. 17).[29]

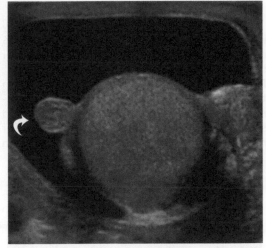

Fig. 16. Torsion of the appendix testis. A 13-year-old boy who presented to the emergency room with acute testicular pain. Transverse gray-scale US image shows a round hyperechoic mass (curved arrow) with tiny central hypoechoic areas adjacent to the left testes and epididymis with a reactive hydrocele and mild scrotal wall thickening. Mild reactive increased flow was seen within the adjacent testis and epididymis on color Doppler US evaluation (not shown). Color Doppler US evaluation of the torsed appendix testes is of limited value, because internal flow is usually not demonstrated within a normal testicular appendage.

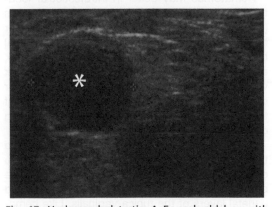

Fig. 17. Undescended testis. A 5-week-old boy with a single testis within the scrotum on physical examination. Transverse US image of the right inguinal region shows a markedly hypoechoic structure consistent with an undescended testicle (asterisk).

The major complications of cryptorchidism are malignant degeneration, infertility, torsion, and bowel incarceration because of an associated indirect inguinal hernia.[1,30] There is a risk ratio of malignancy of 2.5 to 8 in the undescended testis. Seminoma is the most common malignancy in the cryptorchid testis. Orchiopexy of the cryptorchid testis is usually performed in patients between 1 and 10 years of age; orchiectomy is considered for postpubertal patients. Orchiopexy does not change the risk of malignant degeneration of the once cryptorchid testis, but it does allow easier surveillance. If malignancy does occur in one testis, prompting unilateral orchiectomy, the remaining contralateral testis remains at high risk for the development of cancer.[1]

SCROTAL TRAUMA

Scrotal trauma accounts for less than 1% of all trauma-related injuries because of the anatomic location and mobility of the scrotum. The peak occurrence of scrotal trauma is in the age range of 10 to 30 years.[31] Mechanisms of trauma include blunt, penetrating, thermal, and degloving injuries, of which blunt trauma is the most common. The right testis is injured more often than the left one because of its greater propensity to be trapped against the pubis or inner thigh.[32,33] Rapid and accurate diagnosis is necessary to guide treatment and prevent loss of the testis.

US is the first-line imaging modality for scrotal trauma, and US findings are crucial in clinical decision making.[34–37] US manifestations include fluid collections (intratesticular, epididymal, or scrotal hematoma; hydrocele; and hematocele) and testicular disruption (fracture and rupture) as well as vascular injury.

Hematomas may occur in intratesticular locations (**Fig. 18**) or in the extratesticular soft tissues (**Fig. 19**), such as the scrotal wall, epididymis, or between the testes. Hematomas are usually focal but may be multiple, hyperechoic (acute bleeding), or hypoechoic (as the hemorrhage ages) and lack vascularity. The fluid in a hematoma may appear complex and be heterogeneous. Hematomas of the scrotal wall may appear as focal thickening of the wall or as fluid collections within the wall.

Up to 50% of acquired hydroceles are due to trauma[38] and hydroceles may occur in up to 25% of patients with major trauma.[39] Hematoceles are complex collections that separate the visceral and parietal layers of the tunica vaginalis. Like hematomas, they are acutely echogenic and become more complex and more hypoechoic with age; fluid-fluid levels or low-level internal echoes may also be seen.[1]

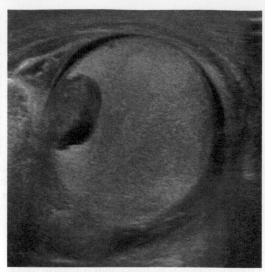

Fig. 18. Intratesticular hematoma. A 21-year-old man who presented with history of blunt trauma to the scrotum. Transverse US image shows a heterogeneous mass with a crescentic peripheral area of hypoechogenicity in the right testis, consistent with an intratesticular hematoma in setting of testicular trauma. Marked scrotal wall edema is also present. Subsequent imaging (not shown) confirmed resolution of the hematoma. (*Courtesy of* Dr Paul Nikolaidis, Northwestern University, Chicago, IL.)

US is an essential diagnostic tool in the early identification of testicular rupture. More than 80% of ruptured testes can be salvaged if surgical repair is performed within 72 hours of testicular injury.[40] Findings of a heterogeneous echotexture within the testis, testicular contour abnormality, and disruption of the tunica albuginea are considered sensitive and specific for the diagnosis of testicular rupture in the setting of scrotal trauma (**Fig. 20**). In

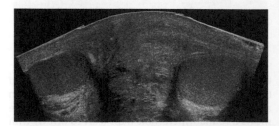

Fig. 19. Extratesticular hematoma. A 33-year-old man who presented after scrotal injury sustained when playing soccer. Extended field-of-view US image shows a hyperechoic mass in the scrotum located between the normal left and right testes, consistent with an extratesticular hematoma in setting of testicular trauma. Mild scrotal wall edema is also present. (*Courtesy of* Dr Paul Nikolaidis, Northwestern University, Chicago, IL.)

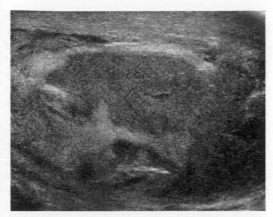

Fig. 20. A 24-year-old man who presented following blunt trauma to the scrotum. Longitudinal US image shows markedly heterogeneous echotexture in the posterior and inferior aspect of the testis. There are associated significant testicular contour abnormality and disruption of the tunica albuginea, findings classic for testicular rupture. (*Courtesy of* Dr Paul Nikolaidis, Northwestern University, Chicago, IL.)

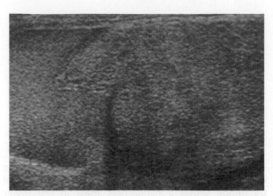

Fig. 21. Testicular fracture. A 32-year-old man with a history of high-speed motor vehicle accident. Longitudinal US image of the left testicle shows discontinuity of the normal testicular parenchyma along with a linear hypoechoic band consistent with a testicular fracture.

one series of patients with blunt trauma, a sensitivity of 100% and a specificity of 93.5% were noted for the diagnosis of testicular rupture on the basis of US findings of a heterogeneous echotexture and contour abnormality.[34] In addition, an absence of normal vascularity within the testis may help characterize a rupture. A heterogeneous echotexture may also be seen in the presence of intratesticular hematomas without a tunica albuginea rupture; therefore, it should not be considered indicative of testicular rupture unless it is accompanied by an observed tunica albuginea disruption or testicular contour irregularity.[41]

In patients with a large extratesticular hematocele, however, US may be of limited use for evaluating the tunica albuginea. Surgical exploration should be performed in such patients, irrespective of the presence or absence of definitive US signs of testicular rupture.[42]

Testicular fracture refers to a break or discontinuity in the normal testicular parenchyma. A testicular fracture line is identified at US as a linear hypoechoic and avascular area within the testis, a finding that may or may not be associated with a tunica albuginea rupture (Fig. 21). A fracture line is rare and is seen in only approximately 17% of cases. Color Doppler imaging plays a significant role in guiding management in such cases. The presence of vascularity in the testicular parenchyma is indicative of its salvageability; often, only débridement along the line of fracture is required while the vascular parenchyma is preserved.[42]

MALIGNANT TESTICULAR LESIONS

Testicular tumors are divided into those derived from germ cells, gonadal stromal cells, along with lymphoma, leukemia, and metastases. Germ cell tumors compose 90% to 95% of testicular tumors and are divided into seminoma and nonseminomatous germ cell tumors (NSGTCTs), each with different treatments and prognosis.[1]

Seminoma

Seminomas are the most common testicular malignancy and compose approximately 35% to 50% of germ cell tumors. Seminomas occur in men, with an average age of 40, approximately 5 to 10 years older than men with other germ cell tumors of the testes. They are usually unilateral and range in size from small well-defined lesions to large masses that replace the entire testicle.[3] Seminomas are sensitive to radiation and chemotherapy and have the best prognosis of the germ cell tumors.[1] On US, seminomas are homogeneously hypoechoic (Fig. 22) and usually limited by the tunica albuginea, corresponding to their smooth homogenous appearance on gross examination.[1,3] Large seminomas can have a more heterogeneous appearance.[3] Seminomas may be lobulated or multinodular and can have cystic spaces, which may be appreciated on US.[1,3]

Nonseminomatous Germ Cell Tumors

NSGCTs occur in a younger population compared with seminomas, with an average age at presentation of 30.[1] NSGCTs usually have multiple histologic morphologies and the US features are reflected by the proportionality of each of the

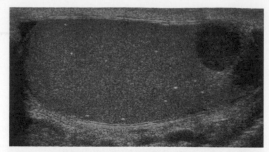

Fig. 22. Seminoma. A 27-year-old man presenting with a palpable mass in the right testis. Longitudinal US image shows a hypoechoic mass in the lower pole of the right testis. Microlithiasis is also present throughout the testicle. Pathology postorchiectomy confirmed a seminoma. (*Courtesy of* Dr Paul Nikolaidis, Northwestern University, Chicago, IL.)

histologies. On US, NSGCTs are heterogeneous, have irregular margins, have cystic components, and may contain echogenic foci, which represent hemorrhage, calcification, or fibrosis (Fig. 23). NSGCTs include embryonal carcinoma, yolk sac tumor, choricocarcinoma, and teratoma.[1,4]

Embryonal carcinoma affects men ages 25 to 35 years and is usually smaller in size than seminomas at presentation but more aggressive. Embryonal carcinoma is found in its pure form in 2% to 3% of all testicular tumors, composing 87% of mixed germ cell tumors.[4] US typically shows a poorly defined, hypoechoic lesion with an inhomogeneous echotexture.[1]

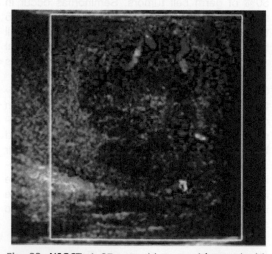

Fig. 23. NSGCT. A 37-year-old man with a palpable mass in the right testis. Transverse color Doppler US image shows a hypoechoic mass with irregular margins in the right testis with mild internal vascularity. The patient had a high β–human chorionic gonadotropin level and this mass was found to be NSGCT on orchiectomy.

Yolk sac tumors, also known as endodermal sinus tumors or infantile embryonal carcinomas, are usually seen in patients less than 5 years of age. α-Fetoprotein is used as a tumor marker for these tumors.[1] In adults, yolk sac tumors usually present as part of a mixed germ cell tumor.[4] On US, yolk sac tumors are inhomogeneous and can have echogenic foci related to hemorrhage.[1]

Choriocarcinoma is a rare germ cell tumor, seen in 16% of mixed germ cell tumors and in less than 1% of patients in its pure form. It presents in boys and men between the ages of 10 and 30 years of age, histologically is composed of cytotrophoblastic and syncytiotrophoblastic cells, and results in elevation of human chorionic gonadotropin, which is used as a tumor marker.[1,4] Choriocarcinomas have malignant behavior and metastasize to the lungs, liver, gastrointestinal tract, and brain; they have the worst prognosis of all the germ cell tumors.[4] Choriocarcinomas are characterized by cystic and solid components, which correspond to areas of hemorrhagic necrosis seen at histopathologic examination.[1]

Pure teratomas are the second most common germ cell tumor in children and usually present before age 4. In adults, the pure form is rare; however, approximately 50% of all mixed germ cell tumors have elements of teratomas.[1,4] Teratomas consist of the 3 germ layers, endoderm, mesoderm, and ectoderm, and can consist of adult and fetal tissues; in children the mature form is considered benign; however, in adults it is always considered malignant. On US, teratomas are large well circumscribed and inhomogeneous.[1,4] Cysts are common and depending on the contents may be anechoic or complex.[4] The presence of echogenic foci relate to calcifications, cartilage, immature bone, and fibrosis.[1]

Leukemia and Lymphoma

Testicular lymphomas constitute between 1% and 9% of all testicular neoplasms and 1% of non-Hodgkin lymphomas. Although uncommon in general, they are the most common testicular malignancy in men 60 years of age and older. Testicular lymphoma may be the primary and only manifestation of malignant lymphoma, the initial sign of generalized disease, or may occur during the clinical course of a patient with established lymphoma. Secondary involvement of the testis in patients with lymphoma is far more common than primary testicular lymphoma.[43] Primary leukemia of the testes is rare but the testes are commonly the site of extramedullary relapse after chemotherapy-induced remission. The testis is a sanctuary organ because of the blood-gonad barrier that inhibits the accumulation of chemotherapeutic agents. This phenomenon is most commonly described in children with acute lymphoblastic leukemia.[44,45] Recurrence of testicular lymphoma is an important consideration in patients with testicular enlargement and should be differentiated from inflammatory processes.

Gray-scale US of lymphoma and leukemia typically shows diffuse or focal regions of decreased echogenicity with maintenance of the normal ovoid testicular shape.[46] Asynchronous involvement of the contralateral testis is more common than in other testicular tumors and occurs in 8.5% to 18% of cases. Involvement of the spermatic cord and epididymis is more characteristic of lymphoma than a seminoma. Gray-scale US may show homogeneously hypoechoic testes or single or, more often, multiple hypoechoic lesions of various sizes (**Fig. 24**). Striated hypoechoic bands with parallel hyperechoic lines radiating peripherally from the mediastinum testis have also been described. Color Doppler US shows increased vascularity regardless of the size of the lesion.[1]

Differential diagnosis for the sonographic appearance of lymphoma includes most primary testicular tumors along with focal orchitis. Testicular hypervascularity without associated epididymal hyperemia is more suggestive of a neoplastic process than of orchitis.[47]

MISCELLANEOUS TUMORS
Metastases to the Testis

Overall, metastatic disease involving the testes is an unusual occurrence and most frequently exists in the context of widely disseminated malignancy.

Invariably, these lesions are discovered at post-mortem examination, having been a subclinical abnormality during the course of illness. In a small proportion of cases, however, metastatic testicular lesions are discovered clinically in patients with known malignancy, although they rarely account for the initial clinical presentation of an extratesticular malignancy. The frequency of individual tumors metastasizing to the testes is highly variable. Review of the literature yields little definite agreement, although lymphoma seems the most common primary tumor, spreading to the testes in less than 3% of cases.[48] These patients are also more likely to have diffuse bilateral gonadal disease. Prostate and bronchial malignancies are also documented, accounting for approximately 35% and 20%, respectively, of cases of testicular metastasis in one review. The incidence of testicular melanoma metastases (**Fig. 25**) seems to vary widely, ranging from 2% in one case series of 248 patients to 41% in a 22-patient cohort.[49]

Mesenchymal Tumors

Mesenchymal tumors of the testes, both benign and malignant, are rare and include leiomyomas, neurofibromas, adenomatoid tumors, and hemangiomas. Sarcomas include osteosarcoma, fibrosarcoma, leiomyosarcomas, Kaposi sarcoma, and rhabdomyosarcoma. Imaging findings are nonspecific (**Fig. 26**). Intratesticular adenomatoid tumors are benign neoplasms less commonly reported than adenomatoid tumors of the epididymis.[1]

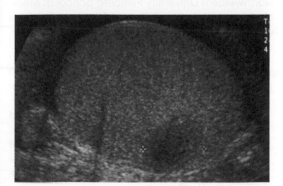

Fig. 24. Lymphoma. A 45-year-old man with abdominal non-Hodgkin lymphoma. Longitudinal US image of the left testicle revealed a hypoechoic testicular mass consistent with patient's known lymphoma. Color Doppler US (not shown) demonstrated increased vascularity of the lesion.

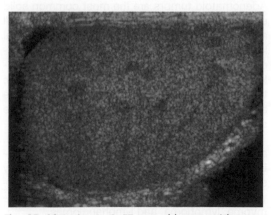

Fig. 25. Metastases. A 57-year-old man with metastatic malignant melanoma. Transverse US image of the right testis shows multiple solid hypoechoic masses consistent with metastases from patient's known melanoma. (*Courtesy of* Dr Paul Nikolaidis, Northwestern University, Chicago, IL.)

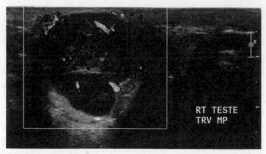

Fig. 26. Leiomyosarcoma. A 62-year-old man with a palpable mass in the right hemicrotum. Color Doppler US image shows a predominantly hyperechoic mass separate from the right testis with mildly increased flow. This lesion was surgically removed and pathology confirmed a leiomyosarcoma.

OTHER EXTRATESTICULAR MASSES
Tumors of the Spermatic Cord

Benign tumors account for 75% of spermatic cord masses and are mostly lipomas. The remainder of the tumors are sarcomas, with rhabdomyoma and sarcoma the most common tumors. These tumors are usually seen in the pediatric population and can be large (up to 20 cm) at presentation. Five-year survival is 75% despite frequent retroperitoneal lymph node metastases. Tumors of smooth muscle origin are the second most common tumors in this region seen in patients between 40 to 70 years of age. The majority of these (70%) are leiomyomas and the remainder are leiomyosarcomas. Other malignant tumors of the spermatic cord are liposarcoma, fibrosarcoma, myxochondrosarcoma, and malignant fibrous histiocytoma.[1]

Epididymal Tumors

Adenomatoid tumors are the most common solid epididymal tumors. Patients can present at all ages in adulthood. These are usually incidental lesions, palpated either by a patient or by a physician during physical examination; they are painless masses. US appearance is variable (Fig. 27); thus, these tumors are usually resected. There are no reported cases of metastases or recurrence after surgical excision.

Other tumors, such as papillary cystadenoma, are rare and often associated with von Hippel-Lindau disease. On US, these lesions are usually solid and less than 2 cm in size. Other rare epididymal tumors include leiomyoma, lipoma, rhabdomyoma, lymphoma, and lymphangiomas.[1]

SUMMARY

US of the scrotum is a commonly performed examination for palpable masses and acute

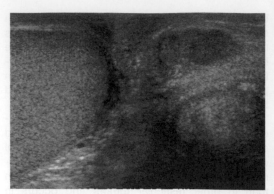

Fig. 27. Adenomatoid tumor. A 33-year-old man with a palpable mass. Transverse US image demonstrates a homogeneous hypoechoic extratesticular mass anterior to the left testes, within the epididymis. The mass was surgically removed and pathology confirmed an adenomatoid tumor.

scrotum. Radiologists play a key role in diagnosing and appropriately guiding management of true emergencies, such as torsion, while avoiding surgery in conditions, such as torsion of the appendix testis. For evaluation of focal lesions and masses, US helps decide whether a lesion is intratesticular or extratesticular and if it is solid or cystic. Often, US appearances of several entities may be characteristic, such as tubular ectasia of the rete testis. Knowledge of US technique and normal and pathologic US findings along with Doppler findings is essential for accurate diagnosis and for guiding appropriate management.

ACKNOWLEDGMENTS

The authors would like to acknowledge Paul Nikolaidis, MD, Associate Professor of Radiology, Northwestern University Feinberg School of Medicine for contributing images of tunica albuginea cyst, testicular hematomas, testicular rupture, seminoma, metastasis, and adenomatoid tumor.

REFERENCES

1. Dogra VS, Gottlieb RH, Oka M, et al. Sonography of the scrotum. Radiology 2003;227:18–36.
2. Woodward PF, Schwab CM, Sesterhenn IA. From the archives of the AFIP extratesticular scrotal masses: radiologic-pathologic correlation. Radiographics 2003;23:215–40.
3. Dogra VS, Gottlieb RH, Rubens DJ, et al. Benign intratesticular cystic lesions: US features. Radiographics 2001;21:S273–81.
4. Woodward PJ, Sohaey R, O'Donoghue MJ, et al. From the archives of the AFIP: tumors and tumorlike

lesions of the testis: radiologic-pathologic correlation. Radiographics 2002;22:189–216.

5. Brown DL, Benson CB, Doherty FJ, et al. Cystic testicular mass caused by dilated rete testis: sonographic findings in 31 cases. AJR Am J Roentgenol 1992;158:1257–9.

6. Martinez-Berganza MT, Sarria L, Cozculluela R, et al. Cysts of the tunica albuginea: sonographic appearance. AJR Am J Roentgenol 1998;170:183–5.

7. Gittleman AM, Perlmutter S, Hutchinson A, et al. Milk of calcium in a tunica albuginea cyst. J Ultrasound Med 2002;21:673–6.

8. Moghe PK, Brady AP. Ultrasound of testicular epidermoid cysts. Br J Radiol 1999;72:942–5.

9. Atchley JT, Dewbury KC. Ultrasound appearance of testicular epidermoid cysts. Clin Radiol 2002;55:493–502.

10. Dogra VS, Gottlieb RH, Rubens DJ, et al. Testicular epidermoid cysts: sonographic features with histopathologic correlation. J Clin Ultrasound 2001;29:192–6.

11. Nair R, Abbaraju J, Rajbabu K, et al. Tubular ectasia of the rete testis: a diagnostic dilemma. Ann R Coll Surg Engl 2008;90:1–3.

12. Colangelo SM, Fried K, Hyacinthe LM, et al. Tubular ectasia of the rete testis: an ultrasound diagnosis. Urology 1995;45:532–4.

13. Older RA, Watson LR. Tubular ectasia of the rete testis: a benign condition with a sonographic appearance that may be misinterpreted as malignant. J Urol 1994;152:477–8.

14. Black JA, Patel A. Sonography of the abnormal extratesticular space. AJR Am J Roentgenol 1996;167:507–11.

15. Ravichandran S, Smith R, Cornford PA, et al. Surveillance of testicular microlithiasis? Results of an UK based national questionnaire survey. BMC Urol 2006;6:8.

16. De Luis Pastor E, Villanueva Marcos A, Zudaire Díaz-Tejeiro B, et al. Scrotal ultrasonography: pearls, patterns, and errors. Actas Urol Esp 2007;31:895–910.

17. Luker GD, Siegel MJ. Color Doppler sonography of the scrotum in children. AJR Am J Roentgenol 1994;163:649–55.

18. Siegel MJ. The acute scrotum. Radiol Clin North Am 1997;35:959–76.

19. Farriol VG, Comella XP, Agromayor EG, et al. Grayscale and power Doppler sonographic appearances of acute inflammatory diseases of the scrotum. J Clin Ultrasound 2000;28:67–72.

20. Gordon LM, Stein SM, Ralls PW. Traumatic epididymitis: evaluation with color Doppler sonography. AJR Am J Roentgenol 1996;166:1323–5.

21. Patriquin HB, Yazbeck S, Trinh B, et al. Testicular torsion in infants and children: diagnosis with Doppler sonography. Radiology 1993;188:781–5.

22. Backhouse K. Embryology of testicular descent and maldescent. Urol Clin North Am 1982;9:315–25.

23. Zerin J, DiPietro M, Grignon A, et al. Testicular infarction in the newborn: ultrasound findings. Pediatr Radiol 1990;20:329–30.

24. Hawtrey CE. Assessment of acute scrotal symptoms and findings: a clinician's dilemma. Urol Clin North Am 1998;25:715–23.

25. Brown SM, Casillas VJ, Montalvo BM, et al. Intrauterine spermatic cord torsion in the newborn: sonographic and pathologic correlation. Radiology 1990;177:755–7.

26. Caesar RE, Kaplan GW. Incidence of the bellclapper deformity in an autopsy series. Urology 1994;44:114–6.

27. Burks DD, Markey BJ, Burkhard TK, et al. Suspected testicular torsion and ischemia: evaluation with color Doppler sonography. Radiology 1990;175:815–21.

28. Luker GD, Siegel MJ. Scrotal US in pediatric patients: comparison of power and standard color Doppler US. Radiology 1996;198:381–5.

29. Johansen TE, Larmo A. Ultrasonography in undescended testes. Acta Radiol 1988;29:159–63.

30. Docimo SG, Silver RI, Cromie W. The undescended testicle: diagnosis and management. Am Fam Physician 2000;62:2037–44.

31. Munter DW, Faleski EJ. Blunt scrotal trauma: emergency department evaluation and management. Am J Emerg Med 1989;7:227–34.

32. Mevorach RA. Scrotal trauma. WebMD Web site. Available at: http://www.emedicine.com/med/topic2857.htm. Published April 15, 2002. Accessed January 7, 2012.

33. Mulhall JP, Gabram SG, Jacobs LM. Emergency management of blunt testicular trauma. Acad Emerg Med 1995;2:639–43.

34. Buckley JC, McAninch JW. Use of ultrasonography for the diagnosis of testicular injuries in blunt scrotal trauma. J Urol 2006;175:175–8.

35. Howlett DC, Marchbank ND, Sallomi DF. Ultrasound of the testis. Clin Radiol 2000;55:595–601.

36. Gross M. Rupture of the testicle: the importance of early surgical treatment. J Urol 1969;101:196–7.

37. Jeffrey RB, Laing FC, Hricak H, et al. Sonography of testicular trauma. AJR Am J Roentgenol 1983;141:993–5.

38. Krone KD, Carroll BA. Scrotal ultrasound. Radiol Clin North Am 1985;23:121–39.

39. Bree RL, Hoang DT. Scrotal ultrasound. Radiol Clin North Am 1996;34:1183–205.

40. Lupetin AR, King W 3rd, Rich PJ, et al. The traumatized scrotum: ultrasound evaluation. Radiology 1983;148:203–7.

41. Cohen HL, Shapiro ML, Haller JO, et al. Sonography of intrascrotal hematomas simulating testicular rupture in adolescents. Pediatr Radiol 1992;22:296–7.

42. Bhatt S, Dogra VS. Role of US in testicular and scrotal trauma. Radiographics 2008;28:1617–29.

43. Zicherman J, Weissman D, Gribbin C, et al. Primary diffuse large B-cell lymphoma of the epididymis and testis. Radiographics 2005;25:243–8.

44. Lupetin A, King W, Rich P, et al. Ultrasound diagnosis of testicular leukemia. Radiology 1983;146: 171–2.

45. Moorjani V, Mashankar A, Goel S, et al. Sonographic appearance of primary testicular lymphoma. AJR Am J Roentgenol 1991;157:1225–6.

46. Subramanyam B, Horii S, Hilton S. Diffuse testicular disease: sonographic features and significance. AJR Am J Roentgenol 1985;145:1221–4.

47. Mazzu D, Jeffrey RB Jr, Ralls PW. Lymphoma and leukemia involving the testicles: findings on gray-scale and color Doppler sonography. AJR Am J Roentgenol 1995;164:645–7.

48. Doll DC, Weiss RB. Malignant lymphoma of the testis. Am J Med 1986;81:515–24.

49. Robertson E, Baxter G. Bilateral testicular metastases in malignant melanoma. BMUS 2010;18:86–8.

Imaging of the Retroperitoneum

Ajit H. Goenka, MD, Shetal N. Shah, MD,
Erick M. Remer, MD*

KEYWORDS

- Retroperitoneal space
- Multidetector computed tomography
- Magnetic resonance imaging • Sarcoma
- Retroperitoneal fibrosis • Neoplasms

The retroperitoneum is the compartmentalized space bounded anteriorly by the posterior parietal peritoneum and posteriorly by the transversalis fascia. It extends from the diaphragm superiorly to the pelvic brim inferiorly. This article discusses clinically relevant anatomy of the abdominal retroperitoneal spaces, their cross-sectional imaging evaluation with computed tomography (CT) and magnetic resonance (MR) imaging, and the imaging features of common retroperitoneal pathologic processes.

IMAGING ANATOMY OF THE ABDOMINAL RETROPERITONEUM

The abdominal retroperitoneum is divided by fascial planes into the anterior and posterior pararenal spaces and the perirenal (or perinephric) space.

Compartments

Anterior pararenal space

The anterior pararenal space is confined by the posterior parietal peritoneum anteriorly, the anterior renal fascia posteriorly, and the lateroconal fascia laterally. It contains the ascending and the descending colon (pericolonic component), the duodenum, and pancreas (pancreaticoduodenal component).

Perirenal space

The perirenal space is confined by the anterior renal fascia (Gerota fascia) and posterior renal fascia (Zuckerkandl fascia), which together comprise the renal fascia. It contains the kidneys, renal vessels, adrenal glands, renal pelves, proximal ureters, perirenal lymphatics, and perirenal fat.

Posterior pararenal space

The posterior pararenal space is confined by the posterior renal fascia anteriorly, by the transversalis fascia posteriorly, and by the psoas muscle medially. It continues laterally external to the lateroconal fascia as the properitoneal fat of the abdominal wall. Inferiorly, the posterior pararenal space is open to the pelvis,[1,2] and superiorly, it continues as a thin subdiaphragmatic layer of extraperitoneal fat. It almost always contains only fat.

Interfascial planes

The traditional tricompartmental anatomy described earlier does not completely explain the spread of fluid collections or tumors in the retroperitoneum. It is now believed that the perirenal fasciae are multilaminated structures with potentially expandable interfascial planes. These planes are represented by the retromesenteric, retrorenal, lateroconal, and combined interfascial planes.[3] Knowledge of the anatomy and interconnections of these interfascial planes can facilitate understanding of the extent

Disclosures: Nothing to disclose.
Funding support: None.
Section of Abdominal Imaging, Imaging Institute, Cleveland Clinic, 9500 Euclid Avenue – Hb6, Cleveland, OH 44195, USA
* Corresponding author.
E-mail address: remere1@ccf.org

Radiol Clin N Am 50 (2012) 333–355
doi:10.1016/j.rcl.2012.02.004
0033-8389/12/$ – see front matter © 2012 Elsevier Inc. All rights reserved.

and pathways of retroperitoneal disease spread. On CT and MR imaging, retroperitoneal fascial planes are usually detected when there is an abundance of retroperitoneal fat. Fascia measuring greater than 3 mm is considered thickened and is a sensitive, although nonspecific, sign of a retroperitoneal pathologic process.[4–6]

CT and MR Imaging of the Retroperitoneum

In general, CT is the workhorse for evaluating retroperitoneal disease, whereas MR imaging is more often used as a problem-solving tool. CT examination is typically from the lung bases to the symphysis pubis after the use of both oral and intravenous contrast media, with 3-mm to 5-mm slice thickness sections acquired during the portal venous phase of enhancement. MR protocols typically contain T1-weighted images (to assess high-signal-intensity fat or hemorrhage, lymphadenopathy, and tumoral vascular invasion) and fat-suppressed T2-weighted images (to assess lymphadenopathy, muscle invasion by a disease process, cystic change or necrosis, fluid collections, bone marrow edema). Venous-phase contrast-enhanced T1-weighted images are particularly useful for differentiating solid from nonenhancing cystic or necrotic lesions, the extent of disease, and the presence and nature of vascular thrombosis or encasement.[7–11]

PATHOLOGIC CONDITIONS

The retroperitoneum can be involved by a wide spectrum of diseases. For the purpose of this article, they are divided into neoplastic and nonneoplastic processes.

Neoplastic Processes

The neoplasms in the retroperitoneum can be further categorized into 4 important groups: (1) mesodermal neoplasms, (2) neurogenic tumors, (3) germ cell, sex cord, and stromal tumors, and (4) lymphoid neoplasms. Diagnosis of these tumors begins with affirmation of their retroperitoneal location and then determination of whether the lesion is primarily retroperitoneal or is arising secondarily from a retroperitoneal organ. Anterior displacement of retroperitoneal organs or vessels strongly suggests that a lesion is retroperitoneal (**Fig. 1**). On the other hand, rounded rather than beaked edges of an adjacent organ (negative beak sign) with a crescentic deformation (negative embedded organ sign) by the tumor suggest a primary retroperitoneal tumor.[12,13]

Mesodermal Neoplasms

Soft tissue sarcomas are rare mesenchymal neoplasms that account for less than 1% of adult malignancies. However, about 15% of them originate in the retroperitoneum.[14,15] Most retroperitoneal neoplasms are malignant, and one-third of malignant retroperitoneal neoplasms are sarcomas.[16,17] They typically present in the sixth and seventh decades of life and are often large at the time of presentation because the loose connective tissue in the retroperitoneum provides little resistance to their growth.[18] Sarcomas typically develop de novo, with the exception of malignant peripheral nerve sheath tumors (MPNST), which can arise from neurofibromas.[19]

Cross-sectional imaging plays an important role in defining the extent of the primary tumor, evaluating direct involvement of adjacent organs and vessels,

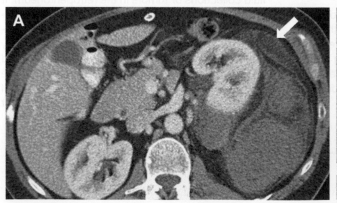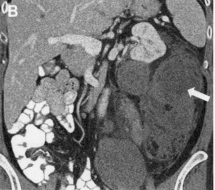

Fig. 1. Well-differentiated liposarcoma in a 53-year-old woman. Contrast-enhanced CT (*A*, axial; *B*, coronal) shows large heterogeneous mass with macroscopic fat (*arrow* in *A*) and enhancing, soft tissue components (*arrow* in *B*). Notice the anterior rotational displacement of kidney, a sign of retroperitoneal location, and negative organ embedded sign, an indication of primary retroperitoneal location.

and detection of distant metastases. In general, extensive vascular involvement, peritoneal implants, and distant metastatic disease suggest unresectability.[17] Moreover, imaging evidence of tumor necrosis suggests a high-grade component and portends a poor prognosis.[20] It is also possible to narrow the differential diagnosis of a retroperitoneal mass based on certain imaging characteristics (Table 1) in combination with the pattern of involvement and demographics. Nevertheless, histologic sampling using percutaneous cross-sectional imaging is typically necessary to establish a definite diagnosis. Imaging is also a component of the GTNM system (G, histologic grade; T, size; N, nodes; and M, metastases) that is often used for staging retroperitoneal sarcomas.[19]

Complete surgical resection is the treatment of choice for primary as well as for recurrent retroperitoneal sarcomas. It is the also single most important independent prognostic factor for survival followed only by histologic grade.[17,21–23] Overall, regional lymphadenopathy is uncommon in soft tissue sarcomas, with a frequency of less than 4% at presentation, and less than one-third of patients have metastases at presentation.[23]

Liposarcoma

Liposarcoma accounts for 40% of retroperitoneal sarcomas and is the most common type.[17,24] It originates from primitive mesenchymal cells and not from adipocytes.[25] The World Health Organization divides liposarcomas into 5 subtypes: well-differentiated, myxoid, dedifferentiated, round-cell, and pleomorphic (Table 2).[19] The most important cause of morbidity and mortality in patients with retroperitoneal liposarcoma is local disease recurrence, whereas the rate of distant metastases, usually to liver and lungs, is less than 10%.[15,17,26,27]

Table 1 Salient imaging features of sarcomas	
Well-differentiated liposarcoma	Macroscopic fat; fat-fluid level
IVC leiomyosarcoma	Necrotic mass having caval and extracaval components with or without metastases
MFH	Extensive hemorrhage, absence of fat or central necrosis; bowl-of-fruit sign
Myxoid liposarcoma, MFH	Myxoid stroma
Dedifferentiated liposarcoma	Calcification, ossification, macroscopic fat

Table 2 Features of liposarcoma subtypes	
Well-differentiated	Low metastatic potential; low-grade histology; high local recurrence (~100%); 10% eventually dedifferentiate
Dedifferentiated	Worst prognosis; calcification or ossification may be seen (30%)
Myxoid	25% may not contain fat; pseudocystic appearance on unenhanced images from the myxoid component; MFH has similar appearance
Pleomorphic and round-cell	Least common subtype, aggressive lesions with little or no macroscopic fat

Well-differentiated liposarcoma Well-differentiated liposarcoma is the most common subtype of liposarcoma. On cross-sectional imaging, it contains components that are similar in attenuation and signal intensity to macroscopic fat. Because of a paucity of intratumoral vessels, there is usually little or no contrast enhancement of the fatty component of this tumor.[28] However, streaky zones of enhancing fibrous or sclerotic components are usually evident.[29] Areas of necrosis and calcification tend to be uncommon in all liposarcomas.[26] The main differential diagnoses on imaging studies include a lipoma (Box 1) or a large exophytic renal angiomyolipoma. Features that suggest an angiomyolipoma are the presence of a renal parenchymal defect from which the mass arises, enlarged intratumoral arteries, and the presence of other angiomyolipomas.[30]

Other liposarcomas Myxoid liposarcoma is the second most common subtype.[25] It is described as pseudocystic because the myxoid component appears of water-attenuation or fluid-signal intensity

Box 1 Features that favor well-differentiated liposarcoma over lipoma
Large size (>10 cm)
Nodular or globular components
Thick septa (>2 mm)
Soft tissue components
Low proportional fat composition (<75% fat in mass)

on noncontrast images. However, it tends to show a characteristic gradual, heterogeneous, and often incomplete pattern of internal enhancement on delayed contrast-enhanced images because of slow, progressive accumulation of contrast within the extracellular space.[12,31] Occasionally, a fatty component at the margin of a mass may simulate extraperitoneal fat and may be missed. These tumors with peripheral fat may be confused with other myxoid-containing retroperitoneal tumors such as malignant fibrous histiocytoma (MFH) or neurogenic tumors. Dedifferentiated liposarcoma contains a well-differentiated lipogenic component and a nonlipogenic (dedifferentiated) component. Therefore, it can appear as a nonlipomatous mass within, adjacent to, or encompassing a fatty mass (Figs. 2 and 3).[29] The nonlipomatous component has a similar appearance to a high-grade fibrosarcoma or an MFH. Pleomorphic and round-cell liposarcoma are the least common subtypes and tend to present as heterogeneous tumors with little or no macroscopic fat, often indistinguishable from other malignant soft tissue masses.[32] They are aggressive tumors, with high tendency toward local recurrence and metastasis.[25]

Leiomyosarcoma

Leiomyosarcoma is the second most common retroperitoneal sarcoma (30%), with two-thirds of all retroperitoneal leiomyosarcomas occurring in women.[17,26] It is also the most common intraluminal venous neoplasm and the most common primary tumor of the inferior vena cava (IVC). Tumors involving the IVC may be completely external to the IVC lumen (approximately two-thirds) (Fig. 4), have both intraluminal and extraluminal components (approximately one-third) (Fig. 5), or may be purely intraluminal (5%). Purely intraluminal types occur primarily in women

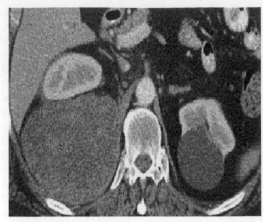

Fig. 3. Dedifferentiated liposarcoma in an 86-year-old woman. Axial contrast-enhanced CT shows a predominantly soft tissue attenuating posterior pararenal mass.

(80%–90% of patients), and present at a younger age (mean age 50 years).[33] Presenting symptoms and resectability of IVC leiomyosarcoma are variable and often depend on the segment of IVC involved. Tumors involving the upper segment (intrahepatic IVC and above) can present with Budd-Chiari syndrome; midsegment tumors may present with right upper quadrant colic or renal insufficiency caused by tumor extension into renal veins; and lower segment tumors may present with lower extremity edema. Midsegment and lower-segment tumors may be resectable, whereas upper-segment tumors tend to be unresectable.[34,35]

Leiomyosarcomas are typically well-circumscribed lesions that often contain necrosis and hemorrhage.[36] Smaller tumors may lack necrosis. Uncommonly, the tumor presents as a predominantly cystic mass with extensive necrosis.[19]

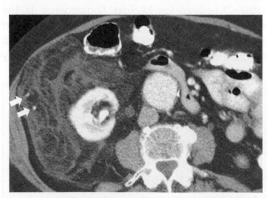

Fig. 2. Dedifferentiated liposarcoma in an 81-year-old woman. Axial contrast-enhanced CT shows a heterogeneous mass with soft tissue swirls encompassing macroscopic fat; note the foci of calcification (arrows).

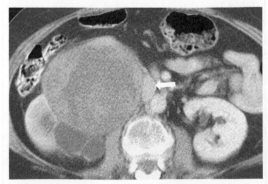

Fig. 4. Leiomyosarcoma in a 66-year-old woman. Axial contrast-enhanced CT shows a heterogeneous right retroperitoneal mass causing ipsilateral obstructive uropathy. The IVC (arrow) is draped along the medial surface of the lesion.

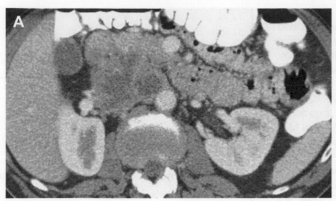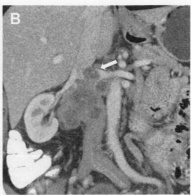

Fig. 5. IVC leiomyosarcoma in a 64-year-old man. Contrast-enhanced CT (*A*, axial; *B*, coronal) shows a necrotic, lobulated mass centered in the IVC with both intraluminal and extraluminal components, features that are pathognomonic for IVC leiomyosarcoma. Note the extension in the left renal vein (*arrow* in *B*).

Initially, adjacent organs are displaced without direct invasion with tumoral growth can become involved. Intracaval leiomyosarcomas are seen as polypoid or nodular masses that are firmly attached to the vessel wall and are most frequently located between the diaphragm and the renal veins. They are soft tissue masses with low to intermediate T1-signal intensity and heterogeneous intermediate to high T2-signal intensity. Fat and calcification are not typically seen. The degree of enhancement depends on the amount of muscular and fibrous components; it is usually delayed compared with the enhancement of the surrounding skeletal muscle.[29,33,36,37] Because of the typically slow growth of the tumor, extensive retroperitoneal collaterals can form.[13] It can be difficult to differentiate bland tumefactive thrombus from a neoplasm. However, expansion of the vascular lumen, evidence of feeding vessels during the arterial phase, and enhancing components are the signs that favor a neoplastic cause.[29]

MFH

MFH is the third most common retroperitoneal sarcoma (15%)[26] and has a male predominance (two-thirds).[38] There are distinct histologic subtypes of MFH: storiform-pleomorphic (most common), myxoid (second most common), giant cell, inflammatory, and angiomatoid.[19] On CT, MFH is a large, relatively well-circumscribed soft tissue mass that spreads along fascial planes and between muscle fibers. It has low to intermediate T1-signal intensity and heterogeneously increased T2-signal intensity relative to muscle.[26,27,29] The bowl-of-fruit sign is a mosaic of mixed low, intermediate, and high T2-signal intensity that correlates with the presence of intratumoral solid components, cystic degeneration, hemorrhage, myxoid stroma, and fibrous tissue.[39] The sign has also been described in other nonretroperitoneal tumors such as synovial sarcoma and Ewing sarcoma. Extensive intratumoral hemorrhage and intratumoral calcifications (20%) may also be seen.[29,39,40]

Perivascular epithelioid cell tumor

Perivascular epithelioid cell tumors (PEComas) are benign mesenchymal tumors of varying malignant potential that are composed of distinctively perivascular epithelioid cells (**Fig. 6**).[41] The cells express melanocytic markers (melan-A, microphthalmia transcription factor) and smooth muscle markers (HMB-45, actin). Angiomyolipomas, lymphangioleiomyomatosis, clear-cell sugar tumors, clear-cell myomelanocytic tumors, sarcoma of perivascular cells, and pigmented melanotic tumors are included in this group.[18]

Desmoid tumor

Desmoid tumor (also known as deep fibromatosis, aggressive fibromatosis, or well-differentiated fibrosarcoma) accounts for less than 1% of

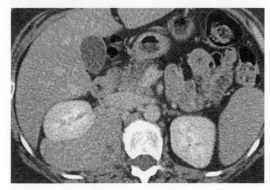

Fig. 6. PEComa in a 44-year-old woman. Axial contrast-enhanced CT shows a minimally heterogeneous soft tissue mass in the posterior pararenal space.

retroperitoneal tumors.[18] It is an estrogen-dependent tumor that is more common in young women, with a peak occurrence in the third decade.[42,43] It can be associated with familial polyposis coli and Gardner syndrome. Desmoids may be single or multiple. They generally have well-defined borders, but may be infiltrative. On CT, they have attenuation equivalent to muscle or greater after contrast administration.[44] On MR, early-stage lesions are cellular and have high T2-signal intensity, but with loss of cellularity and collagen deposition, the lesion becomes hypointense. Moderate to marked enhancement is shown on contrast-enhanced images.[18] They are locally aggressive lesions with high recurrence rate (50%), even after wide surgical excision.[45]

Germ Cell, Sex Cord, and Stromal Tumors

Primary retroperitoneal extragonadal germ cell tumor

Primary retroperitoneal extragonadal germ cell tumors (EGCTs) are hypothesized to arise from primordial midline germ cell remnants of the genital ridge that fail to migrate properly.[26,46,47] However, in general, most retroperitoneal germ cell tumors (GCTs) are metastases from a gonadal primary.[46,48,49] Therefore, every male with a potential retroperitoneal EGCT should be evaluated to exclude a coexistent primary testicular neoplasm (Fig. 7). Retroperitoneal EGCTs may be seminomatous or nonseminomatous (Table 3). On CT and MR imaging, primary EGCTs are typically large, midline, enhancing masses that are of low to intermediate T1-signal intensity and intermediate to high T2-signal intensity relative to skeletal muscle. A midline location favors primary EGCT over that

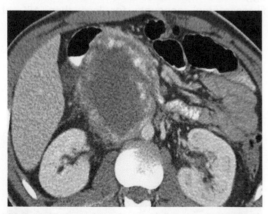

Fig. 7. Metastatic mixed germ cell tumor in a 21-year-old man. Axial contrast-enhanced CT shows a centrally necrotic paramidline retroperitoneal mass. Scrotal ultrasound showed an asymptomatic burnt-out tumor primary in the right testis.

Table 3	
Salient features of primary EGCTs	
Seminomatous Germ Cell Tumors	**Nonseminomatous Germ Cell Tumors**
Usually, no increase of tumor markers	Associated with increased tumor markers
Better survival (88%)	Low survival (63%)
Homogeneous in attenuation and signal intensity	Heterogeneous masses with areas of cystic necrosis or hemorrhage

of metastatic lymphadenopathy from a primary testicular neoplasm.[26,46,47] Prognosis for and treatment of primary EGCT is equivalent to primary testicular neoplasms with retroperitoneal metastases.[50] Nonseminomatous histology, presence of nonpulmonary visceral metastases, and increased human chorionic gonadotropin level are independent prognostic factors for shorter survival.[51]

Growing teratoma syndrome

Growing teratoma syndrome (GTS) is a clinical term for a retroperitoneal mass consisting of chemorefractory teratomatous elements that is defined by the following criteria: a metastatic lesion that increases in size during chemotherapy in a patient with non-seminomatous germ cell tumor, normalization of tumor markers (α fetoprotein [AFP] or human chorionic gonadotropin), and a predominant composition of mature teratoma at the time of resection.[52] It is a rare phenomenon, with reported rates of 1.9% to 7.6% in published series.[52–54] However, it should be considered in the differential diagnosis of a retroperitoneal metastatic lesion that shows increasing size on serial images in the setting of normal or decreasing tumor markers (Fig. 8). Complete surgical excision is the treatment of choice and carries low risk of subsequent progression.[55]

Primary retroperitoneal teratoma

Primary retroperitoneal teratomas are rare lesions that represent 6% to 11% of primary retroperitoneal tumors.[56,57] Although less than 20% of lesions occur in adults, they have a greater chance of being malignant in adults than in children (14%–26% vs 6%–7%, respectively).[19] AFP[56,57] levels may be increased with malignant teratomas.[56] Imaging appearance is similar to teratomas in other locations. In the retroperitoneum, they tend to be located near the upper poles of the kidneys, with preponderance on the left side.[56,58] Lesions

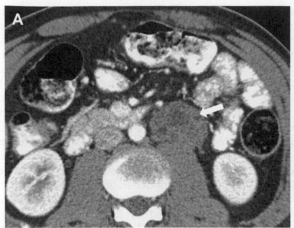
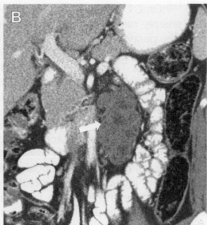

Fig. 8. GTS in a 20-year-old man. Contrast-enhanced CT (CECT) shows a residual solid-cystic left para-aortic mass (*arrow* in A, axial CECT; *arrow* in B, coronal CECT) found after induction chemotherapy for left testicular mixed germ cell tumor with normalization of tumor markers.

may be solid or cystic. Solid teratomas are more frequently malignant and contain immature embryonic tissue in addition to the mature components.[57,59] Calcification can be seen in both benign and malignant tumors.[59] The presence of an internal fat-fluid level is almost pathognomonic of a mature cystic teratoma (**Fig. 9**).[57,60] However, this finding has also been reported in retroperitoneal liposarcoma.[61] A peritoneal fat-fluid level may be a sign of intraperitoneal rupture.[62] Surgical excision is recommended even for benign lesions because significant morbidity may result from continued growth.[63,64]

Neurogenic Tumors

Retroperitoneal neurogenic tumors can originate from the nerve sheath (schwannoma, neurofibroma, MPNST (**Table 4**), ganglionic cells

(ganglioneuroma, ganglioneuroblastoma, neuroblastoma) or from paraganglionic cells (paraganglioma). In toto, they constitute 10% to 20% of primary retroperitoneal tumors in adults.[18]

Schwannoma

Schwannomas are benign nerve sheath tumors of Schwann cell origin that account for up to 4% of all retroperitoneal tumors.[19] They tend to present as asymptomatic, slow-growing, painless soft tissue

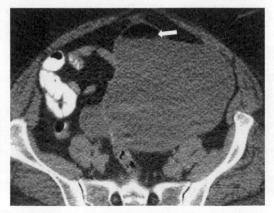

Fig. 9. Mature cystic teratoma in a 58-year-old man. Contrast-enhanced axial CT shows a large lower retroperitoneal mass with an internal fat-fluid level (*arrow*).

Table 4	
Salient features of benign nerve sheath tumors	
Schwannoma	**Neurofibroma**
Heterogeneous attenuation and signal intensity	Relatively homogeneous
Eccentric position in relation to the parent nerve	Centered on and contiguous with the parent nerve
Low-signal-intensity capsule on MR imaging	Nonencapsulated
Composed of Antoni A (cellular) and Antoni B (myxoid) components	Composed of nerve sheath cells, collagenous bundles, and myxoid component
Nerve-sparing surgery is possible	Resection involves excision of the parent nerve
Malignant degeneration is rare	Plexiform neurofibroma may degenerate into MPNST

masses.[65,66] On CT and MR imaging, schwannomas are sharply circumscribed masses, usually located in the paravertebral or presacral retroperitoneum. They are of low to intermediate T1-signal intensity and high T2-signal intensity with solid enhancing components. A target sign consisting of a central low to intermediate T2-signal intensity fibrous tissue surrounded by peripheral high-signal-intensity myxoid tissue may be seen in both schwannomas and neurofibromas. Targetlike central enhancement may also be seen.[67] Larger schwannomas are more likely to undergo degenerative changes, including cyst formation (in up to 66%), calcification, hemorrhage, and hyalinization (Fig. 10).[19,68] Ancient schwannoma refers to a long-standing lesion with advanced degenerative changes.[69,70] Schwannomas are treated by surgical excision or enucleation, particularly if large or symptomatic.

Neurofibroma

Neurofibromas are benign nerve sheath tumors that represent 5% of all benign soft tissue neoplasms.[70] Approximately one-third of patients with a solitary neurofibroma have neurofibromatosis type 1 (NF-1), and almost every patient with multiple or plexiform neurofibromas has NF-1.[67] Neurofibromas associated with NF-1 present in a younger age group (first 2 decades), are multifocal, larger (>5 cm), and are more likely to be associated with neurologic symptoms than those in unaffected patients.

Neurofibromas usually have a fusiform shape that is oriented longitudinally along the course of the parent nerve. Associated muscle atrophy in the particular nerve distribution may be seen. A split-fat sign may be seen as a rim of fat that surrounds the tumor that originates from an intramuscular nerve.[70] As with other spinal nerve or nerve sheath tumors, a dumbbell shape is seen with spinal nerve root neurofibromas that extend through and enlarge a neural foramen.[29,39,71] In

NF-1, a characteristic bag-of-worms appearance may be seen when a large conglomerate of infiltrative masses of innumerable neurofibromas diffusely thicken a parent nerve and extend into multiple nerve branches.[19] Plexiform neurofibromas in the retroperitoneum are typically bilateral and symmetric in a parapsoas or presacral location and follow the distribution of the lumbosacral plexus (Fig. 11).[72]

Neurofibromas are soft tissue attenuation masses on CT and show low T1-signal intensity but variably high T2-signal intensity. A target sign, myxoid degeneration, or a whorled appearance consisting of linear or curvilinear low signal intensity caused by Schwann cell bundles and collagen fibers in a background of high signal intensity may also be seen on T2-weighted images.[39,70] Contrast enhancement is variable. Targetlike central enhancement may be encountered on CT or MR imaging.[67]

Plexiform neurofibromas, symptomatic neurofibromas, and neurofibromas that are suspected to have malignant degeneration are surgically resected along with underlying parent nerves.[70]

MPNST

MPNSTs include malignant schwannoma, neurogenic sarcoma, and neurofibrosarcoma[67] and represent 5% to 10% of soft tissue sarcomas. About 50% of patients with MPNST have NF-1. Conversely, around 2% to 5% of patients with NF-1 develop MPNST, typically from preexisting neurofibromas.[70,73,74] MPNSTs in patients with NF-1 tend to present early (third decade) and have a higher histologic grade and larger size than those that develop de novo.[19] Previous radiation exposure is another risk factor for the development of MPNST.[70,74] MPNSTs tend to be large, heterogeneous masses with central necrosis or calcification (Fig. 12). They may show poorly defined margins or associated edema or may

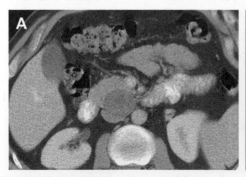
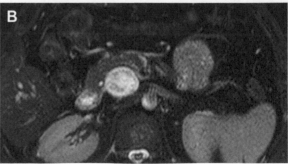

Fig. 10. Schwannoma in a 56-year-old man. (A) Contrast-enhanced axial CT shows a relatively homogeneous, well-circumscribed mass interposed between the aorta and the IVC. On T2-weighted image (B), the lesion shows a targetoid pattern of hyperintensity. Small schwannomas tend to be homogeneous but larger lesions can show a spectrum of degenerative changes.

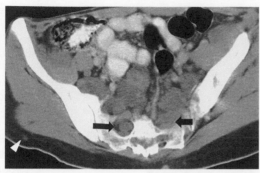

Fig. 11. Plexiform neurofibroma in a 30-year-old woman with NF-1. Contrast-enhanced axial CT shows bilateral retroperitoneal soft tissue masses with extension along the spinal nerve roots and expansion of the involved sacral neural foramina (*arrows*). Note the subcutaneous neurofibroma (*arrowhead*).

expand neural foramina. However, these features may also be seen with benign neural tumors. Therefore, imaging differentiation from benign tumors is not always reliable.[19] The most important finding that should raise suspicion of MPNST is rapid enlargement of a tumor mass, particularly if associated with spontaneous and unremitting pain.[75,76] Complete surgical resection is the treatment of choice and is the most important factor influencing patient survival. Local recurrence and distant metastatic disease are common. In patients with NF-1, MPNSTs have a particularly aggressive course and poor prognosis (15% survival at 5 years).[70,74]

Ganglioneuroma
Ganglioneuromas are benign tumors that arise from the sympathetic ganglia in the 20-year to 40-year age group and represent 5% to 10% of primary

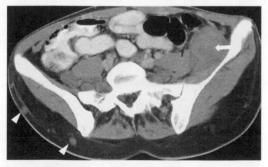

Fig. 12. Malignant peripheral nerve sheath tumor (PSNT) in the same patient as in Fig. 11. Contrast-enhanced axial CT shows new heterogeneity in the preexisting plexiform neurofibroma. This change and the development of unremitting pain in the left lower quadrant prompted a biopsy that revealed MPNST (*arrow*). Note the subcutaneous neurofibromas (*arrowheads*).

retroperitoneal tumors.[67,77] They often present as asymptomatic masses. However, approximately 57% of ganglioneuromas may be functional and produce catecholamines or androgenic hormones.[78] They typically are well-defined, longitudinally oriented, paravertebral soft tissue masses that tend to surround major blood vessels with little or no luminal narrowing, usually do not result in osseous changes, and only infrequently extend into the neural foramina (**Fig. 13**).[18] Discrete punctate calcifications (20%–30%) may be present, and contrast enhancement is variable.[79] On MR, ganglioneuromas have homogeneous T1-hypointensity and variable T2-signal intensity. Like the nerve sheath tumors, a whorled appearance may be seen on T2-weighted images. Imaging differentiation from the malignant ganglionic tumors may be challenging. Metastases and younger age group favor the latter. The prognosis of ganglioneuromas is good after surgical resection.[67]

Paraganglioma
In the abdomen, paragangliomas occur most frequently at the renal hila and in the organs of Zuckerkandl, which are located in the para-aortic region near the inferior mesenteric artery origin.[80] Up to 40% of paragangliomas are malignant, compared with 10% of adrenal pheochromocytomas. Malignancy is recognized by locally aggressive behavior or metastatic spread to sites that do not have paraganglia such as lymph nodes, bone, lung, or liver.[13,81] Paragangliomas may be functional in up to 60% of patients and produce symptoms caused by catecholamine secretion. In affected patients, detection of increased urinary catecholamines is the most efficacious way of characterizing an abdominal mass as a paraganglioma. However, there is poor correlation between the functional activity and the degree of malignancy.[82,83]

On CT, paragangliomas are enhancing, well-circumscribed, soft tissue masses (**Fig. 14**) that contain necrosis (40%), punctate calcification (15%), or intratumoral hemorrhage.[27,67,83,84] Intravenous administration of nonionic iodinated contrast material even without α-adrenergic blockage is now considered safe in patients with paraganglioma.[85] On MR imaging, they show low to intermediate T1-signal intensity and moderately high T2-signal intensity relative to skeletal muscle. They are hypervascular tumors that enhance briskly.[13] Because of its high sensitivity compared with scintigraphy (metaiodobenzylguanidine), imaging with CT or MR imaging is recommended if there is a high index of suspicion and the tumor is not found with scintigraphy.[86–89] Whenever possible, paragangliomas are treated with complete surgical resection. The limitations of

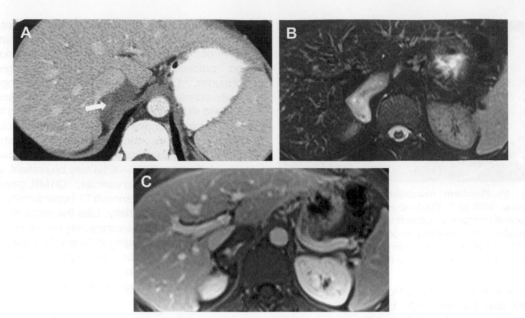

Fig. 13. Ganglioneuroma. (*A*) Contrast-enhanced axial CT shows a well-circumscribed, minimally enhancing, soft tissue mass in the retrocaval space (*arrow*) that is displacing the vessels without encasement. (*B*) Axial true fast imaging with steady-state free precession image shows the lesion to be hyperintense and shows minimal enhancement on postgadolinium image (*C*).

histopathologic criteria in predicting malignant behavior, the long natural history of the disease, and a high propensity for subsequent metastasis make extended follow-up necessary.[90]

Lymphoid Neoplasms

Retroperitoneal lymph nodes are generally present in a perivascular distribution about the aorta, IVC, and iliac vessels. Lymphoma, which is the most common retroperitoneal malignancy, and metastatic disease are the most common causes of abdominopelvic lymphadenopathy.[91] Imaging differentiation between metastatic and reactive lymph nodes is based on size criteria, specifically short-axis dimension. Size criteria are location based: the upper limit of normal in the retrocrural space is 6 mm, in the retroperitoneum is 10 mm, and in the pelvis is 15 mm.[92–94] Relying on size criteria alone diminishes sensitivity to metastatic normal-sized lymph nodes. The presence of multiple, borderline-enlarged lymph nodes, in the 8-mm to 10-mm range, should be viewed with suspicion for an underlying pathologic process (eg, chronic lymphocytic leukemia) (**Fig. 15**). Most normal lymph nodes have an oval shape with a preserved fatty hilum, whereas malignant lymph nodes are often rounded.[94,95]

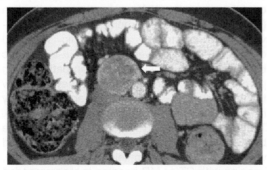

Fig. 14. Paraganglioma in a 30-year-old woman with heart failure and evidence of hormonal secretion. Contrast-enhanced axial CT shows a mass at the organ of Zuckerkandl (*arrow*). Laparoscopic excision confirmed the diagnosis of paraganglioma.

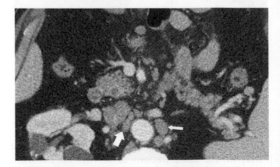

Fig. 15. Chronic lymphocytic leukemia in an 84-year-old man with microscopic hematuria. Contrast-enhanced axial CT urogram shows multiple borderline-enlarged retroperitoneal (*arrows*) nodes, which prompted investigations that led to the diagnosis of chronic lymphocytic leukemia.

Lymphoma

Lymphoma typically begins as local lymph node enlargement and then spreads through lymphatics to adjacent lymph nodes, commonly in the retroperitoneum, and sometimes systemically.[26,96] Conglomerate nodal masses may form and characteristically infiltrate the perinephric spaces of the retroperitoneum.[26] Whereas abdominal Hodgkin lymphoma (HL) tends to be confined to the spleen and retroperitoneum with spread of disease to contiguous lymph nodes, non-Hodgkin's lymphoma (NHL) more commonly involves discontiguous nodal groups and extranodal sites.[97,98]

On CT, nodal and extranodal lymphoma typically has homogeneous soft tissue attenuation, which is the main distinguishing factor from other neoplasms.[29] Necrosis and calcification are uncommon before therapy. Sometimes, the aorta seems to be immersed in the tumor, giving the floating aorta or CT angiogram sign (Fig. 16). This sign is characteristic of lymphoma and is generally not seen in other retroperitoneal disorders such as sarcomas or neurogenic tumors.[13] On MR imaging, lymphoma typically has intermediate to slightly high T1-signal intensity and high T2-signal intensity relative to muscle. Lymphomatous nodal masses may develop low T2-signal intensity after treatment, which represents nonviable tumor or fibrosis. However, assessment of residual tumor is confounded by the presence of edema, granulation tissue, hemorrhage, or immature fibrosis, which may give rise to high T2-signal intensity up to 12 months after therapy.[99]

Metastatic lymphadenopathy

Malignant neoplasms tend to spread initially to their regional nodal groups. However, because of complex intercommunications among regional groups of lymph nodes, lymphadenopathy may involve several contiguous or even widely separated nodal chains.[19] Most common nonlymphomatous neoplasms that lead to retroperitoneal lymphadenopathy are renal cell carcinoma, testicular carcinoma, cervical carcinoma, and prostatic carcinoma. Carcinomas of the bladder, prostate, cervix, uterus, and the anorectum initially spread to the pelvic nodes (Fig. 17). On the other hand, testicular, ovarian, and fallopian tube malignancies spread first to the retroperitoneal nodes adjacent to or near the renal hila because of spread along the gonadal vessels and may involve the pelvic nodes by retrograde spread.[94]

NONNEOPLASTIC PROCESSES
Retroperitoneal Fibrosis

Retroperitoneal fibrosis (RPF) is a rare fibrotic reactive process, with a prevalence of about 1 per 200,000.[100] Most patients present during the fifth or sixth decade of life. Although a gamut of underlying causes may be associated with RPF, no identifiable cause may be found in two-thirds of all cases. Such cases of idiopathic RPF are also called Ormond disease. Idiopathic RPF is more common in men (2:1).[101–103]

Cause

The cause of RPF is unclear. Proposed hypotheses include either an immune-mediated reaction to a component of ruptured atherosclerotic plaque such as ceroid[102,103] or an underlying systemic autoimmune process.[100] In up to 15% of individuals, associated fibrotic processes outside the retroperitoneum may be present.[104] Other associations include autoimmune or inflammatory disease

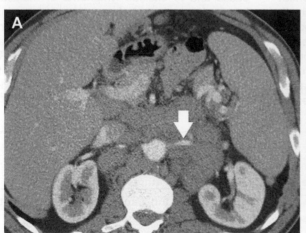
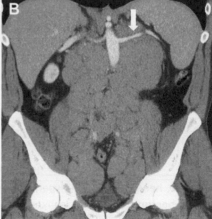

Fig. 16. Lymphoma in a 54-year-old man. Contrast-enhanced axial (A) and coronal (B) CT shows homogeneous, lobulated, minimally enhancing retroperitoneal masses without necrosis or calcification. Major vessels are encased, giving positive CT angiogram sign (arrow) characteristic of lymphoma.

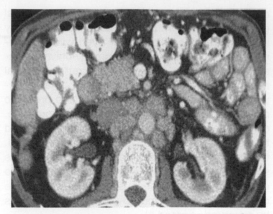

Fig. 17. Metastatic lymphadenopathy in a 54-year-old man with bladder cancer. Contrast-enhanced axial CT with multiple, discrete, enlarged, rounded retroperitoneal lymph nodes.

processes, asbestos exposure, and inflammatory abdominal aortic aneurysms (perianeurysmal fibrosis).[100,105] Ergot derivates such as methysergide (1% patients) and bromocriptine have been associated with a reversible form of RPF that tends to regress on discontinuing these drugs.[101,103] Malignant RPF is an unusual subtype that occurs when small metastatic foci to the retroperitoneum elicit a desmoplastic response.[101] Lymphoma is the most common underlying malignancy, whereas colorectal, breast, prostate, and bladder cancers are other causes.[101,103,106] Other conditions that can lead to RPF are granulomatous infections, nonspecific gastrointestinal inflammation, retroperitoneal hemorrhage, urine extravasation, or previous irradiation or surgery.[100,101,103]

RPF typically originates below the aortic bifurcation at the level of the lumbosacral vertebrae. It then extends superiorly in a periaortic and pericaval distribution toward the renal hila. Typically, the middle third of the ureters is encased and can result in hydroureteronephrosis.[107] However, the fibrotic process may also spread inferiorly to involve the pelvic vessels, rectosigmoid colon, urinary bladder, and other pelvic organs, or anteriorly along the celiac and superior mesenteric arteries.[101,103] Symptoms and signs are related to entrapment and compression of these retroperitoneal structures.

Imaging findings

On CT, RPF has homogeneous soft tissue attenuation. On MR imaging, RPF has low to intermediate T1-signal intensity. The T2-weighted signal intensity and the enhancement pattern of RPF depend on the activity of the disease (**Table 5**).[101,103] The disease progresses from chronic active inflammation to fibrous scarring.[18] The maturation process progresses laterally from the midline. Therefore, the lateral edges of the lesion tend to be T2-hyperintense and enhancing, whereas the central portion tends to be more fibrotic (**Fig. 18**).[102] Factors that favor malignant RPF over idiopathic RPF on imaging are heterogeneous, enhancing soft tissue mass with poorly defined margins, adjacent osseous destruction, high T2-signal intensity in adjacent psoas muscles, or lymphadenopathy (**Fig. 19**).[26,106] On the other hand, malignant lymphadenopathy can be differentiated from RPF by the lobulated appearance of the former and the tendency to displace rather than encase the aorta and the ureters.[101] Moreover, the fibrous tissue in idiopathic RPF is usually not seen between the aorta and the underlying vertebrae, in contrast to that in lymphoma or in disseminated malignancy.[105]

Treatment and prognosis

Corticosteroid therapy is the mainstay of treatment. Tamoxifen has also been used successfully. Ureteral stenting or ureterolysis may be performed when medical therapy is not effective.[105] Biopsies are obtained to exclude a malignant or infectious cause and to exclude lymphoma or metastatic lymphadenopathy, before therapy is instituted.[102,103] RPF that is secondary to infection is treated with specific antimicrobial therapy, and steroids are contraindicated.[100] Idiopathic RPF carries a favorable prognosis. However, the mean survival of patients with malignant RPF is 3 to 6 months after diagnosis.[103,108]

Table 5
Signal intensity and enhancement of RPF

RPF	T2-Signal Intensity	Enhancement	Pathophysiology
Immature, benign	Hyperintense	Present	Inflammatory edema > cellularity
Mature, benign, or after steroid therapy	Isohypointense	Relatively less	Decrease in edema
Malignant RPF	Heterogeneously hyperintense	Present	Hypercellularity > edema

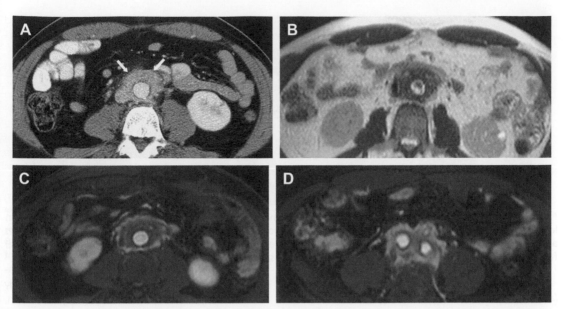

Fig. 18. RPF in a 64-year-old man who presented with nonspecific abdominal pain. (*A*) Contrast-enhanced axial CT shows an enhancing rim of soft tissue around the infrarenal aorta (*arrows*). Note sparing of retroaortic prevertebral space. (*B*) Axial T2-weighted image shows the soft tissue to be hypointense. (*C*) Contrast-enhanced axial T1 fat-suppressed gradient recalled echo shows the lesion to be centrally hypoenhancing with enhancement of the peripheral margins. There was extension along the origin of the common iliac arteries (*D*). (*Courtesy of* Paul Nikolaidis, MD, Northwestern University, Chicago, IL.)

Retroperitoneal Fluid Collections

Retroperitoneal fluid collections tend to be confined by the fascial planes or adhesions unless they are large, rapidly developing, or infected.[4,109] The imaging appearance of any retroperitoneal fluid collection depends on the content of collection and whether infection is present. Infected or proteinaceous collections may have high attenuation on CT, high T1-weighted signal intensity, nonenhancing internal debris, and a thick, enhancing rim.

Hemorrhage/hematoma

Retroperitoneal hemorrhage may be spontaneous, posttraumatic, or secondary to other causes.[4,26,109,110] Spontaneous hemorrhage classically originates in the posterior pararenal space (**Fig. 20**) and may extend into the properitoneal fat, pelvis, psoas muscle, or the abdominal wall musculature.[109] Traumatic hemorrhage tends to be largely confined to the retroperitoneal interfascial planes, and tends to be clinically uncontrollable when extension into the subfascial plane is visualized.[111] Most bleeding caused by ruptured abdominal aortic aneurysms tends to be confined by the psoas space, but may extend into the left posterior interfascial retrorenal plane. On the other hand, hemorrhage from the IVC often bleeds directly into the right posterior interfascial retrorenal plane.[107]

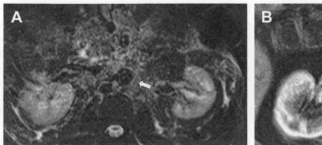
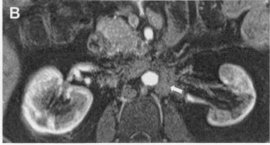

Fig. 19. Malignant RP fibrosis. 54-year-old man with heterogeneous, incomplete rind of soft tissue around the aorta. Lesion is hyperintense on short-tau inversion recovery image (*arrow* in *A*) and shows postgadolinium enhancement (*arrow* in *B*). Biopsy showed metastatic adenocarcinoma.

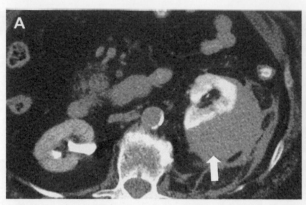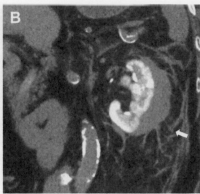

Fig. 20. Retroperitoneal hematoma in a 70-year-old woman who developed an acute decrease in hemoglobin level after a cerebral angiogram for subarachnoid hemorrhage. Noncontrast CT (*A*, axial; *B*, coronal) shows a left perinephric hematoma with extension along the retrorenal interfascial plane (*arrow* in *A*), lateral conal fascia, and along the bridging septae of the perinephric space (*arrow* in *B*).

Acute clotted hematoma has higher attenuation (45–80 HU) than does pure fluid (0–20 HU) or non-clotted or chronic hemorrhage (25–45 HU). These differences are the basis for the sentinel clot sign, in which areas of higher attenuation (acute hematoma) indicate the anatomic sites of hemorrhage origination.[112] Because MR imaging is typically not performed to evaluate for a hyperacute or acute hemorrhage, most hematomas seen on MR imaging are either subacute or chronic.[19] A subacute hematoma may show 2 outer characteristic layers of signal intensity: a thin peripheral rim with low signal intensity on all pulse sequences corresponding to hemosiderin and an inner peripheral high T1-signal intensity zone caused by methemoglobin. This appearance of a concentric ring sign is pathognomonic for a subacute hematoma.[113] A hematocrit effect (layering signal intensities or attenuations) may also be seen, especially in the setting of anticoagulation therapy or coagulopathy.[114,115] Active contrast extravasation on CT or MR imaging indicates ongoing arterial hemorrhage and indicates a need for immediate supportive, angiographic, or surgical intervention.[116]

The main imaging differential diagnostic consideration is a hemorrhagic tumor. The latter typically has enhancing soft tissue components.[26]

Lymphocele

Lymphoceles are fluid-filled cystic collections, without an epithelial lining, that usually occur at least 3 to 4 weeks after radical lymphadenectomy (up to 30% patients) or renal transplantation (up to 18% patients).[117–119] They appear as well-circumscribed water-attenuation or water-signal intensity lesions usually adjacent to surgical clips. Negative attenuation values caused by lipid content, internal septa, or mural calcification may be seen.[120] Percutaneous or surgical drainage is performed for symptomatic lymphoceles, sometimes in conjunction with sclerotherapy.[121]

Urinoma

A urinoma is an encapsulated collection of chronically extravasated urine. Urinomas are usually found in the perirenal spaces, sometimes with extension into the interfascial planes. Common causes include urinary obstruction (most common), abdominopelvic trauma, surgery, or diagnostic instrumentation.[1,4,109,122] On imaging, an urinoma is seen as a water-attenuation or water-signal intensity collection. However, the attenuation and the signal intensity can increase progressively on contrast-enhanced images because of leakage of the contrast-enhanced urine, which is the direct evidence of urine leak (Fig. 21).[64]

Inflammatory collections

Infectious fluid collections in the retroperitoneum are typically subacute and are most often caused by gram-negative bacilli. Most inflammatory fluid collections originate in the anterior pararenal space from extraperitoneal portions of the gastrointestinal tract (Fig. 22), with acute pancreatitis being one of the most common causes. Posterior pararenal space collections are usually caused by extension of infection from another space. Perirenal inflammatory fluid collections are most often secondary to renal infections.[123] Inflammatory fluid collections (in particular those related to acute pancreatitis) can access the posterior interfascial retrorenal plane, the transversalis fascia, and the abdominal wall. Fluid may also traverse the midline through the anterior interfascial retromesenteric plane, may spread inferiorly to the pelvic retroperitoneum through the combined interfascial plane, or may extend superiorly along the diaphragm to

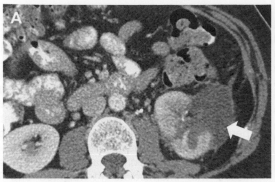
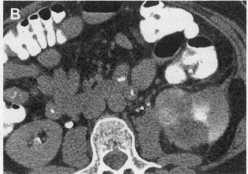

Fig. 21. Urinoma in a 54-year-old woman; status after left laparoscopic partial nephrectomy for renal cell carcinoma. (*A*) Contrast-enhanced axial CT shows a well-circumscribed fluid collection around the kidney (*arrow*). On delayed contrast-enhanced axial CT (*B*), progressive accumulation of contrast is seen in the perinephric fluid collection, indicating that this represents a urinoma.

enter the mediastinum.[4,111,124,125] On imaging, inflammatory collections appear as localized, complex collections that show water or increased-attenuation fluid, variable T1-signal intensity, intermediate to high T2-signal intensity, and thick, peripheral rim of enhancement. Layering debris, gas bubbles, or a gas-fluid level may also be seen. The presence of gas increases the specificity for the diagnosis of an abscess.[26,126]

Psoas muscle fluid collections
Fluid collections related to the psoas muscle are located in the retrofascial space posterior to the transversalis fascia.[127] Common sources of infection that may result in psoas collections include

gastrointestinal disease (most common), renal disease, or extension from lumbar osteomyelitis (**Fig. 23**).[19] Primary psoas abscesses are more likely to occur in immunocompromised patients, with up to 90% caused by *Staphylococcus aureus*. In developing countries, tuberculosis is an important cause of psoas abscess.[128,129] The imaging appearance is similar to any other abscess in the retroperitoneum. Secondary findings of psoas

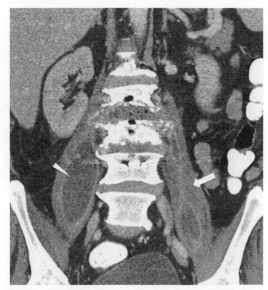

Fig. 22. Coloretroperitoneal fistula in a 45-year-old man with a history of Crohn disease. Contrast-enhanced axial CT shows a linear soft tissue tract extending from the splenic flexure through the anterior renal fascia, the lateral conal fascia (*arrowhead*), perinephric space, and into the lateral abdominal wall (*arrow*). A rim enhancing fluid collection is present in the subcutaneous tissue of the left flank consistent with an abscess.

Fig. 23. Bilateral psoas abscesses in a 71-year-old man with multisystem organ dysfunction of unclear cause. Contrast-enhanced coronal CT shows bilateral rim enhancing fluid collection in the psoas muscles and inflammatory stranding in the retroperitoneal fat adjacent to the psoas muscles (*arrowhead*). There was contiguity of this infectious process with L2 to L3 vertebral bodies, resulting in infective spondylodiskitis (*arrow*).

muscle enlargement and edema, bone destruction, and infiltration and loss of surrounding fat planes may be present.[1,129] Prime differential considerations include a psoas muscle hematoma or a malignancy with cystic components. In distinction, hematomas have high attenuation on CT and a peripheral rim of high signal intensity on T1-weighted imaging secondary to methemoglobin (concentric rim sign as described earlier) may be associated with a hematocrit effect, and are typically associated with psoas muscle enlargement.[1,113,129] These findings, coupled with a history of trauma or anticoagulation therapy, are often diagnostic. On the other hand, solid enhancing tissue favors a malignancy involving the psoas muscle.[107]

Pneumoretroperitoneum

Retroperitoneal gas is most often the result of bowel perforation. It can originate from the duodenum (**Fig. 24**) or the ascending, descending, or rectosigmoid portions of the colon. Other causes include superinfected necrotizing pancreatitis, necrotizing fasciitis, abscess formation, percutaneous biopsy, epidural anesthesia, extracorporeal shock-wave lithotripsy, hydrogen peroxide wound irrigation, or inferior extension of mediastinal air.[107]

MISCELLANEOUS RETROPERITONEAL CONDITIONS

Xanthogranulomatosis/Erdheim-Chester Disease

Xanthogranulomatosis refers to the masslike accumulation of non-Langerhans lipid-laden histiocytes. It is an idiopathic process, with a variable clinical course and a predisposition for the retroperitoneum. When multiple organs are involved, it is called Erdheim-Chester disease.[130,131] On CT and MR imaging, mildly enhancing infiltrative soft tissue with intermediate T1-weighted and T2-weighted signal intensity relative to skeletal muscle is typically seen.[132,133] Circumferential periaortic involvement with associated bilateral symmetric perirenal space involvement but with sparing of the IVC and pelvic ureters are features that differentiate it from RPF (**Fig. 25**).[132] Erdheim-Chester disease may be associated with osteosclerosis, periostitis, partial epiphyseal involvement, and medullary infarction of the long bones.[134]

Extramedullary Hematopoiesis

Extramedullary hematopoiesis (EMH) may rarely be seen in the retroperitoneum. On CT and MR imaging, EMH appears as multiple, bilateral, homogeneous soft tissue masses with

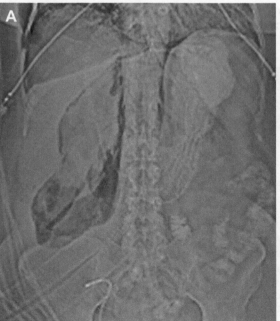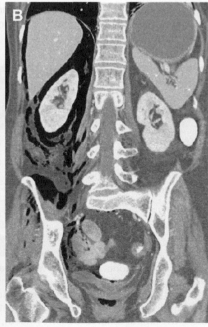

Fig. 24. Pneumoretroperitoneum in a 61-year-old woman with Crohn disease; status after endoscopic dilation of the duodenal strictures. (*A*) Scout image from a CT scan shows an air collection overlying the right paravertebral region. (*B*) Contrast-enhanced coronal CT shows this air to represent extensive right pneumoretroperitoneum caused by duodenal perforation.

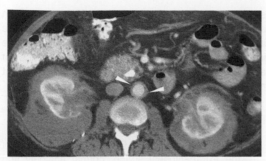

Fig. 25. Erdheim-Chester disease in a 45-year-old man. Contrast-enhanced axial CT shows bilateral, symmetric perinephric rinds of soft tissue and periaortic involvement (*arrowheads*) with sparing of IVC and ureters (*not seen*); there was histiocytic infiltration of multiple organs outside the abdomen as well.

intermediate signal intensity on T1-weighted imaging, intermediate to high signal intensity on T2-weighted imaging relative to skeletal muscle, and variable enhancement.[135–137] Calcification and osseous destruction are usually not present. After blood transfusion therapy, lesions tend to shrink and develop massive iron deposition, with resultant loss of enhancement.[135] Liver and splenic masses may be concurrently seen, as are skeletal changes caused by chronic anemia or myelofibrosis.[137]

Lipoma

Retroperitoneal lipomas are rare, but are the most common benign tumors of the retroperitoneum.[91] They usually appear during periods of weight gain and are composed of large, mature adipocytes, not significantly different from the normal adult fat. They typically have homogeneous fat attenuation and signal intensity on all pulse sequences and do not enhance.[138] However, up to 31% lipomas may have enhancing nonadipose areas caused by fat necrosis and associated dystrophic changes.[19] In the latter cases, a well-differentiated liposarcoma is a close imaging differential (see **Box 1**).

Fat Necrosis

Retroperitoneal fat necrosis can present as a palpable abdominal mass, mimic other abdominal masses, including retroperitoneal liposarcoma, and rarely lead to ureteral obstruction. The most common cause of retroperitoneal fat necrosis is acute pancreatitis.[139–142] On imaging, it appears as a predominantly fat attenuating or fat signal intensity lesion that may also contain foci of enhancing soft tissue or calcification. The distribution is typically peripancreatic but there

may be extension into the mesenteric root, transverse mesocolon, and omentum in severe disease.[143] Fat necrosis tends to remain stable in size or shrink with time.

RETROPERITONEAL NONPARENCHYMAL CYSTS AND CYSTIC LESIONS
Lymphangioma

A retroperitoneal lymphangioma is a developmental malformation that is caused by failure of communication of retroperitoneal lymphatic tissue with the main lymphatic vessels.[144] Retroperitoneal lymphangioma accounts for 1% of all retroperitoneal neoplasms, is more common in men, and can occur in any age group.[144,145] It characteristically appears as a fluid-attenuation or fluid-signal intensity, elongated, thin-walled, multiseptate cystic mass that typically insinuates between the structures (**Fig. 26**). The presence of lymph fluid, chyle, may give rise to negative attenuation values or high T1-signaal and intermediate T2-signal intensity. The presence of septa, compression of intestinal loops, and the lack of fluid in dependent recesses or mesenteric leaves are features used to differentiate lymphangiomas from ascites.[64] Surgical excision is the treatment of choice for symptomatic lesions.[18,145]

Cystadenoma and Cystadenocarcinoma

Cystadenoma is a rare primary epithelial retroperitoneal tumor of unclear histogenesis,[146] which most often occurs in women who have normal ovaries, usually in the fifth decade of life. It can be mucinous or serous and there are several clinicopathologic subtypes. CT and MR imaging show a well-defined, unilocular, homogeneous cystic

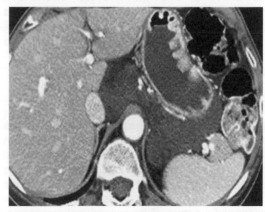

Fig. 26. Lymphangioma. Contrast-enhanced axial CT shows a low-attenuation cystic mass that insinuates between peritoneal and retroperitoneal structures and shows little to no enhancement.

mass. Internal septae, papillary projections, or solid enhancing components may be present in cystadenocarcinoma. Surgical resection is recommended even for benign lesions because of the risk of malignant transformation.[147,148]

Bronchogenic Cyst

Retroperitoneal bronchogenic (foregut) cysts are rare and most of them are found in the paramidline upper retroperitoneum adjacent to the diaphragmatic crura. They appear as sharply marginated, thin-walled, cystic lesions. However, fluid-fluid levels caused by complex internal contents, mural calcification, layering milk of calcium, and rim enhancement may be seen.[149–151]

Extralobar Pulmonary Sequestration

Subdiaphragmatic retroperitoneal localization of pulmonary sequestration can occur in up to 15% of cases.[152] On CT and MR imaging, a nonspecific, well-circumscribed, low-attenuation mass with low T1-weighted and high T2-weighted signal intensity is generally seen, sometimes with foci of cystic change or calcification. Contrast enhancement is variable, but is usually peripheral in distribution. Feeding systemic arterial branches to retroperitoneal extralobar pulmonary sequestrations are not usually well visualized on cross-sectional imaging, which makes a prospective diagnosis difficult.[152–155]

Nonpancreatic Pseudocyst

Nonpancreatic pseudocysts develop because of failure of resorption of previous hematomas or abscesses. Histologically, they are similar to pancreatic pseudocysts and have no epithelial lining.[156,157] On CT and MR imaging, they are thin-walled or thick-walled cystic lesions that may show high attenuation or high T1-weighted or T2-weighted signal intensity because of hemorrhagic, proteinaceous, or purulent contents. There may be a fluid-fluid level, internal septae, calcifications or peripheral enhancement.[156–158]

SUMMARY

The retroperitoneum has been described as a "hinterland of straggling mesenchyme, with vascular and nervous plexuses, weird embryonic rests and shadowy fascial boundaries."[19,159] The prospective diagnosis of a retroperitoneal disease poses a profound clinical challenge because of the nonspecific nature of its consequent symptoms. On the other hand, cross-sectional imaging techniques have significantly contributed to our understanding of retroperitoneal anatomy and the broad spectrum of diseases that occur. Although a precise imaging diagnosis may not be possible in every patient, the identification and accurate interpretation of the imaging characteristics of a lesion can guide a reasonable line of subsequent management.

REFERENCES

1. Korobkin M, Silverman PM, Quint LE, et al. CT of the extraperitoneal space: normal anatomy and fluid collections. AJR Am J Roentgenol 1992; 159(5):933–42.
2. Dodds WJ, Darweesh RM, Lawson TL, et al. The retroperitoneal spaces revisited. AJR Am J Roentgenol 1986;147(6):1155–61.
3. Lee SL, Ku YM, Rha SE. Comprehensive reviews of the interfascial plane of the retroperitoneum: normal anatomy and pathologic entities. Emerg Radiol 2010;17(1):3–11.
4. Gore RM, Balfe DM, Aizenstein RI, et al. The great escape: interfascial decompression planes of the retroperitoneum. AJR Am J Roentgenol 2000; 175(2):363–70.
5. Parienty RA, Pradel J. Radiological evaluation of the peri- and pararenal spaces by computed tomography. Crit Rev Diagn Imaging 1983;20(1): 1–26.
6. Parienty RA, Pradel J, Picard JD, et al. Visibility and thickening of the renal fascia on computed tomograms. Radiology 1981;139(1):119–24.
7. Cyran KM, Kenney PJ. Leiomyosarcoma of abdominal veins: value of MRI with gadolinium DTPA. Abdom Imaging 1994;19(4):335–8.
8. Elsayes KM, Staveteig PT, Narra VR, et al. Retroperitoneal masses: magnetic resonance imaging findings with pathologic correlation. Curr Probl Diagn Radiol 2007;36(3):97–106.
9. Low RN, Semelka RC, Worawattanakul S, et al. Extrahepatic abdominal imaging in patients with malignancy: comparison of MR imaging and helical CT in 164 patients. J Magn Reson Imaging 2000; 12(2):269–77.
10. Low RN, Semelka RC, Worawattanakul S, et al. Extrahepatic abdominal imaging in patients with malignancy: comparison of MR imaging and helical CT, with subsequent surgical correlation. Radiology 1999;210(3):625–32.
11. Low RN, Sigeti JS. MR imaging of peritoneal disease: comparison of contrast-enhanced fast multiplanar spoiled gradient-recalled and spin-echo imaging. AJR Am J Roentgenol 1994; 163(5):1131–40.
12. Nishino M, Hayakawa K, Minami M, et al. Primary retroperitoneal neoplasms: CT and MR imaging findings with anatomic and pathologic diagnostic clues. Radiographics 2003;23(1):45–57.

13. Sanyal R, Remer EM. Radiology of the retroperitoneum: case-based review. AJR Am J Roentgenol 2009;192(6):S112–7 [quiz: S118–21].
14. Jemal A, Siegel R, Ward E, et al. Cancer statistics, 2006. CA Cancer J Clin 2006;56(2):106–30.
15. Shibata D, Lewis JJ, Leung DH, et al. Is there a role for incomplete resection in the management of retroperitoneal liposarcomas? J Am Coll Surg 2001;193(4):373–9.
16. Herman K, Kusy T. Retroperitoneal sarcoma–the continued challenge for surgery and oncology. Surg Oncol 1998;7(1–2):77–81.
17. Lewis JJ, Leung D, Woodruff JM, et al. Retroperitoneal soft-tissue sarcoma: analysis of 500 patients treated and followed at a single institution. Ann Surg 1998;228(3):355–65.
18. Rajiah P, Sinha R, Cuevas C, et al. Imaging of uncommon retroperitoneal masses. Radiographics 2011;31(4):949–76.
19. Torigian DA, Ramchandani P. The retroperitoneum. In: Haaga JR, Dogra VS, Forsting M, et al, editors. CT and MRI of the whole body. 5th edition. Philadelphia: Mosby Elsevier; 2009. p. 1953–2040.
20. Gustafson P, Herrlin K, Biling L, et al. Necrosis observed on CT enhancement is of prognostic value in soft tissue sarcoma. Acta Radiol 1992;33(5):474–6.
21. Makela J, Kiviniemi H, Laitinen S. Prognostic factors predicting survival in the treatment of retroperitoneal sarcoma. Eur J Surg Oncol 2000;26(6):552–5.
22. Pirayesh A, Chee Y, Helliwell TR, et al. The management of retroperitoneal soft tissue sarcoma: a single institution experience with a review of the literature. Eur J Surg Oncol 2001;27(5):491–7.
23. Swallow CJ, Catton CN. Local management of adult soft tissue sarcomas. Semin Oncol 2007;34(3):256–69.
24. Cormier JN, Pollock RE. Soft tissue sarcomas. CA Cancer J Clin 2004;54(2):94–109.
25. Sung MS, Kang HS, Suh JS, et al. Myxoid liposarcoma: appearance at MR imaging with histologic correlation. Radiographics 2000;20(4):1007–19
26. Engelken JD, Ros PR. Retroperitoneal MR imaging. Magn Reson Imaging Clin N Am 1997;5(1):165–78.
27. Lane RH, Stephens DH, Reiman HM. Primary retroperitoneal neoplasms: CT findings in 90 cases with clinical and pathologic correlation. AJR Am J Roentgenol 1989;152(1):83–9.
28. Arkun R, Memls A, Akalin T, et al. Liposarcoma of soft tissue: MRI findings with pathologic correlation. Skeletal Radiol 1997;26(3):167–72.
29. Neville A, Herts BR. CT characteristics of primary retroperitoneal neoplasms. Crit Rev Comput Tomogr 2004;45(4):247–70.
30. Israel GM, Bosniak MA, Slywotzky CM, et al. CT differentiation of large exophytic renal angiomyolipomas and perirenal liposarcomas. AJR Am J Roentgenol 2002;179(3):769–73.
31. Jelinek JS, Kransdorf MJ, Shmookler BM, et al. Liposarcoma of the extremities: MR and CT findings in the histologic subtypes. Radiology 1993;186(2):455–9.
32. Kim T, Murakami T, Oi H, et al. CT and MR imaging of abdominal liposarcoma. AJR Am J Roentgenol 1996;166(4):829–33.
33. Hartman DS, Hayes WS, Choyke PL, et al. From the archives of the AFIP. Leiomyosarcoma of the retroperitoneum and inferior vena cava: radiologic-pathologic correlation. Radiographics 1992;12(6):1203–20.
34. Deshmukh H, Prasad SR, Patankar T, et al. Internal mammary artery pseudoaneurysms complicating chest wall infection in children: diagnosis and endovascular therapy. Clin Imaging 2001;25(6):396–9.
35. Kieffer E, Alaoui M, Piette JC, et al. Leiomyosarcoma of the inferior vena cava: experience in 22 cases. Ann Surg 2006;244(2):289–95.
36. McLeod AJ, Zornoza J, Shirkhoda A. Leiomyosarcoma: computed tomographic findings. Radiology 1984;152(1):133–6.
37. La Fianza A, Alberici E, Meloni G, et al. Extraperitoneal pelvic leiomyosarcoma. MR findings in a case. Clin Imaging 2000;24(4):224–6.
38. Kransdorf MJ. Malignant soft-tissue tumors in a large referral population: distribution of diagnoses by age, sex, and location. AJR Am J Roentgenol 1995;164(1):129–34.
39. Nishimura H, Zhang Y, Ohkuma K, et al. MR imaging of soft-tissue masses of the extraperitoneal spaces. Radiographics 2001;21(5):1141–54.
40. Ko SF, Wan YL, Lee TY, et al. CT features of calcifications in abdominal malignant fibrous histiocytoma. Clin Imaging 1998;22(6):408–13.
41. Prasad SR, Sahani DV, Mino-Kenudson M, et al. Neoplasms of the perivascular epithelioid cell involving the abdomen and the pelvis: cross-sectional imaging findings. J Comput Assist Tomogr 2007;31(5):688–96.
42. Castellazzi G, Vanel D, Le Cesne A, et al. Can the MRI signal of aggressive fibromatosis be used to predict its behavior? Eur J Radiol 2009;69(2):222–9.
43. Kreuzberg B, Koudelova J, Ferda J, et al. Diagnostic problems of abdominal desmoid tumors in various locations. Eur J Radiol 2007;62(2):180–5.
44. Einstein DM, Tagliabue JR, Desai RK. Abdominal desmoids: CT findings in 25 patients. AJR Am J Roentgenol 1991;157(2):275–9.
45. Dinauer PA, Brixey CJ, Moncur JT, et al. Pathologic and MR imaging features of benign fibrous soft-tissue tumors in adults. Radiographics 2007;27(1):173–87.

46. Choyke PL, Hayes WS, Sesterhenn IA. Primary extragonadal germ cell tumors of the retroperitoneum: differentiation of primary and secondary tumors. Radiographics 1993;13(6):1365–75 [quiz: 1377–8].

47. Ueno T, Tanaka YO, Nagata M, et al. Spectrum of germ cell tumors: from head to toe. Radiographics 2004;24(2):387–404.

48. Comiter CV, Renshaw AA, Benson CB, et al. Burned-out primary testicular cancer: sonographic and pathological characteristics. J Urol 1996; 156(1):85–8.

49. Hayashi T, Mine M, Kojima S, et al. Extragonadal germ cell tumor followed by metachronous testicular tumor. A case report. Urol Int 1996;57(3): 194–6.

50. Gutierrez Delgado F, Tjulandin SA, Garin AM. Long term results of treatment in patients with extragonadal germ cell tumours. Eur J Cancer 1993;29A(7): 1002–5.

51. Bokemeyer C, Droz JP, Horwich A, et al. Extragonadal seminoma: an international multicenter analysis of prognostic factors and long term treatment outcome. Cancer 2001;91(7):1394–401.

52. Logothetis CJ, Samuels ML, Trindade A, et al. The growing teratoma syndrome. Cancer 1982;50(8): 1629–35.

53. Andre F, Fizazi K, Culine S, et al. The growing teratoma syndrome: results of therapy and long-term follow-up of 33 patients. Eur J Cancer 2000; 36(11):1389–94.

54. Jeffery GM, Theaker JM, Lee AH, et al. The growing teratoma syndrome. Br J Urol 1991; 67(2):195–202.

55. Spiess PE, Kassouf W, Brown GA, et al. Surgical management of growing teratoma syndrome: the M. D. Anderson cancer center experience. J Urol 2007;177(4):1330–4 [discussion: 1334].

56. Wang RM, Chen CA. Primary retroperitoneal teratoma. Acta Obstet Gynecol Scand 2000;79(8): 707–8.

57. Panageas E. General diagnosis case of the day. Primary retroperitoneal teratoma. AJR Am J Roentgenol 1991;156(6):1292–4.

58. Engel RM, Elkins RC, Fletcher BD. Retroperitoneal teratoma. Review of the literature and presentation of an unusual case. Cancer 1968;22(5): 1068–73.

59. Davidson AJ, Hartman DS, Goldman SM. Mature teratoma of the retroperitoneum: radiologic, pathologic, and clinical correlation. Radiology 1989; 172(2):421–5.

60. Engel IA, Auh YH, Rubenstein WA, et al. Large posterior abdominal masses: computed tomographic localization. Radiology 1983;149(1):203–9.

61. Kurosaki Y, Tanaka YO, Itai Y. Well-differentiated liposarcoma of the retroperitoneum with a fat-fluid level: US, CT, and MR appearance. Eur Radiol 1998;8(3):474–5.

62. Ferrero A, Cespedes M, Cantarero JM, et al. Peritonitis due to rupture of retroperitoneal teratoma: computed tomography diagnosis. Gastrointest Radiol 1990;15(3):251–2.

63. Gatcombe HG, Assikis V, Kooby D, et al. Primary retroperitoneal teratomas: a review of the literature. J Surg Oncol 2004;86(2):107–13.

64. Yang DM, Jung DH, Kim H, et al. Retroperitoneal cystic masses: CT, clinical, and pathologic findings and literature review. Radiographics 2004;24(5): 1353–65.

65. Hayasaka K, Tanaka Y, Soeda S, et al. MR findings in primary retroperitoneal schwannoma. Acta Radiol 1999;40(1):78–82.

66. Li Q, Gao C, Juzi JT, et al. Analysis of 82 cases of retroperitoneal schwannoma. ANZ J Surg 2007; 77(4):237–40.

67. Rha SE, Byun JY, Jung SE, et al. Neurogenic tumors in the abdomen: tumor types and imaging characteristics. Radiographics 2003;23(1): 29–43.

68. Takatera H, Takiuchi H, Namiki M, et al. Retroperitoneal schwannoma. Urology 1986;28(6):529–31.

69. Loke TK, Yuen NW, Lo KK, et al. Retroperitoneal ancient schwannoma: review of clinico-radiological features. Australas Radiol 1998;42(2):136–8.

70. Lin J, Martel W. Cross-sectional imaging of peripheral nerve sheath tumors: characteristic signs on CT, MR imaging, and sonography. AJR Am J Roentgenol 2001;176(1):75–82.

71. Hughes MJ, Thomas JM, Fisher C, et al. Imaging features of retroperitoneal and pelvic schwannomas. Clin Radiol 2005;60(8):886–93.

72. Bass JC, Korobkin M, Francis IR, et al. Retroperitoneal plexiform neurofibromas: CT findings. AJR Am J Roentgenol 1994;163(3):617–20.

73. Woodruff JM. Pathology of tumors of the peripheral nerve sheath in type 1 neurofibromatosis. Am J Med Genet 1999;89(1):23–30.

74. Leroy K, Dumas V, Martin-Garcia N, et al. Malignant peripheral nerve sheath tumors associated with neurofibromatosis type 1: a clinicopathologic and molecular study of 17 patients. Arch Dermatol 2001;137(7):908–13.

75. Hrehorovich PA, Franke HR, Maximin S, et al. Malignant peripheral nerve sheath tumor. Radiographics 2003;23(3):790–4.

76. Korf BR. Malignancy in neurofibromatosis type 1. Oncologist 2000;5(6):477–85.

77. Singh KJ, Suri A, Vijjan V, et al. Retroperitoneal ganglioneuroma presenting as right renal mass. Urology 2006;67(5):1085.e7–8.

78. Otal P, Mezghani S, Hassissene S, et al. Imaging of retroperitoneal ganglioneuroma. Eur Radiol 2001; 11(6):940–5.

79. Lonergan GJ, Schwab CM, Suarez ES, et al. Neuroblastoma, ganglioneuroblastoma, and ganglioneuroma: radiologic-pathologic correlation. Radiographics 2002;22(4):911–34.

80. Remer EM, Miller FH. Imaging of pheochromocytomas. In: Blake MA, Boland GW, editors. Adrenal imaging. Totowa (NJ): Humana Press; 2009. p. 109–27.

81. Pommier RF, Vetto JT, Billingsly K, et al. Comparison of adrenal and extraadrenal pheochromocytomas. Surgery 1993;114(6):1160–5 [discussion: 1165–6].

82. Goldstein DS, Eisenhofer G, Flynn JA, et al. Diagnosis and localization of pheochromocytoma. Hypertension 2004;43(5):907–10.

83. Hayes WS, Davidson AJ, Grimley PM, et al. Extraadrenal retroperitoneal paraganglioma: clinical, pathologic, and CT findings. AJR Am J Roentgenol 1990;155(6):1247–50.

84. Lee KY, Oh YW, Noh HJ, et al. Extraadrenal paragangliomas of the body: imaging features. AJR Am J Roentgenol 2006;187(2):492–504.

85. Bessell-Browne R, O'Malley ME. CT of pheochromocytoma and paraganglioma: risk of adverse events with i.v. administration of nonionic contrast material. AJR Am J Roentgenol 2007;188(4):970–4.

86. Brink I, Hoegerle S, Klisch J, et al. Imaging of pheochromocytoma and paraganglioma. Fam Cancer 2005;4(1):61–8.

87. Plouin PF, Gimenez-Roqueplo AP. Pheochromocytomas and secreting paragangliomas. Orphanet J Rare Dis 2006;1:49.

88. Rufini V, Calcagni ML, Baum RP. Imaging of neuroendocrine tumors. Semin Nucl Med 2006;36(3): 228–47.

89. Shapiro B, Sisson JC, Shulkin BL, et al. The current status of meta-iodobenzylguanidine and related agents for the diagnosis of neuro-endocrine tumors. Q J Nucl Med 1995;39(4 Suppl 1):3–8.

90. Hruby G, Lehman M, Barton M, et al. Malignant retroperitoneal paraganglioma: case report and review of treatment options. Australas Radiol 2000;44(4):478–82.

91. Barker CD, Brown JJ. MR imaging of the retroperitoneum. Top Magn Reson Imaging 1995;7(2): 102–11.

92. Balfe DM, Mauro MA, Koehler RE, et al. Gastrohepatic ligament: normal and pathologic CT anatomy. Radiology 1984;150(2):485–90.

93. Dorfman RE, Alpern MB, Gross BH, et al. Upper abdominal lymph nodes: criteria for normal size determined with CT. Radiology 1991;180(2): 319–22.

94. Einstein DM, Singer AA, Chilcote WA, et al. Abdominal lymphadenopathy: spectrum of CT findings. Radiographics 1991;11(3):457–72.

95. Coakley FV, Hricak H. Imaging of peritoneal and mesenteric disease: key concepts for the clinical radiologist. Clin Radiol 1999;54(9):563–74.

96. Healy JC, Reznek RH. The peritoneum, mesenteries and omenta: normal anatomy and pathological processes. Eur Radiol 1998;8(6):886–900.

97. Blackledge G, Best JJ, Crowther D, et al. Computed tomography (CT) in the staging of patients with Hodgkin's Disease: a report on 136 patients. Clin Radiol 1980;31(2):143–7.

98. Neumann CH, Robert NJ, Canellos G, et al. Computed tomography of the abdomen and pelvis in non-Hodgkin lymphoma. J Comput Assist Tomogr 1983;7(5):846–50.

99. Rahmouni A, Tempany C, Jones R, et al. Lymphoma: monitoring tumor size and signal intensity with MR imaging. Radiology 1993;188(2):445–51.

100. Vaglio A, Salvarani C, Buzio C. Retroperitoneal fibrosis. Lancet 2006;367(9506):241–51.

101. Amis ES Jr. Retroperitoneal fibrosis. AJR Am J Roentgenol 1991;157(2):321–9.

102. Gilkeson GS, Allen NB. Retroperitoneal fibrosis. A true connective tissue disease. Rheum Dis Clin North Am 1996;22(1):23–38.

103. Kottra JJ, Dunnick NR. Retroperitoneal fibrosis. Radiol Clin North Am 1996;34(6):1259–75.

104. Oguz KK, Kiratli H, Oguz O, et al. Multifocal fibrosclerosis: a new case report and review of the literature. Eur Radiol 2002;12(5):1134–8.

105. Geoghegan T, Byrne AT, Benfayed W, et al. Imaging and intervention of retroperitoneal fibrosis. Australas Radiol 2007;51(1):26–34.

106. Arrive L, Hricak H, Tavares NJ, et al. Malignant versus nonmalignant retroperitoneal fibrosis: differentiation with MR imaging. Radiology 1989;172(1): 139–43.

107. Torigian DA, Ramchandani P. Retroperitoneum. In: Haaga JR, Dogra VS, Forstring M, et al, editors. CT and MRI of the whole body. New York: Mosby Elsevier; 2000. p. 484–90.

108. Vivas I, Nicolas AI, Velazquez P, et al. Retroperitoneal fibrosis: typical and atypical manifestations. Br J Radiol 2000;73(866):214–22.

109. Alexander ES, Colley DP, Clark RA. Computed tomography of retroperitoneal fluid collections. Semin Roentgenol 1981;16(4):268–76.

110. Danaci M, Kesici GE, Kesici H, et al. Coumadin-induced renal and retroperitoneal hemorrhage. Ren Fail 2006;28(2):129–32.

111. Ishikawa K, Tohira H, Mizushima Y, et al. Traumatic retroperitoneal hematoma spreads through the interfascial planes. J Trauma 2005;59(3):595–607 [discussion: 607–8].

112. Orwig D, Federle MP. Localized clotted blood as evidence of visceral trauma on CT: the sentinel clot sign. AJR Am J Roentgenol 1989; 153(4):747–9.

113. Hahn PF, Saini S, Stark DD, et al. Intraabdominal hematoma: the concentric-ring sign in MR imaging. AJR Am J Roentgenol 1987;148(1):115–9.

114. Federle MP, Jeffrey RB Jr. Hemoperitoneum studied by computed tomography. Radiology 1983;148(1):187–92.

115. Federle MP, Pan KT, Pealer KM. CT criteria for differentiating abdominal hemorrhage: anticoagulation or aortic aneurysm rupture? AJR Am J Roentgenol 2007;188(5):1324–30.

116. Shanmuganathan K, Mirvis SE, Sover ER. Value of contrast-enhanced CT in detecting active hemorrhage in patients with blunt abdominal or pelvic trauma. AJR Am J Roentgenol 1993;161(1):65–9.

117. Braun WE, Banowsky LH, Straffon RA, et al. Lymphoceles associated with renal transplantation: report of fifteen cases and review of the literature. Proc Clin Dial Transplant Forum 1973;3:185–9.

118. Petru E, Tamussino K, Lahousen M, et al. Pelvic and paraaortic lymphocysts after radical surgery because of cervical and ovarian cancer. Am J Obstet Gynecol 1989;161(4):937–41.

119. Schweizer RT, Cho S, Koutz Kountz SL, et al. Lymphoceles following renal transplantation. Arch Surg 1972;104(1):42–5.

120. vanSonnenberg E, Wittich GR, Casola G, et al. Lymphoceles: imaging characteristics and percutaneous management. Radiology 1986;161(3): 593–6.

121. Zuckerman DA, Yeager TD. Percutaneous ethanol sclerotherapy of postoperative lymphoceles. AJR Am J Roentgenol 1997;169(2):433–7.

122. Titton RL, Gervais DA, Hahn PF, et al. Urine leaks and urinomas: diagnosis and imaging-guided intervention. Radiographics 2003;23(5):1133–47.

123. Capitan Manjon C, Tejido Sanchez A, Piedra Lara JD, et al. Retroperitoneal abscesses–analysis of a series of 66 cases. Scand J Urol Nephrol 2003; 37(2):139–44.

124. Ishigami K, Khanna G, Samuel I, et al. Gas-forming abdominal wall abscess: unusual manifestation of perforated retroperitoneal appendicitis extending through the superior lumbar triangle. Emerg Radiol 2004;10(4):207–9.

125. Ishikawa K, Idoguchi K, Tanaka H, et al. Classification of acute pancreatitis based on retroperitoneal extension: application of the concept of interfascial planes. Eur J Radiol 2006;60(3):445–52.

126. Callen PW. Computed tomographic evaluation of abdominal and pelvic abscesses. Radiology 1979; 131(1):171–5.

127. Simons GW, Sty JR, Starshak RJ. Retroperitoneal and retrofascial abscesses. A review. J Bone Joint Surg Am 1983;65(8):1041–58.

128. Muttarak M, Peh WC. CT of unusual iliopsoas compartment lesions. Radiographics 2000;20(Spec No): S53–66.

129. Paley M, Sidhu PS, Evans RA, et al. Retroperitoneal collections–aetiology and radiological implications. Clin Radiol 1997;52(4):290–4.

130. Eble JN, Rosenberg AE, Young RH. Retroperitoneal xanthogranuloma in a patient with Erdheim-Chester disease. Am J Surg Pathol 1994;18(8):843–8.

131. Veyssier-Belot C, Cacoub P, Caparros-Lefebvre D, et al. Erdheim-Chester disease. Clinical and radiologic characteristics of 59 cases. Medicine (Baltimore) 1996;75(3):157–69.

132. Dion E, Graef C, Haroche J, et al. Imaging of thoracoabdominal involvement in Erdheim-Chester disease. AJR Am J Roentgenol 2004;183(5): 1253–60.

133. Fortman BJ, Beall DP. Erdheim-Chester disease of the retroperitoneum: a rare cause of ureteral obstruction. AJR Am J Roentgenol 2001;176(5):1330–1.

134. Dion E, Graef C, Miquel A, et al. Bone involvement in Erdheim-Chester disease: imaging findings including periostitis and partial epiphyseal involvement. Radiology 2006;238(2):632–9.

135. Tsitouridis J, Stamos S, Hassapopoulou E, et al. Extramedullary paraspinal hematopoiesis in thalassemia: CT and MRI evaluation. Eur J Radiol 1999; 30(1):33–8.

136. Vlahos L, Trakadas S, Gouliamos A, et al. Retrocrural masses of extramedullary hemopoiesis in beta-thalassemia. Magn Reson Imaging 1993;11(8):1227–9.

137. Mesurolle B, Sayag E, Meingan P, et al. Retroperitoneal extramedullary hematopoiesis: sonographic, CT, and MR imaging appearance. AJR Am J Roentgenol 1996;167(5):1139–40.

138. Kransdorf MJ, Bancroft LW, Peterson JJ, et al. Imaging of fatty tumors: distinction of lipoma and well-differentiated liposarcoma. Radiology 2002; 224(1):99–104.

139. Andac N, Baltacioglu F, Cimsit NC, et al. Fat necrosis mimicking liposarcoma in a patient with pelvic lipomatosis. CT findings. Clin Imaging 2003;27(2):109–11.

140. Haynes JW, Brewer WH, Walsh JW. Focal fat necrosis presenting as a palpable abdominal mass: CT evaluation. J Comput Assist Tomogr 1985;9(3):568–9.

141. Ross JS, Prout GR Jr. Retroperitoneal fat necrosis producing ureteral obstruction. J Urol 1976; 115(5):524–9.

142. Takao H, Yamahira K, Watanabe T. Encapsulated fat necrosis mimicking abdominal liposarcoma: computed tomography findings. J Comput Assist Tomogr 2004;28(2):193–4.

143. Jeffrey RB, Federle MP, Laing FC. Computed tomography of mesenteric involvement in fulminant pancreatitis. Radiology 1983;147(1):185–8.

144. Davidson AJ, Hartman DS. Lymphangioma of the retroperitoneum: CT and sonographic characteristic. Radiology 1990;175(2):507–10.

145. Konen O, Rathaus V, Dlugy E, et al. Childhood abdominal cystic lymphangioma. Pediatr Radiol 2002;32(2):88–94.

146. Kaku M, Ohara N, Seima Y, et al. A primary retro-peritoneal serous cystadenocarcinoma with clinically aggressive behavior. Arch Gynecol Obstet 2004;270(4):302–6.

147. Lee SA, Bae SH, Ryoo HM, et al. Primary retroperitoneal mucinous cystadenocarcinoma: a case report and review of the literature. Korean J Intern Med 2007;22(4):287–91.

148. Pennell TC, Gusdon JP Jr. Retroperitoneal mucinous cystadenoma. Am J Obstet Gynecol 1989;160(5 Pt 1):1229–31.

149. Buckley JA, Siegelman ES, Birnbaum BA, et al. Bronchogenic cyst appearing as a retroperitoneal mass. AJR Am J Roentgenol 1998;171(2):527–8.

150. McAdams HP, Kirejczyk WM, Rosado-de-Christenson ML, et al. Bronchogenic cyst: imaging features with clinical and histopathologic correlation. Radiology 2000;217(2):441–6.

151. Liang MK, Yee HT, Song JW, et al. Subdiaphragmatic bronchogenic cysts: a comprehensive review of the literature. Am Surg 2005;71(12):1034–41.

152. Hernanz-Schulman M, Johnson JE, Holcomb GW 3rd, et al. Retroperitoneal pulmonary sequestration: imaging findings, histopathologic correlation, and relationship to cystic adenomatoid malformation. AJR Am J Roentgenol 1997;168(5):1277–81.

153. Furuno T, Morita K, Kakizaki H, et al. Laparoscopic removal of a retroperitoneal extralobar pulmonary sequestration in an adult. Int J Urol 2006;13(2):165–7.

154. Kopecky KK, Bodnar A, Morphis JG, et al. Subdiaphragmatic pulmonary sequestrian simulating metastatic testicular cancer. Clin Radiol 2000;55(10):794–6.

155. Baker EL, Gore RM, Moss AA. Retroperitoneal pulmonary sequestration: computed tomographic findings. AJR Am J Roentgenol 1982;138(5):956–7.

156. de Perrot M, Brundler M, Totsch M, et al. Mesenteric cysts. Toward less confusion? Dig Surg 2000;17(4):323–8.

157. Stoupis C, Ros PR, Abbitt PL, et al. Bubbles in the belly: imaging of cystic mesenteric or omental masses. Radiographics 1994;14(4):729–37.

158. Ros PR, Olmsted WW, Moser RP Jr, et al. Mesenteric and omental cysts: histologic classification with imaging correlation. Radiology 1987;164(2):327–32.

159. Goodwin WE, Fonkalsrud EW, Goldman R, et al. Diagnostic problems in retroperitoneal disease. Ann Intern Med 1966;65(1):160–84.

Index

Note: Page numbers of article titles are in **boldface** type.

A

Absolute percentage washout
  and adrenal imaging, 223
  and pheochromocytomas, 233
ACC. See *Adrenocortical carcinoma.*
Acute pyelonephritis
  and renal lesions, 246, 247
ADC. See *Apparent diffusion coefficient.*
Adenocarcinoma
  and bladder neoplasms, 307–309
  ureteric, 288, 289
Adenomas
  and adrenal imaging, 219–223
Adrenal adenoma
  and dual-energy computed tomography, 201
Adrenal cysts
  and adrenal imaging, 226, 227
Adrenal imaging
  and absolute percentage washout, 223
  and adenomas, 219–223
  and adrenal-to-spleen chemical shift ratio, 222
  and adrenocortical carcinoma, 235, 236
  and benign lesions, 219–227
  and collision tumors, 230
  and cysts, 226, 227
  and diffusion-weighted imaging, 236, 237
  and dual-energy computed tomography, 237–239
  and emerging technologies, 236–239
  and 18F-fluorodeoxyglucose positron emission
    tomography, 230, 231, 234, 236
  and ganglioneuromas, 236
  and hemangiomas, 227–236
  and hemorrhage, 225, 226
  and infection, 236
  and lymphoma, 230, 231
  and metastasis, 227–236
  and multiple endocrine neoplasia, 231, 235
  and myelolipoma, 223–225
  and neuroblastomas, 236
  and pheochromocytomas, 231–235
  and relative percentage washout, 223
Adrenal imaging: a comprehensive review, **219–243**
Adrenal lesions
  benign, 219–227
  and chemical shift imaging, 221, 222
  management of, 220
Adrenal masses
  and chemical shift imaging, 237
Adrenal metastasis

  and opposed-phase imaging, 229
Adrenal neoplasms
  syndromes associated with, 232
Adrenal-to-spleen chemical shift ratio
  and adrenal imaging, 222
Adrenocortical carcinoma, 235, 236
Advanced ultrasonography
  and harmonic imaging, 212, 213
Advances in uroradiologic imaging in children, **207–218**
AML. See *Angiomyolipoma.*
Angiomyolipoma
  and genitourinary imaging, 250
  and renal lesions, 250
Apparent diffusion coefficient mapping
  and diffusion-weighted imaging, 236–237
Applications of dual-energy CT in urologic imaging:
    an update, **191–205**
APW. See *Absolute percentage washout.*
Aspergillosis
  renal, 263, 264
ASR. See *Adrenal-to-spleen chemical shift ratio.*
Autoimmune pancreatitis
  and renal lesions, 247

B

Bladder neoplasms
  and adenocarcinoma, 307–309
  benign, 303–305
  and computed tomographic urography,
    301, 302, 304
  imaging techniques for, 301–303
  and leiomyoma, 303
  and leiomyosarcoma, 310–312
  and lymphoma, 312
  malignant, 305–314
  and metastases, 312, 313
  and neurofibromas, 304, 305
  and paragangliomas, 303, 304
  and small cell tumors, 309, 310
  and squamous cell carcinoma, 306, 307
  staging of, 305
  and transitional cell carcinoma, 305–308
  and urothelial carcinoma, 305, 306
Bronchogenic cyst
  retroperitoneal, 350

C

Calculi
  ureteral, 282, 283

0033-8389/12/$ – see front matter © 2012 Elsevier Inc. All rights reserved.

radiologic.theclinics.com

Moving?

Make sure your subscription moves with you!

To notify us of your new address, find your **Clinics Account Number** (located on your mailing label above your name), and contact customer service at:

Email: journalscustomerservice-usa@elsevier.com

800-654-2452 (subscribers in the U.S. & Canada)
314-447-8871 (subscribers outside of the U.S. & Canada)

Fax number: 314-447-8029

**Elsevier Health Sciences Division
Subscription Customer Service
3251 Riverport Lane
Maryland Heights, MO 63043**

*To ensure uninterrupted delivery of your subscription,
please notify us at least 4 weeks in advance of move.

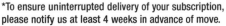

Printed and bound by CPI Group (UK) Ltd, Croydon, CR0 4YY
DX/03/2024
9781455744640

Printed and bound by CPI Group (UK) Ltd, Croydon, CR0 4YY

03/10/2024

01040356-0010